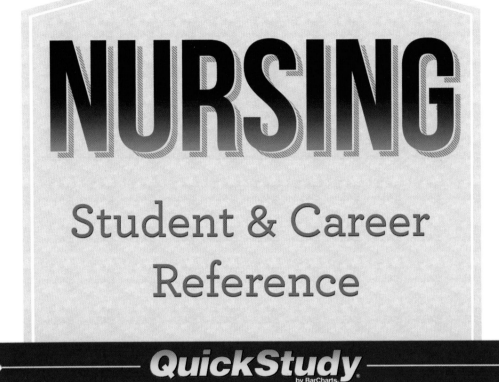

NURSING

Student & Career Reference

QuickStudy
by BarCharts.

Edited by

Julie Henry, RN, MPA

BarCharts, Inc.
Boca Raton, Florida

BarCharts, Inc.
6000 Park of Commerce Boulevard, Suite D
Boca Raton, FL 33487
www.quickstudy.com

© 2013 BarCharts, Inc.
ISBN-13: 978-1-423-22045-9
ISBN-10: 1-423-22045-5

The following illustrations by Vincent Perez (perezstudio.com) have been reprinted with permission: stethoscope placement for auscultating heart sounds, 22; stethoscope placement for auscultating lung sounds, 29; decubitus ulcer staging, 36; mid-deltoid, ventrogluteal, and vastus lateralis injections, 151; Z-track technique, 151.

Art direction, design, and layout: Dale A. Nibbe
Additional illustrations: Cathie Richards

Printed in the United States

Contents

Introduction   01

1
Ethics & Responsibility   03

5
Medical Math   109

2
Nursing Assessment   13

6
Pharmacology   119

3
Nursing Procedures   53

7
Medication Administration
& Laboratory Values   143

4
Nursing Chemistry   79

8
Specialty Nursing   161

Contents

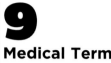

9

Medical Terminology, Abbreviations & Acronyms   185

Appendix C
Periodic Table of Elements   253

10

Getting a Job in the Field   225

Appendix D
NCLEX-RN Study Guide   257

Appendix A
Wound Healing   231

List of Contributors   283

Appendix B
Math Review   235

Index   285

Introduction

When I first started thinking about becoming a nurse, I had visions of walking around in my white uniform saving lives here and there as I went about my day. Someone would call out, "I need a nurse," and I'd go rushing into the room just in time to save the patient from certain death. Needless to say, my nursing career wasn't quite as glamorous as I'd anticipated. There were mounds of paperwork to fill out (I didn't see that coming). I cleaned up messes that most people should be grateful they never have to see. And, unfortunately, patients did sometimes die. It's the nature of the business.

Although the job may not always live up to expectations, nurses are, without a doubt, one of the most important members of the health care team. They are often in the best position to see what's going on with each patient on a day-to-day basis and to intervene if something is wrong. And nurses do, in fact, save lives, even if it isn't always in quite the way I'd envisioned. For example, the following nursing interventions may save someone's life:

- Noticing that something is "not quite right" with the patient and alerting the physician
- Speaking up when a treatment or medication seems to be contraindicated
- Catching a potential medication or other medical error before it reaches the patient
- Insisting on a "time out" before a surgical procedure to verify that you have the correct patient, correct procedure, and correct surgical site
- Noticing early signs of infection and alerting the physician
- Catching adverse medication reactions and intervening early
- Picking up on signs of a possible transfusion reaction and stopping the transfusion

Nursing can be a stressful career, but it can also be extremely rewarding, even when dealing with death. When I was working in a nursing home early in my career, I met an older man named Al. He was a resident on the skilled nursing unit. Al was lucid, so when I was caring for him, he would talk to me about his life. He told me about his wife (the only woman he ever loved) who had passed away years earlier and about his career at the post office. One day, Al told me he was ready to die. "I want to see my wife again," he said. "But I don't think my kids are ready to let me go yet. I don't think they'll understand."

I had met Al's children. They loved their dad, and I knew they wanted the best for him. "Why don't you give them a chance?" I asked. "Tell them what you just told me." I honestly don't know if he ever did.

One Friday afternoon as I was getting ready to leave for the weekend, I went into Al's room to see if he needed anything. He asked me if I was working that weekend. I told him I was not. "I'm really glad I got to know you," he said.

At the time, I didn't think too much about what he had just said, but I was pleased that he had said it. "I'm glad I got to know you, too," I replied. "See you on Monday."

When I got to work on Monday, Al was in a coma. On Tuesday morning, he died. My coworkers were expecting me to be upset, but I wasn't. Although I knew I would miss him, I was glad to know that when the time came, Al was ready to go. I was also happy that he had said good-bye to me before he died.

That's my favorite nursing story. One day, you'll have a similar story to tell.

My mother always told me that it takes a special person to be a nurse. She was right. Nursing not only requires knowledge and skill but also patience and compassion. The first two you can learn; the other two can only come from within.

The purpose of this book is to provide you with real-world knowledge that will prepare you for the reality of a nursing career. It includes nursing assessment techniques, step-by-step instruction for procedural skills, and information about medication administration, pharmacology, medical math, chemistry, and medical terminology. It also includes information about nursing ethics, specialty nursing, and choosing a career path. There are also helpful appendices, including a review for those who are preparing to take the NCLEX-RN exam.

ETHICS & RESPONSIBILITY

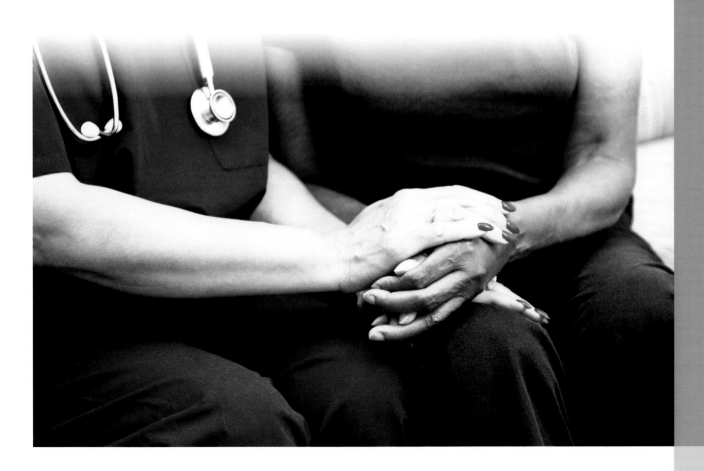

Introduction

There are certain basic principles that every nurse should know before delving into the physical aspects of caring for patients. These principles will help you become a good leader and make the best possible decisions for your patients. This chapter includes the following topics:

- Accountability
- Nursing ethics
- Professional boundaries
- Infection prevention and control
- Nursing care delivery models
- Standards of practice
- Evidence-based practice
- Critical thinking
- Collaboration
- Leadership
- Delegation
- Patient advocacy
- Mentoring
- Membership in professional nursing organizations

Accountability

> Nurses are both morally and legally accountable for their actions and for the omission of necessary actions.

Many people use the words *responsibility* and *accountability* interchangeably. However, the two words have very different meanings: responsibility is a duty or obligation; accountability is being answerable for one's actions. Areas of accountability that are specific to nursing include the following:

- Interventions (nursing care)
- Outcomes (results)
- Costs (expenditures)

Nursing Ethics

Nurses frequently encounter ambiguity in practice, as values and beliefs conflict in complex clinical situations. Examples of ethical dilemmas in nursing practice may include the following:

- Quality of life versus quantity of life
- The patient's best interests versus organizational rules
- Knowledge versus beliefs
- Truth versus deception

Ethical decisions should be based on the following principles:

> Nursing depends on scientific knowledge of health and illness, the perception of human experiences, an understanding of the unique individuality of each person, and the capacity to make choices involving moral dilemmas.

- Patients have the right to make health care decisions for themselves, even if you do not agree with their decisions.
- Individual autonomy should not interfere with the rights, health, or well-being of others.
- All patients should have the individual freedom to make rational and unconstrained decisions.
- Patients have the right to be treated equally, regardless of race, ethnicity, gender, marital status, sexual orientation, medical diagnosis, social standing, economic level, or religious belief.
- Nurses should refrain from providing ineffective treatments or acting with malice toward patients.

- Nurses should not intentionally deceive or mislead patients unless the truth would seriously harm the patient, cause stress or distress, or place the patient's well-being at risk.
- Communications between the nurse and patient are privileged and may not be discussed or divulged to third parties.
- Limits can be placed on confidentiality when maintaining it may jeopardize the safety or well-being of others.

Ethical Decision Making

The steps of ethical decision making are as follows:

1. Collect, analyze, and interpret the data; important issues to consider may include the following:
   a. The patient's wishes
   b. The family's wishes
   c. The physical or emotional problem causing the dilemma
   d. The physician's beliefs about the patient's condition
   e. Your own values and beliefs
   f. The mental competency of the patient
2. Consider your options:
   a. List all the possible courses of action to resolve the dilemma.
   b. Consider input from outside sources, including colleagues, supervisors, review committees, and experts in the field of ethics.
3. Analyze the advantages and disadvantages of each course of action:
   a. List the consequences of each course of action.
   b. Completely evaluate the advantages and disadvantages of each consequence.
   c. Include relevant passages from the American Nurses Association (ANA) Code of Ethics for Nurses in your deliberation process (see below).
   d. Plan your course of action.
4. Make the decision:
   a. Know that not everyone may agree with your decision.
   b. Once the decision has been made, be prepared to live with the consequences.
5. Evaluate the decision and outcome:
   a. Identify the results of the action taken.
   b. Reflect on your moral feeling about your actions.

> Moral distress occurs when one knows what ought to be done but is unable to do so because of internal or external pressures or constraints. Think of your best role model in school, and act in the manner that you know that person would have acted, regardless of the consequences.

ANA Code of Ethics for Nurses

The ANA Code of Ethics for Nurses should serve as a guideline for ethical obligations and duties for every individual who enters the nursing profession. The ANA Code of Ethics for Nurses is available online at www.nursingworld.org.

Professional Boundaries

Nurses are responsible for maintaining professional boundaries. Those boundaries are in place to protect the patient at a time when he or she is vulnerable. To maintain professional boundaries, keep the following guidelines in mind:

- Do not develop personal or sexual relationships with patients.
- Do not engage in flirtatious behavior with patients.
- Do not interfere with or become involved in a patient's personal relationships.
- Do not divulge personal information about yourself to patients.
- Do not accept gifts from patients.

> The difference between a caring relationship and an overinvolved relationship is narrow. You must learn to distinguish between professional and personal interactions.

Hand Hygiene

Hand hygiene is the single most important aspect of infection prevention and control. The Centers for Disease Control and Prevention (CDC) recommends that hand hygiene be performed:

- Before and after direct patient contact
- Before procedures, such as administering intravenous medications
- Before and after contact with vascular access
- Before and after dressing changes
- After contact with blood, body fluids, or contaminated surfaces
- After removing gloves

Hand hygiene can be performed with alcohol-based hand rubs or by washing hands with antimicrobial soap.

Standard Precautions

The CDC developed the following standard precautions to protect against the transmission of infection. Under standard precautions, all blood, body fluids, secretions and excretions, broken skin, and mucous membranes should be treated as potentially infectious.

- Perform hand hygiene in the following situations:
  - Before touching a patient, even if gloves will be worn
  - Before exiting the patient care area after touching a patient or the patient's immediate environment
  - After contact with blood, body fluids or excretions, or wound dressings
  - Prior to performing an aseptic task (e.g., accessing a port, preparing an injection)
  - If hands will be moving from a contaminated body site to a clean body site during patient care
  - After removing gloves
- Wear gloves when there is a potential for contact with blood, body fluids, mucous membranes, nonintact skin, or contaminated equipment.
- Wear a gown to protect skin and clothing during procedures or activities where contact with blood or body fluids is anticipated.
- Wear a face mask, goggles, or a face shield during any procedure where there may be a potential for splashing.

> Make friends with everyone—the housekeeping staff, dietary aides, pharmacy staff, unit secretaries, therapists. Remember their names and thank them often.

Contact Precautions

According to the CDC, the following contact precautions should be applied to patients with stool incontinence, draining wounds, uncontrolled secretions, pressure ulcers, ostomy tubes or bags draining body fluids, or generalized rashes or exanthems:

- Perform hand hygiene before touching the patient and before putting on gloves.
- Wear gloves when touching the patient or the patient's immediate environment or belongings.
- Wear a gown if substantial contact with the patient or his or her environment is anticipated.
- Perform hand hygiene after removing personal protective equipment (PPE); use soap and water when hands are visibly soiled or after caring for patients with known or suspected infectious diarrhea.

Droplet Precautions

CDC guidelines suggest that the following droplet precautions be applied to patients who are known or suspected to be infected with a pathogen that can be transmitted by droplet route:

- Place the patient in a private room with a closed door as soon as possible.
- Utilize PPE:

- ○ Wear a face mask for close contact with the patient.
- ○ Wear gloves, a gown, and goggles if spraying is likely to occur.
- Perform hand hygiene before and after touching the patient and after contact with respiratory secretions or with contaminated objects or materials; use soap and water when hands are visibly soiled.
- Instruct the patient to wear a face mask when exiting the room, to avoid close contact with other patients, and to practice respiratory hygiene and cough etiquette.

Airborne Precautions

According to the CDC, the following airborne precautions should be applied to patients known or suspected to be infected with a pathogen that can be transmitted by airborne route:

- Place the patient in an airborne infection isolation room.
- Wear a fit-tested N-95 or higher-level disposable respirator mask, if available, when caring for the patient.
- Wear gloves, a gown, and goggles if spraying is likely to occur.
- Perform hand hygiene before and after touching the patient and after contact with respiratory secretions or with contaminated objects or materials; use soap and water when hands are visibly soiled.
- Instruct the patient to wear a face mask when exiting the room, to avoid close contact with other patients, and to practice respiratory hygiene and cough etiquette.

Nursing Care Delivery Models

Nursing care delivery models have evolved through the years to meet the challenges of the health care environment. How nursing care is delivered is continually redesigned to meet the changing needs of patients, nurses, and organizations. The underlying objectives of all nursing care delivery models are as follows:

- To assess the patient
- To identify the nursing needs of the patient
- To provide the necessary nursing care

Factors to be considered in evaluating the choice of a nursing care delivery model include the following:

- Number of nurses available
- Fiscal resources
- Staff buy-in
- Expected outcomes

Models of Nursing Care Delivery

- **Case method:** A nurse is assigned to provide complete care for a patient or group of patients for a defined time period.
  - ○ This method is based on a holistic philosophy.
  - ○ However, it is often considered inefficient and costly because one nurse provides all the care to the patient.
- **Functional:** A variety of caregivers are assigned to perform specific tasks or functions for each patient.
  - ○ The functional method is based on the allocation of tasks or functions (e.g., one nurse gives all medications, another does all treatments, and still another caregiver gives all baths).
  - ○ Task completion is emphasized over patient care.
  - ○ Fragmentation of care and unmet patient needs may result.
  - ○ This method may also lead to the lack of an ongoing nurse-patient relationship and the absence of continuity of care.

- **Team:** A team that is made up of licensed and unlicensed providers is assigned to deliver care under the direction of a team leader.
  - The team leader delegates tasks and activities and provides some direct patient care.
  - Nursing services are provided to more patients, which improves continuity of care while relieving nurses from doing simple, routine tasks.
  - Communication is complex; for example, the caregiver reports to the team leader, who shares information with the next team leader, making the information subject to interpretation by each person in the chain.
- **Primary:** A single nurse has sole responsibility for assessing patient needs, developing a plan of care, and evaluating the patient's response to the plan of care.
  - Decision making is decentralized.
  - The nurse provides care to the patient when possible.
  - A therapeutic relationship is established between the nurse and the patient.
  - Because this type of nursing care delivery is very dependent on the nurse, it is perceived to be a costly model.
- **Case management:** This is an integrated system of care that uses a multidisciplinary team approach in a variety of care settings.
  - Care is organized around the patient, promoting continuity and cost-effectiveness.
  - The contributions of the members of the interdisciplinary team are recognized.
  - This method is used in hospitals:
    - To facilitate and integrate the contributions of the interdisciplinary team
    - To facilitate quality and cost-effective care
    - With a variety of care delivery systems
  - This method is used across the continuum:
    - To provide episodic services, which are initiated and completely related to events specific to a condition or patient need. The type of service depends on the patient populations served. It includes preventive teaching and intervention, acute care and discharge monitoring, and follow-up education and lifestyle modification, with the goal of preventing hospital admission in an at-risk population.
  - This method is used in the community:
    - After hospital discharge. Patients are assessed, counseled, reminded of follow-up appointments, and referred for additional services as needed.

Standards of Practice

A standard of practice, also known as a *standard of care*, is an established practice that is considered to be the norm. Standards of clinical practice:
- Provide direction for clinical practice.
- Provide a framework for the evaluation of nursing practice.
- Define the profession's accountability to the public.
- Clarify the specific functions and activities of the nurse.

Evidence-Based Practice

Evidence-based practice (EBP) is the process by which nurses make clinical decisions using the best available research findings. Competencies that are important to EBP include the following:
- Skill and knowledge in interpreting and using research
- The ability to apply evidence to clinical practice
- The ability to evaluate the effectiveness of evidence-based interventions

Nursing practice should be evidence based in order to improve clinical practice and patient outcomes and to raise standards of care.

Critical Thinking

Critical thinking is engaging in a purposeful cognitive activity directed toward establishing a plan of action. A critical thinker actively gathers, processes, and evaluates information to validate existing knowledge and to create new knowledge. Critical thinking requires:

- A broad educational foundation
- Common sense
- Experience
- A knowledge of one's own limitations and biases
- An ability to gather and evaluate quality data
- An ability to suspend judgment until all evidence is gathered and evaluated
- A willingness to challenge the status quo

Strategies for developing critical thinking skills include the following:

- Reflecting on your own experiences and on the experiences of others
- Questioning, analyzing, and reflecting on the rationale(s) for decisions
- Rehearsing multiple scenarios before making a decision
- Exploring alternatives
- Reflecting on what could be done to improve or change a situation

Collaboration

To be successful, nurses must build collaborative relationships with their colleagues in other disciplines. Collaboration fosters collegial working relationships with other health care providers and contributes to patient safety. Elements of a collaborative relationship may include the following:

- Communication skills
- Mutual respect
- Reciprocal trust
- Shared feedback
- Ethical decision making
- Effective conflict management
- Enhanced problem-solving skills

> Engaging with colleagues makes the job easier and ultimately improves patient outcomes and well-being.

Leadership

Leadership is the ability to influence others. There are a variety of different leadership styles, including the following:

- **Autocratic leaders** make decisions without consulting anyone else, which can demotivate and alienate staff.
- **Democratic or participative leaders** make decisions by consulting the team, which improves the sharing of ideas and experiences.
- **Laissez-faire or nondirective leaders** exercise little control over the team, leaving staff to sort out roles and tackle work without leadership participation in the process.
- **Paternalistic leaders** act as "parental figures" and believe in the need to support staff.
- **Situational leaders** offer direction and support that varies with the maturity or skill set of the group.
- **Caring leaders** recognize the importance of caring and compassion in the practice of nursing.

Leadership Skills

Good leaders use a number of different skills, which may include the following:

- **Coaching:** Helping employees build confidence and motivation
- **Delegating:** Giving responsibility to employees to carry out plans and make task decisions
- **Empowerment:** Giving others a sense of achievement, belonging, and self-esteem
- **Intuition:** Having a feel for the environment and the needs and desires of others
- **Self-understanding:** Building on one's strengths and working on one's weaknesses
- **Valuing congruence:** Understanding and accepting the objectives of the organization and the values of employees and being able to reconcile them

Leadership Competencies

Effective leaders frequently possess the following competencies:

- Achievement and ambition
- Ability to learn from adversity
- High dedication to the job
- Sound analytic and problem-solving skills
- Ability to work with people
- High level of creativity and innovation

Leadership Challenges

There are some challenges to being a good leader, including the following:

- Limited access to health care services
- Limited resources for providing care
- The need to provide care for a large number of underinsured or uninsured individuals and families

Delegation

Delegation is the transfer of responsibility from one individual to another while retaining accountability for the outcome. The application of effective principles of delegation is essential to patient safety. Activities considered appropriate for delegation are those:

- That frequently recur in the daily care of a patient or group of patients
- That do not require nursing judgment
- That do not require complex or multidimensional application of the nursing process
- For which the results are predictable and the potential risk is minimal
- That use a standard or unchanging procedure

Delegation should include the following components:

- Matching the complexity of the activity with the competencies of the person to whom you are delegating each task
- Clearly communicating activities to be performed, patient-specific instructions, and expected results or potential complications
- Clearly identifying constraints and boundaries; for example, should the person:
  - Wait to be told what to do?
  - Ask what to do?
  - Recommend what should be done and then act?
  - Act and then report results immediately?
  - Initiate action and then report periodically?
- Providing adequate support, including being available to answer questions
- Monitoring and evaluating performance, and intervening if necessary
- Taking steps to remedy failure to meet standards
- Ensuring proper documentation

> When possible, include people in the delegation process; allow them to help make decisions about what tasks are to be delegated to them and when.

Patient Advocacy

Patient advocacy involves looking out for your patients' best interests. Nurses advocate on behalf of their patients by using their professional power to influence behaviors or decisions. Effective advocates should be willing to do the following:

- Question the physician when something does not seem quite right.
- Adequately inform patients and families about decisions regarding their health care.
- Recognize that the rights and values of the patient and family take precedence when they conflict with those of health care providers.
- Be aware that potential conflicts may occur, which could require consultation, confrontation, or negotiation.
- Be assertive when necessary.

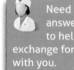
Therapeutic care of your patients can be summed up in one word: respect. Regardless of how they treat you and others, respect that they are precious lives. Respect that they could be going through the worst time of their lives. Respect that they may not have the mental energy to graciously handle the dependent position they are in.

Mentoring

Mentoring is the act of sharing your knowledge and skills with someone who is less experienced. Nurses often act as mentors to nursing students and to other nurses. A good mentor will possess the following skills:

- A willingness to share his or her knowledge and skills
- The ability to adapt to any situation
- The foresight to ask thoughtful questions
- Active listening skills
- The ability to provide constructive feedback

Mentoring can lead to:

- Development of new skills and knowledge
- Generation of creative ideas
- Improved self-awareness
- Career progress

Need some help or an answer to a question? Offer to help a busy nurse in exchange for spending some time with you.

Membership in Professional Nursing Organizations

Professional nursing organizations function at local, regional, and national levels. The purpose of these organizations is to:

- Establish common values and norms.
- Promote professional parameters of practice, education, administration, and research.
- Provide educational opportunities.

Types of Nursing Organizations

- National nursing organizations:
  - American Nurses Association (ANA)
  - National League for Nursing (NLN)
- Specialty-specific nursing organizations:
  - American Association of Critical-Care Nurses (AACN)
  - Association of periOperative Registered Nurses (AORN)
  - Association of Rehabilitation Nurses (ARN)
  - Association of Women's Health, Obstetric, and Neonatal Nurses (AWHONN)
  - Emergency Nurses Association (ENA)
  - Society of Pediatric Nurses (SPN)
- Special-interest nursing organizations:
  - National Black Nurses Association (NBNA)
  - National Association of Hispanic Nurses (NAHN)
  - American Assembly for Men in Nursing (AAMN)

Professional nursing organizations provide support and a sense of professional community, which together create a reliable foundation for lasting success.

NURSING ASSESSMENT

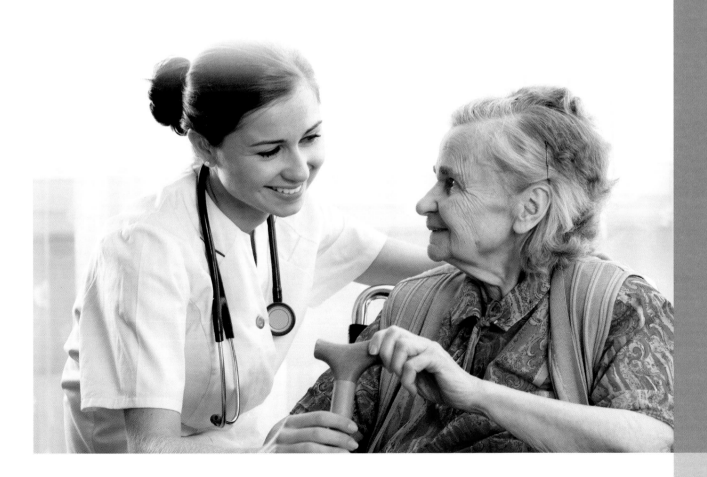

Introduction

The nursing assessment is the process by which a nurse investigates the physical, psychosocial, and spiritual needs of a patient through the collection of subjective and objective data. It generally follows an account of the patient's current illness. Nurses use assessment to:

- Obtain baseline data.
- Identify and manage patient problems.
- Make clinical judgments.
- Evaluate the effectiveness of nursing care.

Components of the Nursing Process

- **Assessment:** The physical, psychosocial, and spiritual needs of a patient are investigated through the collection of subjective and objective data.
- **Analysis (a.k.a. diagnosis):** The data collected during the assessment phase are analyzed to determine the plan of care.
- **Planning:** The data from the assessment and analysis phases of the nursing process are used to develop measurable goals and outcomes (i.e., nursing interventions).
- **Implementation:** The nursing interventions are put into practice.
- **Evaluation:** The outcomes of the nursing interventions are measured.

Assessment Techniques

Inspection

Inspection is the careful examination of the patient as a whole, as well as of each body system, using the visual, auditory, and olfactory senses to gather information. Inspection:

- Looks at the color, shape, symmetry, and position of body parts
- Should be purposeful and systematic; body parts should be compared bilaterally throughout the entire examination
- Requires good lighting to visually inspect the body without distortion or shadows

Palpation

Palpation is the technique of using touch to gather information about the temperature, turgor, texture, moisture, size, shape, consistency, location, and tenderness of an organ or body part.

- Palpation can be **light** (using inward pressure to depress the skin and underlying structures approx. ½ inch) or **deep** (using inward pressure to depress the skin and underlying structures approx. 1 inch).
- The patient should be provided with privacy, and the nurse should have warm hands and short fingernails. Any areas of tenderness should be palpated last.
- During palpation, make sure you assess:
  - Consistency of tissues
  - Alignment and intactness of structures
  - Symmetry of body parts or movements
  - Transmission of fine vibrations

Percussion

Percussion is the art of striking one object with another to create sound to assess the location, size, and density of underlying tissues. The sound changes as you move from one area to the next. Percussion is done with the middle finger of the dominant hand tapping on the middle finger of the nondominant hand while the nondominant palm is on the body.

- The nondominant hand is placed on the area to be percussed, with fingers slightly separated.

- The dominant hand is used to deliver the striking force by exerting a sharp downward wrist movement so that the tip of the middle finger of the dominant hand strikes the joint of the middle finger on the nondominant hand.
- There are five types of percussion sounds:
  - **Tympany:** Loud; drumlike sound
  - **Resonance:** Moderate to loud; low-pitched, hollow sound
  - **Hyperresonance:** Very loud; low-pitched, booming sound
  - **Flatness:** Soft, high-pitched, flat sound
  - **Dullness:** Soft to moderate; high-pitched, thud-like sound

Percussion Sounds & Potential Causes		
Percussion Sound	**Where Normally Heard**	**Potential Cause**
Tympany	Abdomen	Normal
Resonance	Chest	Healthy lungs
Hyperresonance	Chest	Chronic obstructive pulmonary disease (COPD), asthma, pneumothorax
Flatness	Solid areas	Muscle or bone, severe pneumonia
Dullness	Liver or heart	Pneumonia, tumor, pleural effusion

Auscultation

Auscultation is the act of listening to sounds produced by the body using a stethoscope. Auscultation is performed for the purposes of examining the circulatory system, respiratory system, and gastrointestinal (GI) system.

- Sounds must be isolated for proper identification and evaluation.
- The stethoscope has a diaphragm, which detects high-pitched sounds best, and a bell, which detects low-pitched sounds best. There are several types of stethoscopes:
  - **Acoustic stethoscope:** Operates on the transmission of sound from the chest piece through air-filled hollow tubes to the listener's ears. The chest piece usually consists of two sides that can be placed against the patient for sensing sound: a diaphragm (plastic disc) and a bell (hollow cup). If the diaphragm is placed on the patient, body sounds vibrate the diaphragm, creating acoustic pressure waves that travel up the tubing to the listener's ears. If the bell is placed on the patient, the vibrations of the skin directly produce acoustic pressure waves that travel up to the listener's ears.
  - **Electronic stethoscope or stethophone:** Amplifies and emits audible sounds that are magnified through an amplifier to earphones and may be broadcast through loudspeakers; the results are less precise than the results of an acoustic stethoscope.
  - **Fetal stethoscope, fetoscope, or Pinard stethoscope:** An acoustic stethoscope shaped like a listening trumpet. It is placed against the abdomen of a pregnant woman to listen to the heart sounds of the fetus.
- Four characteristics of sounds should be noted:
  - Pitch
  - Loudness
  - Quality
  - Duration

> Auscultation is a skill that requires substantial clinical experience, a fine stethoscope, and good listening skills. High-pitched tones are best heard with the diaphragm of the stethoscope; low-pitched tones are best heard with the bell of the stethoscope.

The Nursing Interview & History

A nursing interview is a structured interview done prior to the physical examination. The nursing interview identifies:

- Actual or potential health problems
- Patient support systems
- Teaching needs
- Referral needs

A comprehensive nursing history is obtained at the patient's first visit and updated at subsequent visits. Elements of the nursing history include the following:

- Reason for seeking care or health status
- Course of present illness, including symptoms
- Current management of illness
- Past medical history
- Family history
- Social history
- Perception of illness
- Review of systems
  - Current and past health history of each system, including health-promoting practices
  - Signs and symptoms, as well as diseases related to each body system
- Functional assessment (i.e., activities of daily living)
- Perception of health

Analysis of a Symptom: PQRST

Provokes: What makes the symptom better or worse?

Quality: What does it feel like?

Radiation: Where is the symptom, and where does it go?

Severity: How bad does it feel on a scale of 1–10?

Time: When does it occur, how often does it occur, and how long does it last?

Assessment Preparation

Preparation is important in conducting a comprehensive and accurate nursing assessment. Before you begin your assessment, make sure you review the patient's chart. The chart provides a starting point for getting to know your patient and can give you the following information:

- Demographics (the patient's name, age, address, race, occupation, and religious affiliation)
- Lifestyle information
- Potential risk factors
- History of previous illnesses
- Results of previous diagnostic tests
- Recent laboratory values

After you have reviewed the patient's chart, you will want to greet the patient and establish rapport:

- Greet the patient in a friendly, nonthreatening manner.
- Explain your role in the patient's care.
- Share with the patient the purpose of the nursing assessment (e.g., "This assessment will help give us an idea of your overall health status.").

Before entering rooms, take a minute to "center" yourself. Patients do not care what your problems are. They want to know that you are caring for them.

During your nursing assessment, make sure you control the environment:
- Give the patient privacy by drawing the curtain or closing the door.
- Excuse family members so that the patient can speak candidly.

When you are ready to begin, position the patient:
- Ask the patient to put on a loose-fitting gown that provides easy access for inspection and palpation.
- Respect the patient's personal space; stand only as close as you need to be to perform the assessment.
- Ask permission before touching the patient, especially in private or sensitive areas of the body.

General Assessment

Assess general appearance and behavior, posture, gait, hygiene, speech, mental status, height and weight, hearing and visual acuity, vital signs, and nutrition.

Vital Signs (Normal Ranges)					
Age	Blood Pressure (mm Hg)	Pulse Rate (beats/min)	Respiratory Rate (breaths/min)	Temperature	
				°F	°C
Newborn	73/45	110–160	30–50	98.6–99.8	37–37.7
3 yr	90/55	80–125	20–30	98.5–99.5	36.9–37.5
10 yr	96/57	70–110	16–22	97.5–98.6	36.4–37
16 yr	120/80	55–100	15–20	97.6–98.8	36.4–37.1
Adult	120/80	60–100	12–20	96.8–99.5	36–37.5
Older adult (>70 yr)	150/90	60–100	15–25	96.5–97.5	35.8–36.4

Head, Eyes, Ears, Nose & Throat (HEENT) Assessment

Head
- Inspect and palpate for size, shape, and symmetry.
- Assess hair growth, distribution, and texture.
- Use fingertips to palpate for masses of the scalp, ears, face, throat, and neck.
- Palpate maxillary sinuses and frontal sinuses for tenderness or masses; transilluminate to assess whether the sinuses are clear.

Face
- Observe for symmetry of facial features.
- Assess cranial nerves (CN) V and VII (*see* **CN Assessment**, p. 43).

Neck
- Observe the movement of the cervical spine by having the patient rotate his or her head and shrug his or her shoulders against resistance (tests CN XI, spinal accessory).
- Palpate carotid pulses (one at a time).
- Auscultate carotids for bruits and turbulent blood flow.
- Palpate trachea for midline position.
- Palpate thyroid for masses.
- Palpate lymph nodes (pre- and postauricular, occipital, cervical, and submental nodes) for tenderness and swelling.

Eyes

- Inspect lashes, position and symmetry of eyes, and symmetry and size of pupils; inspect and palpate lids.
- Palpate lacrimal sacs for abnormal tearing or purulent excretion from the inner canthus area.
- Inspect:
  - **Sclera:** Normally white to buff colored.
  - **Conjunctiva:** Clear to pink colored, with shiny appearance.
  - **Pupils:** Approx. one-quarter the size of the iris; constrict with light and dilate in the absence of light; observe for symmetrical reactions.
  - **Irises:** Compare for equal color, size, and shape.
- Assess CN III (oculomotor), IV (trochlear), and VI (abducens) (*see* **CN Assessment**, p. 43).
- Assess convergence: As eyes shift from a far object to a near object, pupils should constrict.
- Assess confrontation: Have the patient cover one eye and look straight ahead while you hold your fingers in his or her peripheral fields; then ask the patient to tell you where he or she sees your fingers (e.g., upper left, lower right).
- Assess visual acuity using a Snellen chart for distance and a Rosenbaum chart for near vision.
  - **Snellen chart:** An eye chart used to measure visual acuity at a distance. The traditional Snellen chart is printed with 11 lines of block letters. The first line consists of one very large letter, which may be one of several letters (e.g., E, H, N, or A). Subsequent rows have an increasing amount of letters in decreasing sizes. A patient taking the test covers one eye and then reads aloud the letters of each row, beginning at the top. The smallest row that can be read accurately indicates the patient's visual acuity in the other eye.
  - **Rosenbaum chart:** An eye chart used to measure visual acuity up close. The Rosenbaum chart is held in the patient's hand at a distance of 14 inches. The chart is printed with 10 lines of numbers. The first line consists of a few very large numbers. Subsequent rows have an increasing amount of numbers in decreasing sizes. A patient taking the test covers one eye and then reads aloud the numbers of the smallest row that he or she is able to read. The smallest row that can be read accurately indicates the patient's visual acuity in the other eye.
- Assess extraocular movements (EOMs) by having the patient move the eyes in all directions without moving the head; this tests CN III, IV, and VI.
- Assess pupillary response using **PERRLA** (**p**upils should be **e**qual, **r**ound, and **r**eactive to **l**ight and **a**ccommodation).
  - Pupils should constrict in response to light.
  - Pupils should accommodate (constrict) for near vision.
  - Pupils should dilate (open) for dimness and distance.
- Use an ophthalmoscope to inspect the retina and inner eye structures.
  - **Ophthalmoscope or funduscope:** An instrument used to examine the eye; it consists of a mirror that reflects light into the eye and a central hole through which the eye is examined.

Grading Pupil Size

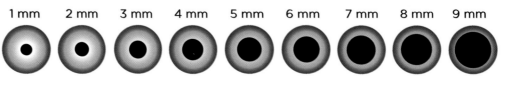

| 1 mm | 2 mm | 3 mm | 4 mm | 5 mm | 6 mm | 7 mm | 8 mm | 9 mm |

Ears

- Inspect and palpate for size, shape, position, discharge, lesions, and alignment. The tops of the ears should line up with the outer corners of the eyes.
- Test hearing acuity using normal voice, whisper test, Weber test, and Rinne test.
- Perform otoscopic examination:
  - The normal eardrum (tympanic membrane [TM]) should be pearly gray in color.
  - An inflamed TM will be reddish pink.
- Assess CN VIII (*see* **CN Assessment**, p. 43).
- Be familiar with equipment for ear assessment:
  - **Otoscope or auriscope:** A device used to look into the ears. The head of the otoscope contains an electric light source and a low-power magnifying lens. The examiner can look through the lens and see inside the ear canal.
  - **Tuning fork:** An acoustic tool that resonates at a specific constant pitch when set vibrating by striking it against a surface or with an object; it emits a musical tone. Tuning forks are used to assess hearing. They are sometimes also used to check vibration sense as part of the peripheral nervous system examination.

Nose

- Observe external structure for shape, size, color, and presence of nasal discharge (note color, amount, and consistency).
- Palpate for masses or deviations; occlude one naris (nostril) at a time and assess for obstructions in the other.

Mouth & Throat

- Inspect for sores, condition of teeth and gums, irritation, or other conditions that could affect the intake of food and liquid.
- Look under tongue for tumors or lesions.
- Assess for unusual breath odors.
- Inspect oropharynx for presence or absence of tonsils, color, swelling, movement of uvula, and presence of gag reflex.

Upper Extremities Assessment

- Inspect skin.
- Test capillary refill.
- Rate muscle strength.
- Assess range of motion (ROM).
- Check deep tendon reflexes.
- Palpate peripheral pulses.

Posterior Thorax Assessment

- Inspect spine for alignment.
- Assess anteroposterior to lateral diameter.
- Assess thoracic expansion.
- Palpate for tactile fremitus.
- Auscultate breath sounds.
- Percuss over costovertebral angles for tenderness.

Anterior Thorax Assessment

- Observe respiratory pattern.
- Inspect jugular veins.
- Palpate respiratory excursion.

- Perform breast examination.
- Auscultate breath sounds.
- Auscultate heart sounds.

Abdominal Assessment
- Palpate the kidneys and spleen.
- Percuss for masses and tenderness.
- Percuss the liver.
- Auscultate for bowel sounds.

Lower Extremities Assessment
- Inspect skin.
- Inspect joints for swelling.
- Assess for Homans sign.
- Assess for pedal and ankle edema.
- Assess ROM.
- Palpate peripheral pulses.
- Palpate joints for swelling.

Cardiovascular Assessment

The primary purpose of the cardiovascular system is to move nutrients, gases, and wastes to and from cells. It encompasses the neck vessels, heart, and peripheral vascular system.

Blood Pressure

Blood pressure (BP) is recorded as two numbers:
- The higher number, or **systolic pressure**, is the maximal contraction of the heart.
- The lower number, or **diastolic pressure**, is the resting pressure in the heart's ventricles.

The difference between the systolic and diastolic pressure, called the **pulse pressure**, represents the force that the heart generates each time it contracts.

> The cardiac cycle has two phases: **systole**, when the ventricles contract and eject blood, and **diastole**, when the ventricles relax and blood fills the ventricles and the coronary arteries.

Adult BP Values		
	Diastolic	Systolic
Normal	<120	<80
Prehypertension	120–139	80–89
Stage 1 hypertension	140–159	90–99
Stage 2 hypertension	≥160	≥100

Neck Vessel Assessment

Assessment of the neck vessels will give you information about the patient's cardio-pulmonary status.

Inspection

The right internal jugular vein is typically the best neck vessel to inspect:
- Position the patient at a 45-degree angle, and turn his or her head slightly away from you.
- Using tangential light, observe the physical appearance and the venous pulsation of the external jugular vein where it passes over the sternomastoid muscle.

Palpation

Palpate the carotid arteries low in the neck to avoid the carotid sinus:

- Locate the internal jugular pulsation, and mark the highest point of pulsation.
- Find the angle of Louis; use two straight lines to mark the intersection, and measure the distance above the sternal angle (2 cm or less is normal).

Auscultation

Auscultate the carotid arteries using the bell of the stethoscope:

- Listen at the angle of the jaw, the midcervical area, and the base of the neck; then ask the patient to hold his or her breath momentarily.
- Listen for carotid bruits (blowing or rushing sounds over the carotid artery). Carotid bruits are usually the result of carotid artery stenosis.

> Palpate the carotid arteries one side at a time to prevent compromising blood flow to the head.

Heart & Pericardium Assessment

Inspection

While the patient is in a supine position, inspect the chest wall, looking for pulsations, heaves, or lifts. The apical pulse may be visible in the fourth or fifth intercostal space (ICS) at the left midclavicular line, known as the **point of maximum impulse (PMI)**.

Palpation

Methodically palpate the pericardium using the palms and fingers. Begin at the apex, and move to the left sternal border and then to the base of the heart.

- The PMI can be felt on palpation.
  - The PMI is normally 2–3 cm in diameter.
  - A large, laterally displaced or diffuse PMI may indicate some form of cardiomegaly.
- No palpable pulsations should be felt over the aortic, pulmonic, or mitral valve.
- There should be no palpable heaves or thrills over the apex.
  - **Heave:** Upward displacement of the chest against the hand; heaves are best felt with the heel of the hand at the sternal border. Heaves have various associations.
  - **Thrill:** A palpable murmur that feels similar to a cat purring; the tips of the fingers may be more sensitive to this vibration. Thrills are always associated with murmurs.

Percussion

Although percussion is used to determine cardiac borders, it is of limited use in assessment of the heart.

Auscultation

Heart sounds produced by valve closure are best heard where blood flows away from the valve instead of directly over the valve. The systolic phase begins with the first heart sound (S1), the closure of the mitral and tricuspid (atrioventricular [AV]) valves. The diastolic phase begins with the second heart sound (S2), the closure of the aortic and pulmonic (semilunar) valves.

The white circled areas on the corresponding figure indicate optimal placement of the stethoscope for auscultating heart sounds. For placement of the stethoscope, think of "APE To Man":

- **Aortic valve:** S2 is louder
- **Pulmonary valve:** S2 is louder
- **Erb's point:** S1 equals S2
- **Tricuspid valve:** S1 is louder
- **Mitral valve (PMI):** S1 is louder

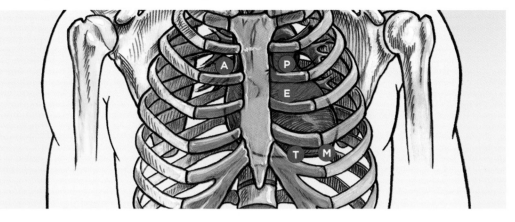

Listen to the blood flow through the cardiac structures. If heart sounds are faint or undetectable, have the patient lean forward or lie on his or her left side to bring the heart closer to the surface of the anterior chest wall.

- **Aortic valve:** Right second ICS sternal border
- **Pulmonic valve:** Left second ICS sternal border
- **Tricuspid valve:** Left fifth ICS sternal border
- **Mitral valve:** Left fifth ICS midclavicular line

Using the diaphragm of the stethoscope, note the following at each area (repeat the auscultation process using the bell of the stethoscope):

- Rate and rhythm
- S1 and S2:
  - S1 is the "lub" sound; S2 is the "dub" sound.
  - S1 is best heard over the mitral valve; S2 is best heard over the aortic valve.
  - S1 is louder than S2 at the apex; S2 is louder than S1 at the base.
  - S1 coincides with carotid pulsation.
- Extra heart sounds or murmurs:
  - S3 (a.k.a. ventricular gallop) is caused by increased blood volume within the ventricle and is best heard with the bell of the stethoscope.
  - S4 (a.k.a. atrial gallop) is caused by blood being forced into a hypertrophic ventricle.
  - Murmurs are turbulence, or a gentle blowing or swooshing sound, caused by a change in the velocity of blood flow, a structural defect in the valves, or an unusual opening in the cardiac chambers.

Grading of Murmurs	
Grade	**Sound**
Grade I	Barely audible
Grade II	Clearly audible but faint
Grade III	Moderately loud; easy to hear with stethoscope
Grade IV	Loud; associated with a thrill palpable on the chest wall
Grade V	Very loud; heard with stethoscope partially lifted off the chest wall
Grade VI	Loudest; heard with entire stethoscope lifted off the chest wall

Normal Electrocardiogram (ECG/EKG) Pattern

Complex	Normal Length of Time	What It Represents
P wave	0.06–11 sec	Depolarization of atria; preparation for contraction
PR interval	0.12–0.2 sec	Time for impulse to spread from atria to ventricles
QRS complex	0.04–0.11 sec	Depolarization of ventricles
QT interval	Up to 0.44 sec	Electrical systole
ST segment	Not measured	Completion of ventricular depolarization
T wave	Not measured	Repolarization of ventricles
U wave	Varies	Sometimes follows T wave; may indicate hypokalemia

Normal Sinus Rhythm

Lead Numbers & Corresponding Views of the Heart

	Lead	View of Heart
Standard limb leads (bipolar)	I	Lateral wall
	II	Inferior wall
	III	Inferior wall
Augmented limb leads (unipolar)	aVR	No specific view
	aVL	Lateral wall
	aVF	Inferior wall
Precordial (chest) leads (unipolar)	V_1	Septal wall
	V_2	Septal wall
	V_3	Anterior wall
	V_4	Anterior wall
	V_5	Lateral wall
	V_6	Lateral wall

Views of the Heart Reflected on a 12-Lead ECG

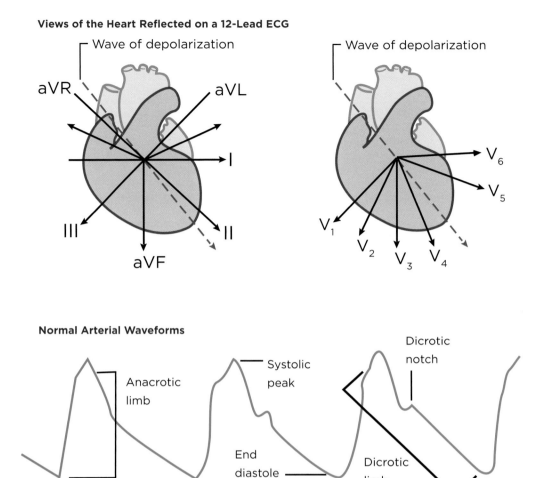

Normal Arterial Waveforms

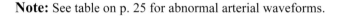

Note: See table on p. 25 for abnormal arterial waveforms.

Cardiac Output

Cardiac Output = Heart Rate × Stroke Volume

Hemodynamic Parameters

Afterload Normal Values

- **Pulmonary vascular resistance (PVR)**
  - **Normal value:** <250 dynes/sec/cm^{-5}
  - [(MPAP – PAOP)/CO] × 80 = PVR
  - **Calculation:** [(Mean Pulmonary Artery Pressure – Pulmonary Artery Occlusion Pressure)/Cardiac Output] × 80 = PVR (right ventricle)
- **Systemic vascular resistance (SVR)**
  - **Normal value:** 800–1500 dynes/sec/cm^{-5}
  - [(MAP – RAP)/CO] × 80 = SVR
  - **Calculation:** [(Mean Arterial Pressure – Right Arterial Pressure)/Cardiac Output] × 80 = SVR (left ventricle)

Abnormal Arterial Waveforms

Abnormality	Possible Causes	Nursing Interventions
Flattened waveform	Hypotension or overdamped waveform	Use sphygmomanometer to check BP; suspect hypotension if reading is low or absent; if reading is high, suspect overdamping; try to aspirate the arterial line and, if successful, flush the line.
Alternating high and low waves in a regular pattern	Ventricular bigeminy	Check the ECG to confirm ventricular bigeminy; for every second beat, the tracing should reflect premature ventricular contractions; look for signs of tamponade in the patient.
Slow upstroke	Aortic stenosis	Check the heart sounds for signs of aortic stenosis; notify the doctor.
Diminished amplitude on inspiration	Paradoxical pulse, possibly caused by lung disease, cardiac tamponade, or constrictive pericarditis	Check the systolic pressure during inspiration and expiration; if the inspiratory pressure is at least 10 mm Hg less than the expiratory pressure, notify the doctor; if you are monitoring pulmonary artery pressure, check for diastolic plateau.
Slightly rounded waveform with consistent variations in systolic height	Patient on ventilator with positive end-expiratory pressure	Regularly check systolic BP; the difference between the highest and lowest systolic pressures should be less than 10 mm Hg.

Contractility Normal Values
- **Right ventricular stroke work index (RVSWI)**
    - **Normal value:** 5–10 g/m^2/beat
    - SVI × (MPAP – CVP) × 0.0136 = RVSWI
    - **Calculation:** Stroke Volume Index × (Mean Pulmonary Artery Pressure – Central Venous Pressure) × 0.0136 = RVSWI
- **Left ventricular stroke work index (LVSWI)**
    - **Normal value:** 50–62 g/m^2/beat
    - SVI × (MAP – PAOP) × 0.0136 = LVSWI
    - **Calculation:** Stroke Volume Index × (Mean Arterial Pressure – Pulmonary Arterial Occlusion Pressure) × 0.0136 = LVSWI

Blood Flow Rate

Flow rate $= \dfrac{\Delta P}{R}$, where ΔP = pressure difference and R = resistance to flow

Mean Arterial Pressure

$$\frac{\left[(\text{Systolic}) + 2(\text{Diastolic})\right]}{3} = \text{MAP}$$

Stroke Symptoms

Sudden onset of:
- Numbness or weakness
- Confusion
- Loss of vision
- Loss of balance
- Severe headache

Cardiac Markers & Serum Enzyme Levels Following Acute Myocardial Infarction				
Enzyme or Marker	Normal	Appears in Serum (hr)	Peaks (hr)	Duration (days)
Myoglobin	12–90 ng/mL	1–2	4–6	1–1½
Cardiac troponin I (cTnI)	<0.6 ng/mL	4–6	14–24	5–14
Cardiac troponin T (cTnT)	<0.1 ng/mL	3–5	12–48	5–14
Creatine phosphokinase/ creatine kinase myocardial specific (CPK/CK-MB2)	<0–7.5 ng/mL	2–6	12–24	2–3

Heart Failure Classifications	
Classification	Symptoms
I	No limitation of physical activity; ordinary physical activity does not cause undue fatigue, palpitation, dyspnea, or anginal pain
II	Slight limitation of physical activity; comfortable at rest; ordinary physical activity results in fatigue, palpitation, dyspnea, or anginal pain
III	Marked limitation of physical activity; comfortable at rest; less than ordinary activity causes fatigue, palpitation, dyspnea, or anginal pain
IV	Inability to carry on any physical activity without discomfort; symptoms of heart failure or the anginal syndrome may be present even at rest; if any physical activity is undertaken, discomfort increases
Note: Based on the New York Heart Association (NYHA) functional classification system.	

Peripheral Vascular Assessment

The peripheral vascular system is the system of intertwining veins and arteries that carry blood to and from the heart and lungs.

Six Ps of Circulatory Checks
Pain
Pallor
Paralysis
Paresthesia
Pulse
Poikilothermia

Edema Rating Scale	
Number	**Corresponding Response**
0	No edema
1+	Barely discernible depression
2+	Deeper depression (less than 5 mm) accompanied by normal foot and leg contours
3+	Deep depression (5–10 mm) accompanied by foot and leg swelling
4+	Even deeper depression (more than 1 cm) accompanied by severe foot and leg swelling

Artery Assessment

When checking pulses, note strength, rate, and symmetry. Rate the strength of each pulse as:

- 0 (absent)
- 1+ (decreased)
- 2+ (normal)
- 3+ (full)
- 4+ (bounding)

Repeat the procedure on the opposite side.

Carotid
See **Neck Vessel Assessment**, p. 20.

Radial & Brachial

- Palpate the radial pulse using the index and middle finger on the inside of the wrist at the base of the thumb. Raise the patient's forearm, and feel for a bounding pulse with the flat of your palm.
- Palpate the brachial pulse using the index and middle fingers on the inside of the arm in the elbow crease. The brachial pulse can be more easily palpated if the arm is slightly hyperextended.

> A normal adult pulse is symmetrical, regular, and between 60 and 90 beats per minute.

Femoral

Palpation
- The femoral pulse can be found in the crease between the upper thigh and the lower pelvic area.
- With the patient lying flat, press deeply about midway between the iliac crest and the groin.

Auscultation
- Use the diaphragm of the stethoscope to listen over the femoral artery for a bruit.

Popliteal, Posterior Tibial & Dorsalis Pedis
- Gently flex the knee, wrap your hands around it, and feel for the popliteal pulse by deep palpation in the midline of the popliteal space.
- Palpate the posterior tibial pulse on the inner ankle behind and below the medial malleolus.
- Palpate the dorsalis pedis pulse on top of the foot in between the base of the big toe and the ankle.
- Palpate the feet to assess vascularity:
  - Warmth
  - Capillary refill
  - Elevation pallor
  - Dependent rubor

> Special attention should be given to signs of chronic arterial or venous insufficiency.

Respiratory Assessment

The primary purpose of the respiratory system is twofold: (1) gas exchange, or the transfer of oxygen and carbon dioxide between the atmosphere and the blood; and (2) the maintenance of the acid-base balance.

Inspection
- Inspect ability to breathe, respiratory rate, chest contour, and chest movement; look for the presence of retractions.
- Evaluate the state of oxygenation by inspecting skin color, level of consciousness, and emotional state.
- Observe the position of the trachea.
- Assess the size and shape of the chest; lateral diameter should be greater than anterior to posterior diameter.
- Determine whether there is uniform and equal expansion of the chest.
- Inspect for chest wall deformities:
  - **Kyphosis:** Curvature of the upper spine, which may lead to hunchback
  - **Scoliosis:** Lateral curvature of the spine
  - **Barrel chest:** A rounded chest that is shaped like a barrel (normal in children; typical of hyperinflation seen in COPD)
  - **Pectus excavatum:** Sternum sunken into the chest
  - **Pectus carinatum:** Sternum protruding from the chest
- Evaluate for signs of respiratory distress:
  - **Cyanosis:** Bluish discoloration of skin and mucous membranes caused by an excessive concentration of reduced hemoglobin in the blood
  - **Pursed-lip breathing:** Breathing in through the nose and out through puckered or pursed lips that is used to increase end-expiratory pressure
  - **Accessory muscle use:** Raising of the shoulders and intercostal retractions with inspiration
  - **Diaphragmatic paradox:** Diaphragm movement that is opposite of the normal direction on inspiration; suspect flail chest in trauma patients
  - **Intercostal retractions:** Retraction of the ICSs from abnormally high negative pressure generated during inspiration
- Evaluate breathing patterns:
  - Rate:
    - **Eupnea:** Normal (12–20 breaths per minute)
    - **Tachypnea:** Increased rate
    - **Bradypnea:** Decreased rate
  - Depth:
    - **Hyperpnea:** Deep, labored breathing
    - **Hyperventilation:** Deep, rapid breathing
    - **Hypoventilation:** Slow, shallow breathing
  - Rhythm:
    - **Apnea:** Brief pause in breathing

- **Cheyne-Stokes respiration:** Alternating periods of shallow and deep breathing; often seen in comatose patients
- **Biot respiration:** Groups of quick, shallow inspirations followed by periods of apnea
- **Kussmaul respiration:** Rapid, deep, labored breathing; often seen in patients with metabolic acidosis, particularly diabetic ketoacidosis

Palpation

Palpate the posterior aspect of the chest for masses, bulges, crepitus, and areas of tenderness:
- Feel for tracheal deviation.
- Feel the posterior, anterior, and lateral thorax for tenderness, masses, or lesions.
- Palpate for crepitus (air leaks into the subcutaneous tissue).
- Evaluate tactile fremitus (palpable vibration); with the ulnar surface of the hand on the chest, ask the patient to say "blue moon," "boy-oh-boy," or "ninety-nine":
  - Vibration should be equal on the right and left side at any location.
  - Decreased fremitus occurs with conditions that obstruct transmission of vibrations (e.g., pneumonia or pleural effusion).
  - Increased fremitus occurs with consolidation or compression of lung tissue.
- Check respiratory expansion: To check if thoracic expansion is equal, place your palms on the patient's chest with your thumbs parallel to each other near the midline; then lightly pinch the skin between your thumbs and ask the patient to take a deep breath. Observe for equal, bilateral expansion.

Percussion

Percuss to determine if underlying tissue is filled with air or other substance:
- Compare the left side to the right side.
- Begin percussing at the apex of the left lung, then move your hands symmetrically, comparing the left to the right side as you move toward the bases.

Auscultation

To auscultate lung sounds, move the diaphragm of your stethoscope according to the numbers on the corresponding figure. There are three normal breath sounds:
- **Bronchial (B) breath sounds:** Loud, harsh, high-pitched; heard over the trachea, bronchi (between clavicles and midsternum), and main bronchus. These sounds are more tubular and hollow-sounding than vesicular sounds but not as harsh as tracheal breath sounds. Expiratory sounds last longer than inspiratory sounds.
- **Bronchovesicular (BV) breath sounds:** Blowing sounds of moderate intensity and pitch; heard in the posterior chest between the scapulae and in the center part of the anterior chest. These sounds are softer than bronchial sounds but have a tubular quality. They are about equal during inspiration and expiration, but differences in pitch and intensity are often more easily detected during expiration.
- **Vesicular (V) breath sounds:** Soft, low-pitched, and breezy; heard over the peripheral lung area; heard throughout most of the lung fields. These sounds are normally heard throughout inspiration, continue without pause through expiration, and then fade away about one-third of the way through expiration.

Stethoscope Placement for Auscultating Lung Sounds

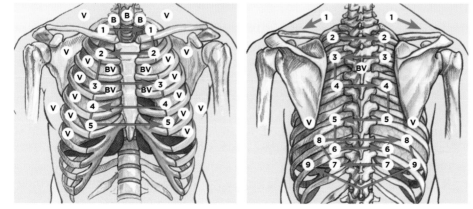

Auscultate to assess air flow through the bronchial tree:
- Work superior to inferior, and compare right to left.
- Auscultate the posterior chest, then the anterior chest.
  - Auscultate the trachea using the diaphragm of the stethoscope.
  - Auscultate the primary bronchi (from T3 to T5) using the diaphragm of the stethoscope.
  - Auscultate the lungs; begin at the apex of each lung (C7) and zigzag downward between ICSs to the bases (about T10) using the diaphragm of the stethoscope.
- Compare the sound being heard with the expected sound at each location to identify adventitious sounds.

Abnormal breath sounds include the absence of sound and the presence of sounds in areas where they are normally not heard; *adventitious* breath sounds refer to extra or additional sounds that are heard over normal breath sounds.

- **Crackles** (a.k.a. **rales**) are caused by fluid in the small airways or by atelectasis. The popping sounds they produce are created when air is forced through respiratory passages that are narrowed by fluid, mucus, or pus. Crackles:
  - Are referred to as discontinuous sounds, as they are intermittent, nonmusical, and brief
  - Most commonly heard on inspiration
  - Are often associated with inflammation or infection of the small bronchi, bronchioles, and alveoli
  - May indicate pulmonary edema or fluid in the alveoli caused by heart failure or adult respiratory distress syndrome (ARDS) if they do not clear after a cough
  - Are often described as fine, medium, or coarse:
    - Fine crackles are soft, high-pitched, and very brief (simulate this sound by rolling a strand of hair between your fingers near your ear or by moistening your thumb and index finger and separating them near your ear).
    - Coarse crackles are somewhat louder, lower in pitch, and longer lasting than fine crackles; they have been described as sounding like opening a Velcro fastener.
    - Medium crackles are between fine and coarse in sound and duration.
- **Wheezes** are caused by air moving through airways narrowed by constriction, swelling of the airway, or partial airway obstruction. They are normally heard continuously during inspiration or expiration or during both inspiration and expiration.
  - Wheezes that are relatively high-pitched and have a shrill or squeaking quality may be referred to as *sibilant rhonchi*; they occur when airways are narrowed (e.g., during an acute asthmatic attack).
  - Wheezes that are lower in pitch with a snoring or moaning quality may be referred to as *sonorous rhonchi*; secretions in large airways, such as those that occur with bronchitis, may produce these sounds, which may clear somewhat with coughing.
- **Pleural friction rubs** are low-pitched, grating, or creaking sounds that occur when inflamed pleural surfaces rub together during respiration; they are more often heard on inspiration than on expiration.
  - The pleural friction rub is easy to confuse with a pericardial friction rub.
  - To determine whether the sound is a pleural friction rub or a pericardial friction rub, ask the patient to hold his or her breath briefly; if the rubbing sound continues, it is a pericardial friction rub because the inflamed pericardial layers continue rubbing together with each heartbeat. A pleural friction rub stops when breathing stops.
- **Stridor** refers to a high-pitched, harsh sound heard during inspiration. Stridor is caused by obstruction of the upper airway; it is a sign of respiratory distress and requires immediate attention.
- **Rhonchi** are characterized by a coarse rattling sound (almost like snoring) on expiration; they are caused by secretions in the bronchial tube.

Detection of adventitious sounds is an important part of the respiratory examination, often leading to diagnosis of cardiac or pulmonary conditions.

The patterns of normal breath sounds are created by the effect of body structures on air moving through airways; breath sounds are described by:
- **Duration:** How long the sound lasts
- **Intensity:** How loud the sound is
- **Pitch:** How high or low the sound is
- **Timing:** When the sound occurs in the respiratory cycle

Adventitious Lung Sounds & Potential Causes

Sound	Characteristics	Lung Problem
Crackles	Popping, cracking, bubbling sound; most commonly heard on inspiration	Pneumonia, pulmonary edema, pulmonary fibrosis, congestive heart failure
Rhonchi	Rattling sound on expiration	Pneumonia, emphysema, bronchitis, bronchiectasis
Wheezes	High-pitched musical sound during both inspiration and expiration (louder)	Emphysema, asthma, foreign bodies, anaphylaxis
Pleural friction rub	Dry, grating sound; most commonly heard on expiration	Pleurisy, pneumonia, pleural infarct
Stridor	High-pitched harsh sound on inspiration	Airway obstruction

Arterial Blood Gas Analysis

Arterial blood gas (ABG) analysis is a measure of how much oxygen and carbon dioxide are in the blood. It is used to evaluate respiratory diseases and conditions, to determine the effectiveness of oxygen therapy, and to evaluate acid-base balance.

Normal ABG Results

Arterial blood pH	7.35–7.45
Partial arterial pressure of oxygen (PAO$_2$)	>80 mm Hg
Partial arterial pressure of carbon dioxide (PACO$_2$)	35–45 mm Hg
Bicarbonate (HCO$_3$)	20–30 mEq/L
Oxygen saturation (SaO$_2$)	94%–100%

Lung Volume & Capacities

	Symbol	Normal Value
Tidal volume	TV or VT	500 mL or 5–10 mL/kg
Inspiratory reserve volume	IRV	3000 mL
Expiratory reserve volume	ERV	1100 mL
Residual volume	RV	1200 mL
Vital capacity	VC	4600 mL
Inspiratory capacity	IC	3500 mL
Functional residual capacity	FRC	2300 mL
Total lung capacity	TLC	5800 mL

Respiratory Tools & Equipment

- **Airway:** A tube or tubelike device that is inserted through the nose or mouth or directly into the trachea to provide an opening for ventilation.
- **Endotracheal tube (ETT):** A tube that is inserted into a patient's trachea to ensure that the airway is not closed off and that air is able to reach the lungs. The ETT is

regarded as the most reliable method for protecting a patient's airway. ETTs come in a number of sizes, ranging from 2 to 10.5 mm in internal diameter. Size is chosen based on the patient's body size, with smaller sizes being used for pediatric and neonatal patients. The choice of ETT size is always a compromise between choosing the largest size to maximize flow and minimize airway resistance and the smallest size to minimize airway trauma.

- **Flowmeter:** An instrument for measuring the amount of air flowing out of the lungs; it is used to determine how well a patient's asthma is being controlled.
- **Laryngoscope:** A rigid instrument used to examine the larynx and to facilitate intubation of the trachea.
- **Nasopharyngeal tube or trumpet:** A tube that is inserted through one nostril to create an air passage between the nose and the nasopharynx. The nasopharyngeal tube is preferable to the oropharyngeal airway in conscious patients because it is better tolerated and less likely to induce a gag reflex.
- **Oropharyngeal airway or oral airway:** A curved piece of plastic inserted over the tongue that creates an air passage between the mouth and the posterior pharyngeal wall. It is used to maintain a patent, or open, airway. An oral airway prevents the tongue from covering (either partially or completely) the epiglottis, which could prevent the patient from breathing.
- **Pressure regulator:** An instrument that is used to reduce the high pressure of oxygen delivered from a cylinder to a lower pressure that is controllable by the flowmeter. Regulators are used to allow high-pressure fluid supply lines or tanks to be reduced to safe and usable pressures for various applications.
- **Suction catheters:** Flexible, long tubes used to remove respiratory secretions from the airway. One end of the suction catheter is connected to a collection container (suction canister) and a device that generates suction. The open end is advanced through the airway (through either an endotracheal or a tracheostomy tube) to remove secretions. The purpose of suctioning is to keep the airway clear of secretions and to prevent plugging.
- **Tracheal tube:** A flexible tube inserted nasally (nasotracheal), orally (orotracheal), or through a tracheotomy into the trachea to provide an airway.

Integumentary Assessment

The integumentary system includes the skin, hair, and nails. The skin protects the body by preventing fluid loss; regulating body temperature; providing sensory perception; excreting impurities; and protecting against infection, exposure, and trauma. The skin is the largest organ in the body; the average adult has more than 20 square feet of skin.
- The skin responds to external changes and reflects internal changes.
- Skin consists of three layers: the epidermis, the dermis, and the subcutaneous tissue.
- Skin carries out seven major functions:
    - Maintaining an internal environment by acting as a barrier to loss of water and electrolytes
    - Protecting the body from external agents that could injure the internal environment
    - Regulating body heat
    - Acting as a sense organ for touch, temperature, and pain
    - Performing self-maintenance and repairing wounds
    - Producing vitamin D
    - Delaying hypersensitivity reaction to foreign substances

Skin Assessment
- Begin with a general inspection, followed by a detailed examination.
- Wear gloves if the patient has any lesions or complains of itching or if mucous membranes are to be examined.

- Inspect for color, texture, tone, and the presence and distribution of lesions.
  - **Normal findings:** Color varies by person but should be uniform, smooth, and toned.
  - **Abnormal findings:** Look for pale, shiny skin of lower extremities; moles with irregular borders or color changes; and localized hemorrhages.
- Inspect for scars or masses; note location, size, and appearance.
- Palpate using the back of the hand to assess for temperature, moisture, and texture.
  - **Normal findings:** Cool to warm, dry, smooth
  - **Unexpected findings:** Lesions, temperature elevation or depression, pedunculation, exudates
- Inspect distribution of hair on the head and body.
- Inspect nails for color, contour, texture, symmetry, and cleanliness.
  - **Normal findings:** Smooth nail plate, nail-base angle of 160 degrees, uniform color
  - **Unexpected findings:** Color change, white spots, cuticle trauma
- Inspect nails for clubbing (loss of normal angle between nail and nail bed because of chronic oxygen deprivation).
- Perform capillary refill test:
  - Press down on nail until it blanches.
  - Release nail and observe for return of pink color; color should return in less than 3 seconds.
  - A delay indicates poor arterial circulation.

> Room and body temperature, as well as vasoconstriction from smoking or peripheral edema, can affect capillary refill.

Abnormal Findings & Potential Causes

Finding	Possible Meaning
Jaundice (yellow discoloration, including sclera)	Liver problem, biliary tract disease
Pale yellow skin tone	Renal problem
Flushed, red face	Excessive ethyl alcohol (EtOH) consumption, fever, localized inflammation, embarrassment
Pale	Circulatory problem

Quick Guide to Skin Assessment

Color	Texture	Turgor (elasticity)	Moisture	Temperature	Lesions
Bruising, discoloration, erythema, pallor, duskiness, jaundice, cyanosis	Thickness, thinness, mobility, roughness, smoothness, fragility	Squeeze skin on patient's forearm to assess: if it returns quickly to its regular shape, turgor is normal; if it returns slowly or remains indented, turgor is abnormal	Excessive dryness, redness, flakiness; excessive moisture or sponginess	Generalized or localized warmth or coolness	Red, pigmented lesions may indicate vascular changes; common disease-indicating lesions are hemangiomas, telangiectases, petechiae, purpura, and ecchymosis

Note: Use both inspection and palpation to examine the skin.

Evaluating Skin Color Variations

Color	Distribution	Possible Cause
Absent	Small, circumscribed areas or generalized	Vitiligo or albinism
Blue	Around lips or generalized	Cyanosis*
Deep red	Generalized	Polycythemia vera
Pink	Local or generalized	Erythema
Tan to brown	Facial patches	Chloasma, pregnancy, or butterfly rash of lupus erythematosus
Tan to brown-bronze	Generalized (unrelated to sun exposure)	Addison disease
Yellow	Sclera or generalized	Jaundice from liver dysfunction**
Yellow-orange	Palms, soles, and face; not sclera	Carotenemia (carotene in blood)

*Bluish gingivae are normal in African American patients.

**Yellow-brown pigmentation of the sclera is normal in African American patients.

Careful assessment of the skin can alert the nurse to cutaneous problems, as well as to systemic diseases.

Primary Lesions & Associated Conditions

Primary Lesion	Appearance	Associated Conditions
Macule	Flat and small (1 cm or less) with color change	Rubeola, rubella, scarlet fever, roseola infantilis
Papule	Elevated, well circumscribed, small (1 cm), colored	Ringworm, psoriasis
Vesicle or blister	Bulging; small (1 cm or less); sharply defined; filled with clear, free fluid	Herpes simplex, varicella, poison ivy, herpes zoster
Bulla	Large (greater than 1 cm) vesicle	Scarlet fever, sunburn
Pustule	Elevated, well circumscribed, small (less than 1 cm), filled with pus	Impetigo, acne, staphylococcus infection
Wheal	Elevated, white to pink edematous lesion that is unstable and associated with itching; evanescent (they appear and disappear quickly)	Mosquito bites, hives
Petechiae	Tiny, reddish-purple, well-circumscribed spots of hemorrhage in the superficial layers of the epidermis	Severe systemic disease, such as meningococcemia, bacterial endocarditis, or nonthrombocytopenic purpura

Secondary Lesions & Associated Conditions

Secondary Lesion	Appearance	Associated Conditions
Scales	Dried fragments of sloughed dead epidermis	Seborrhea, tinea capitis
Crusts	Dried blood, serum, scales, and pus from corrosive lesions	Infectious dermatitis
Excoriation	Mechanical removal of epidermis, leaving dermis exposed	Scratch or scrape of original lesion
Erosion	Loss of some or all of epidermis, leaving a denuded surface	Excessive dryness, chemicals
Ulcer	Destruction and loss of the epidermis, dermis, and possibly subcutaneous layers	Trauma, exposure to heat or cold, problems with blood circulation, irritation from exposure to corrosive material
Fissure	A vertical, linear crack through epidermis and dermis	Candidiasis, dermatitis
Scar	Formation of dense connective tissue	Skin injury
Lichenification	Pronounced thickening of the epidermis and dermis	Chronic scratching or rubbing

Seven Warning Signs of Cancer

Change in bowel or bladder habits

A sore that does not heal

Unusual bleeding or discharge

Thickening or lump in breast or elsewhere

Indigestion or difficulty swallowing

Obvious change in wart or mole

Nagging cough or hoarseness

Decubitus Ulcers

To avoid decubitus ulcers, reposition the patient often and check the patient's skin carefully.

Common Locations for Decubitus Ulcers

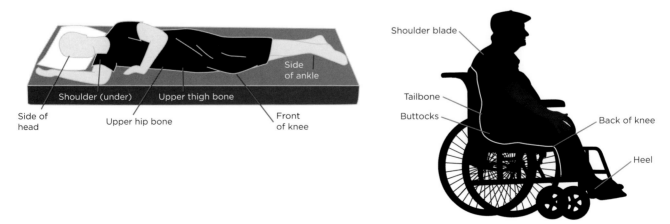

Decubitus Ulcer Staging

Stage	Assessment Findings
Stage I 	Nonblanchable erythema that remains red 30 minutes after pressure has been relieved; epidermis remains intact
Stage II 	Epidermis is broken, lesion is superficial, and there is partial-thickness skin loss
Stage III 	Full-thickness skin loss down through the dermis, which may include subcutaneous tissue
Stage IV 	Full-thickness skin loss extending into supportive structures, such as muscle, tendon, and bone

Decubitus Ulcer Risk Assessment		
Activity	Ambulant without assistance	0
	Ambulant with assistance	1
	Chairfast	2
	Bedfast	3
Mobility: ROM	Full ROM	0
	Moves with minimal assistance	1
	Moves with moderate assistance	2
	Immobile	3
Skin condition	Hydrated and intact	0
	Rashes or abrasions	1
	Decreased turgor, dry	2
	Edema, erythema, pressure ulcers	3
Predisposing disease process	No involvement	0
	Chronic, stable	1
	Acute or chronic, unstable	2
	Terminal	3
Level of consciousness	Alert	0
	Slow verbal response	1
	Responds to verbal or painful stimuli	2
	Absence of response to stimuli	3
Nutritional status	Good (eats 75% or more of food offered)	0
	Fair (eats less than 75% of food offered)	1
	Poor	2
	Unable or refuses, emaciated	3
Incontinence: bladder	None	0
	Occasional	1
	Usually	2
	Total	3
Incontinence: bowel	None	0
	Occasional	1
	Usually	2
	Total	3

Note: Lowest possible score is 0; highest possible score is 24. A higher score means a higher risk for decubitus ulcers.

Gastrointestinal Assessment

The gastrointestinal (GI) system performs the functions of ingestion, digestion, and elimination. Interruptions of any of these functions can quickly affect the patient's nutritional intake and cause acid-base imbalances. When performing a GI assessment, remember that much of the population has preexisting problems; these problems can be exacerbated, and new conditions can develop when illness in other systems occurs.

Abdominal Assessment
Inspection
Inspect all four quadrants of the abdomen for contour, symmetry, abdominal aorta pulsation, and distention.
- A lower-quadrant bulge may indicate a distended bladder.
- A midline bulge may be an umbilical hernia.
- Wavelike movements are normal, especially in thin individuals, but visible rippling waves may indicate an obstruction.
- Abdominal distention can be caused by three factors:
  - **Obesity:** Soft and rounded, with sunken umbilicus
  - **Ascites:** Shiny and glistening skin with an everted umbilicus and dilated, prominent veins
  - **Obstruction:** Visible, marked peristalsis; restlessness; lying with knees flexed; grimacing facial expression; and uneven respirations

> Do not touch the abdomen during inspection, as peristalsis can be stimulated.

Auscultation
Auscultate before palpation and percussion to avoid increasing the frequency of bowel sounds.
- **Bowel sounds** are best heard with the diaphragm of the stethoscope.
  - Begin in the right lower quadrant, near the ileocecal valve, and listen to each quadrant in a clockwise pattern for at least 2 minutes.
  - Note the frequency of bowel sounds.
  - Note the classification of bowel sounds:
    - **Hypoactive:** Infrequent
    - **Normal:** Intermittent at 5–15 times per minute
    - **Hyperactive:** More frequent than normal
  - Note the character and quality of the sounds (high-pitched, gurgling, clicking).
- **Vascular sounds** are best heard with the bell of the stethoscope.
  - Listen over the iliac, aortic, renal, and femoral arteries for vascular sounds, such as bruits, venous hums, and friction rubs.

Percussion
- Percuss all four quadrants of the abdomen.
- Identify the location and size of the internal organs.
- Identify percussion sounds:
  - Tympany is the normally predominant sound as air rises to the surface of the abdominal cavity (e.g., empty stomach or bowel).
  - Hyperresonance is heard with gaseous distention.
  - Dullness is heard over a distended bladder, the liver, adipose tissue, fluid in the abdomen, a feces-filled bowel, or an abdominal mass.

WARNING!
Do not percuss if an abdominal aortic aneurysm is suspected.

Evaluating Nutritional Disorders

System or Region of the Body	Symptom or Sign	Implications
Cardiovascular	Hypotension, tachycardia, edema	Fluid volume deficit, protein deficiency
Eyes	Red conjunctiva; Bitot spots; swelling, dryness, or softening of the corneas; night blindness	Riboflavin or vitamin A deficiency
General	Weight loss, weakness, and lethargy	Decreased calorie intake, increased calorie use, or inadequate absorption or intake of nutrients; electrolyte imbalance; anemia
GI	Ascites	Protein deficiency
Musculoskeletal	Muscle wasting, bow leg, bone pain	Protein, carbohydrate, or fat deficiency; vitamin D or calcium deficiency
Neurologic	Paresthesia, altered mental status	Vitamin B_{12}, thiamine, or pyridoxine deficiency; dehydration
Skin, hair, nails	Rough skin with bumps and scales; flaky, dry skin; sore that will not heal; ridged, brittle, or spoon-shaped nails; dry, thinning hair; ecchymoses or petechiae	Vitamin A, vitamin B complex, linoleic acid, zinc, protein, vitamin C, iron, or vitamin K deficiency
Throat, mouth	Spongy, bleeding, soft gums; red, beefy tongue; magenta tongue; cracks at corner of mouth; swollen neck (goiter)	Vitamin C, vitamin B_{12}, riboflavin, niacin, or iodine deficiency

Palpation

To palpate, have the patient bend the knees to relax the abdominal muscles and identify localized areas of pain or tenderness; palpate the painful or tender areas last.

- Palpate by quadrant and note any muscle guarding, rigidity, tenderness, or masses.
  - **Light palpation:** Detects superficial masses and fluid accumulating in an abdomen that is soft and nontender
  - **Deep palpation:** Detects masses, tenderness, pulsations, and organ enlargement
- Palpate for rebound tenderness.
- Palpate groin for femoral pulse and inguinal nodes.

Rectal Assessment

Inspection

Inspect rectal area (in male or female patient) for hemorrhoids, blood, fissures, scars, lesions, rectal prolapse, or discharge.

Palpation

Palpate for hemorrhoids, masses, and tonicity using a lubricated, gloved index finger. (In some settings, rectal palpation is done only by an advanced practice nurse.)

- Have the patient take a deep breath.
- Gently insert your index finger, and smoothly follow the posterior wall of the rectum.
- Rotate your finger to follow the curve of the rectal wall, which should be smooth and soft.
- Withdraw your finger, and look for stool on the glove, noting color, consistency, and presence of blood.

Genitourinary Assessment

The genitourinary (GU) system consists of the reproductive organs and the urinary system.

Male Genitalia Assessment

Inspection

- Inspect hair distribution in the pubic region.
- Inspect the penis and scrotum.
  - Observe the presence of the dorsal vein in the penis.
  - Note whether the patient is circumcised; if not, see if the foreskin retracts completely.
  - Check for smegma (whitish substance under the foreskin).
  - Note the appearance of the urethral meatus (normally slit-like) and whether there is a discharge.
  - Look for bumps, blisters, redness, and masses; assess the skin underlying the pubic hair.
  - Check the condition of the pigmented pouch, which may appear asymmetrical.
- Ask about history of sexually transmitted diseases.

Palpation

Palpate the scrotal sac; check for pain, masses, and presence of testicles.

Female Genitalia Assessment

Inspection

- Inspect the external genitalia.
  - Spread the labia to visualize the urethral meatus, vaginal orifice, labia majora, labia minora, and clitoris.
  - Look for discharge, ulcerations, and warts on the perineal floor and labia.
- Ask about menstrual history (menarche, regularity, duration, flow, dysmenorrhea, menopause), pain during intercourse, and history of sexually transmitted diseases.

> Internal vaginal examinations are conducted by an advanced practice nurse, a nurse midwife, or a physician.

Palpation

- Palpate the external genitalia.
- Examine the Skene and Bartholin glands, perineum, and perineal muscle strength.
- Check for vaginal bulging.

Breast Examination

The breast examination is a critical part of the GU assessment.

- Inspect for smoothness, dimpling, and color.
- Observe for edema and symmetry of size.
- Observe for nipple inversion or discharge.
- Palpate in concentric circles, noting tissue consistency (soft, firm, or hard).
- Palpate the areola and nipple, then gently compress the nipple and observe for discharge.
- Palpate the axillary lymph nodes.

Urinary Assessment

Inspection

- Assess urinary intake and output.
- Inspect the urethral meatus.

- Ask about potentially abnormal urinary symptoms:
  - Urgency
  - Pain with urination
  - Pelvic or back pain
  - Nocturia
  - Dysuria
  - Incontinence
  - Blood in urine
  - Difficulty in starting or stopping the urinary stream
  - Pain in the testicles
  - Leaking or feeling of full bladder after voiding

Palpation

Palpate the bladder for distention, tenderness, and masses.

Evaluating Urine Color	
Color	**Indications**
Amber or straw color	Normal
Dark yellow or amber (concentrated urine)	Low fluid intake, vomiting or diarrhea causing fluid loss, or acute febrile disease
Dark brown or black	Drugs (e.g., antimalarials, chlorpromazine, or nitrofurantoin) or acute glomerulonephritis
Orange-red to orange-brown	Obstructive jaundice (tea-colored urine), drugs (e.g., phenazopyridine and rifampin), or urobilinuria
Red or red-brown	Hemorrhage, drugs (e.g., doxorubicin), or porphyria
Green-brown	Bile duct obstruction
Cloudy	Inflammation, infection, glomerulonephritis, or vegetarian diet
Colorless or pale straw color (dilute urine)	Anxiety, chronic renal disease, excess fluid intake, diuretic therapy, or diabetes insipidus

Musculoskeletal Assessment

The musculoskeletal system consists of muscles, tendons, ligaments, bones, cartilage, and joints. Its primary function is to produce skeletal movement.

Inspection

- Evaluate the patient's ability to "get up and go."
- Test ROM bilaterally:
  - Test ROM of the upper extremities (shoulders, elbows, wrists, fingers).
  - Test ROM of the lower extremities (hips, knees, ankles, toes).
  - Test ROM of the spine by asking the patient to bend forward and touch his or her toes.
- Note the size, tone, and any involuntary movement of the major muscle groups; compare bilaterally.

Gait, arms, legs, and spine (GALS) are the major components of the musculoskeletal assessment.

- Test the strength of the major muscle groups using a grading scale:
  - **Grade 5:** Full ROM against gravity and full resistance (100% of normal)
  - **Grade 4:** Full ROM against gravity and some resistance (75% of normal)
  - **Grade 3:** Full ROM with gravity (50% of normal)
  - **Grade 2:** Full ROM with gravity eliminated or passive ROM (25% of normal)
  - **Grade 1:** Slight contraction (10% of normal)
- Inspect each joint for size, contour, masses, and deformities.
- Compare one side of the body to the other side; inspect and measure any discrepancies.

Physiologic Effects of Immobility	
System	**Effects**
Neurologic	Sensory deprivation
Cardiovascular	Increased cardiac workload, orthostatic hypotension, formation of thrombus
Urinary	Urinary stasis, urinary tract infection, calculi
Respiratory	Increased respiratory effort, hypostatic pneumonia, altered gas exchange
Integumentary	Decubitus ulcers, skin shearing
Musculoskeletal	Decreased bone density, contractures, muscle atrophy, increased pain
Psychosocial	Anxiety, depression, helplessness, hopelessness, increased dependency
GI	Decreased appetite, constipation, stress ulcers, fecal impaction

Immobility can affect a variety of body systems and functions.

Palpation
- Palpate the length of each extremity; check skin for pretibial (or other) edema.
- Palpate each joint for musculature, bony articulation, and crepitation.
- Palpate for heat, swelling, or tenderness.
- Palpate the length of the spine for musculature, bony articulation, heat, swelling, or tenderness.

Musculoskeletal Pain
Musculoskeletal pain is usually classified as bone, muscle, or joint pain. ROM tests assist in identifying the type of pain.
- **Bone pain:**
    - Is deep, aching, and constant
    - Is unrelated to movement unless fracture is present
- **Muscle pain:**
    - May be related to posture or occur with movement
    - May be accompanied by tremors, twitches, or weakness
    - May produce referred pain
- **Joint pain:**
    - Is tender to palpation
    - May produce referred pain
    - May produce distal pain because of nerve root irritation
    - Is worse with movement and worsens throughout the day

Neurologic Assessment

The neurologic system consists of the central nervous system (CNS) and the peripheral nervous system (PNS).

CNS
The CNS is composed of the brain and spinal cord. It is the part of the nervous system that controls how your body functions.
- The brain collects, integrates, and interprets all stimuli; it also initiates voluntary and involuntary motor activity.
- The spinal cord relays messages to and from the brain.

PNS

The PNS connects the CNS to the extremities and to the other organs in the body. It also controls involuntary actions like breathing and heartbeat. The neurologic assessment consists of tests in four areas:

- Cranial nerves
- Reflexes
- Motor skills
- Sensory system

CN Assessment		
CN	**Function**	**Assessment**
I (olfactory)	Smell	Identify familiar odors with each naris separately
II (optic)	Vision	Snellen chart, examine ocular fundus with ophthalmoscope, assess light reflex
III (oculomotor)	EOM, elevation of eyelid, pupil constriction	Assess EOM with six cardinal positions of gaze, cover/uncover test to assess constriction with light
IV (trochlear)	EOM	Same as CN III
V (ophthalmic branch, maxillary branch, mandibular branch)	Somatic sensations of the face and head, mastication	Palpate temporal and masseter muscles, teeth clenched; test corneal reflex; touch forehead, cheeks, and chin with cotton wisp; symmetrical comparisons; bite down or chew
VI (abducens)	Lateral eye movement	Look to right and left
VII (facial)	Facial expression, taste (anterior two-thirds of tongue), salivation	Smile, frown, puff cheeks, identify tastes, assess for saliva
VIII (vestibular, cochlear)	Equilibrium, hearing	Observe balance, hearing acuity, Weber and Rinne tests
IX (glossopharyngeal)	Taste (posterior one-third of tongue), pharyngeal sensation, swallowing	Identify tastes; test gag reflex, use tongue blade, note rise of uvula with "ahhhh"
X (vagus)	Sensation in pharynx, larynx, esophagus, trachea, external ear, and thoracic and abdominal visceral cavities	Same as CN IX
XI (spinal accessory)	Neck and shoulder movement	Push chin against hand, shrug shoulder(s)
XII (hypoglossal)	Tongue movement	Move tongue side to side against a tongue depressor

Reflex Testing

- Using a reflex hammer, strike a slightly stretched tendon and see if a simple muscle contraction occurs; test the biceps, triceps, brachioradialis, patellar, and Achilles reflexes.
  - **Hyperactive (4+):** Often pathologic; may be associated with disease of the cerebral cortex, brain stem, or spinal cord
  - **Brisker than normal (3+)**
  - **Normal (2+)**
  - **Diminished (1+)**
  - **Absent (0):** Pathologic; associated with upper and lower motor neuron disease or injury
- Evaluate reflexes bilaterally.

Motor Assessment

- Evaluate bilateral muscle strength, balance, and coordination.
- Look for atrophy and abnormal movement or tremors.
  - **Perform passive ROM:** Note any resistance.
  - **Test biceps strength:** Ask the patient to bend his or her forearm by flexing the elbow while you hold the wrists with a slight downward pressure.
  - **Test triceps strength:** Have the patient extend his or her arm while you push against the wrist.
  - **Test upper leg muscle strength:** Have the patient lie flat and flex his or her hip and knee so that the knee is about 8 inches off the bed.
  - **Test lower leg and foot muscle strength:** Have the patient push his or her foot against your hand and then pull the foot against your hand.
- Test balance and coordination:
  - **Balance:** Use the Romberg test: Have the patient stand with feet together and arms at the sides, as if standing at attention. The patient must maintain this position for about 30 seconds with eyes open, and then another 30 seconds with eyes closed.
  - **Coordination:** Have the patient close his or her eyes and touch the index finger to the nose; or have patient perform rapid alternating movements, such as patting the upper thigh with the palm and then the top side of the hand.

Sensory System Assessment

- Have the patient close his or her eyes and tell you when you are touching his or her skin; use different stimuli, such as a cotton ball for light touch and fingertips for pressure.
- Compare one side with the other to identify if sensory perception is bilateral.

Glasgow Coma Scale

The Glasgow Coma Scale (GCS) is a neurologic assessment scale that provides objective measurement of the patient's level of consciousness. The total of the three scores can range from 3 to 15. A patient who is oriented, opens his or her eyes spontaneously, and follows commands scores a 15. A patient in a deep coma would score a 3. The first GCS score becomes the baseline. Future scores indicate trends or changes in neurologic status.

Glasgow Coma Scale

Measure	Response	Score
Eye response	Opens spontaneously	4
	Opens to verbal command	3
	Opens to pain	2
	No response	1
Motor response	Reacts to verbal command; reacts to painful stimuli	6
	Identifies localized pain	5
	Flexes and withdraws	4
	Assumes flexor posture	3
	Assumes extensor posture	2
	No response	1
Verbal response	Is oriented and converses	5
	Is disoriented but converses	4
	Uses inappropriate words	3
	Makes unintelligible sounds	2
	No response	1

Six Neurologic States of Altered Arousal

State	Manifestations
Confusion	Loss of ability to think clearly and quickly; impaired judgment and decision making
Disorientation	Beginning to lose consciousness; disorientation to time progression or place; impaired memory function; lack of self-recognition
Lethargy	Limited spontaneous speech or movement; easily aroused by normal speech or touch; possible disorientation to time, place, or person
Obtundation	Mild to moderate reduction in arousal; limited responsiveness to environment; ability to fall asleep without difficulty with no verbal or tactile stimulation; answers questions with minimal response
Stupor	State of being deeply asleep or unresponsive; difficulty being aroused (motor or verbal response only to intense stimulation); responds to stimulation by withdrawing or grabbing
Coma	Does not display motor or verbal response to environment or stimuli; does not respond to noxious stimuli such as intense pain; no stimulus causes arousal

Psychosocial Assessment

The psychosocial assessment consists of a mental status examination, an assessment of the patient's home environment, an assessment of the patient's community environment, and a spiritual assessment.

Mental Status Examination

The mental status examination assesses the patient's current state of mind and should include the following:

- **Appearance:** Outward characteristics, including age, height, weight, manner of dress, and grooming
- **Attitude:** The patient's approach to the interview process and interaction with the examiner (e.g., cooperative, belligerent, apathetic, fearful)
- **Behavior:** Gestures, mannerisms, facial expressions, gait, tremors, level of activity and arousal
- **Mood and affect:** The current subjective state as described by the patient and the examiner's inferences of the quality of the patient's emotional state based on objective observation (e.g., apathetic, euphoric, depressed, anxious)
- **Speech:** Loudness, rhythm, prosody, intonation, pitch, phonation, articulation, quantity, rate, spontaneity, latency
- **Thought process:** Loose associations, flight of ideas, word salad
- **Thought content:** Delusions, overvalued ideas, obsessions, phobias, preoccupations
- **Perception:** Hallucinations, illusions, dissociative symptoms
- **Cognition:** Level of consciousness, orientation to reality, attention, memory, visual-spatial functioning, language
- **Insight:** Understanding of illness and treatment options
- **Judgment:** Ability to make sound, reasoned, and responsible decisions

Home Environment Assessment

- Ask about family structure, interactions, and support systems.
- Ask about safety issues, including those that may require the use of equipment.

Community Environment Assessment

Ask the patient about his or her community environment, including recreational activities, transportation issues, and potential safety issues.

Spiritual Assessment

Ask about religious affiliations and spiritual beliefs.

Comparing Depression, Delirium & Dementia			
Clinical Feature	**Depression**	**Delirium**	**Dementia**
Onset	Brief or sudden	Sudden, acute	Gradual
Course	Diurnal effects, with symptoms usually worse in morning; fluctuations based on situation (less than with acute confusion)	Short, with diurnal fluctuations in symptoms; symptoms usually worse on waking up, in darkness, or at night	Lifelong; symptoms irreversible and progressive
Progression	Rapid, slow but even, or variable	Abrupt	Slow, uneven

Duration	Minimum of 2 weeks but up to months or years (*Diagnostic and Statistical Manual of Mental Disorders* [DSM]-IV-TR specifies at least 2 weeks for diagnosis)	From hours to 1 month; rarely longer	From months to years
Attention	May decrease temporarily	Decreased	Usually normal
Awareness	Clear	Reduced	Clear
Alertness	Normal	Fluctuates; can be hypervigilant or lethargic	Usually normal
Orientation	Possibly disoriented	Generally impaired but can be reversed	Can be impaired as disease progresses
Thinking	Intact but with hopelessness, helplessness, or self-deprecation	Fragmented, disorganized, and distorted	Impoverished thoughts; impaired judgment; struggles with abstraction; struggles to find words
Perception	Intact; delusions or hallucinations in severe cases	Distorted with hallucinations, delusions, and illusions; trouble distinguishing between misperceptions and reality	Misperceptions usually not present
Memory	Patchy or selective impairment	Immediate and recent memory impaired	Remote and recent memory impaired
Speech	Rapid, slow, or normal	Incoherent, either slow or accelerated	Dysphasia as disease progresses; aphasia
Affect	Depressed, dysphoric mood with detailed and exaggerated symptoms; preoccupied with personal thoughts; insight present; verbal elaboration	Variable irritability, restlessness, and affective anxiety; reversible	Attempts to conceal deficits in intellect; possible personality changes; aphasia; agnosia; lacks insight; superficial, labile, and inappropriate
Psychomotor behavior	Variable, with psychomotor agitation or retardation	Variable; hyperkinetic, hypokinetic, and mixed	Normal; possible apraxia
Sleep-wake cycle	Somnolence or insomnia	Altered	Fragmented

Comparing Depression, Delirium & Dementia (continued)

Mental status testing results	Commonly responds "don't know"; highlights failings; commonly gives up; exerts little effort; appears indifferent toward test and does not attempt to find answer or care	Many errors; distracted	Struggles with test with many "near-miss" answers; family highlights failings; makes great effort to answer questions; often seeks feedback on performance

Pain Assessment

Acute vs. Chronic Pain

Pain Type	Physiologic Evidence	Behavioral Evidence
Acute	Increased respirations, increased pulse, increased BP, dilated pupils, diaphoresis	Restlessness, distraction, worry, distress
Chronic	Normal respirations, pulse, BP, pupil size; no diaphoresis	Reduced or no physical activity, depression or despair, feelings of hopelessness

Visual Analog Pain Scale

Ask the patient to put a mark, such as an X, on the scale to show his or her current level of pain.

No Pain |————————————————| Worst Pain

Numerical Pain Scale

Ask the patient to rate his or her pain from 0 (indicating no pain) to 10 (indicating the worst pain possible). The patient may either say the number or circle the number on the scale.

No Pain   0 1 2 3 4 5 6 7 8 9 10   Worst Pain

Faces Pain Scale

This scale may be helpful to a child or an adult with language barriers. Ask the patient to choose the face that best shows the severity of his or her own pain on a scale of 0–10.

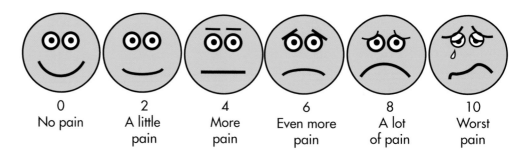

| 0 No pain | 2 A little pain | 4 More pain | 6 Even more pain | 8 A lot of pain | 10 Worst pain |

Post-Assessment

To conclude your patient assessment:

- Ask the patient, "Is there anything else you think it would be important for me to know?"
- Remove drapes and equipment, and allow (or assist) the patient to get dressed.
- Provide patient education as needed.
- Thank the patient for his or her cooperation.
- Arrange for follow-up care or referrals.
- Use your instincts to explore intriguing findings in greater depth.

After the nursing assessment, the information collected must be analyzed and evaluated and the findings documented.

- Identify abnormal findings and changes since prior assessment.
- Cluster findings into logical groups, and localize findings anatomically.
- Consider the quality of the information gathered. Check for:
  - **Reliability:** The ability to produce consistent results under the same conditions
  - **Validity:** The degree to which a test actually measures what it is intended to measure
  - **Sensitivity:** The proportion of people with a disease or condition who test positive for that disease on a given test
  - **Specificity:** The proportion of people without the disease or condition who test negative on a given test

Documentation

Documentation is written evidence of:

- The interaction between and among health professionals, patients, families, and health care organizations
- The administration of tests, procedures, treatments, and patient education
- The patient's response to diagnostic tests, procedures, treatments, and interventions

Systematic documentation is critical because it presents the care administered by nurses in a logical manner, as follows:

- Assessment data identify the patient's specific condition or alterations and provide the foundation of the nursing care plan.
- Risk factors and the identified alteration in health patterns direct the formation of the nursing diagnosis and nursing care priorities.
- Identifying the nursing diagnosis promotes the development of the patient's goals (short term and long term) and expected outcomes and triggers the creation of nursing actions or interventions.
- The plan of care identifies the actions necessary to resolve the nursing diagnosis.
- Implementation, or the act of "nursing," is evidenced by actions the nurse performs to assist the patient in achieving the expected outcomes.

> From a legal perspective, if it is not documented, it was not done.

Documentation requirements differ depending on the health care facility:

- All nursing documentation must reflect the nursing process, the individualized context of the patient, and the nursing situation.
- Nursing documentation must be logical, focused, and relevant to care and must represent each phase of the nursing process.

General Documentation Guidelines

- Make sure you have the correct patient record or chart and that the patient's name and identifying information are on every page of the record.
- Document as soon as the patient encounter is concluded to ensure accurate recall of data.
- Date and time each entry accurately.

When you make a mistake, because every nurse does, do the right thing!
1. Think about your patient first.
2. Correct the mistake.
3. Do not be ashamed to report it.
4. Last, and possibly the most important, forgive yourself.

- Sign each entry with your full legal name and professional credentials.
- Do not leave space between entries.
- If an error is made, use a single line to cross out the error, then date, time, and sign the correction; do not erase or use correction fluid.
- Do not change another person's entry, even if it is incorrect.
- Use quotation marks to indicate direct patient responses.
- Document in chronological order.
- Write legibly.
- Use pens with permanent black ink.
- Document in a complete but concise manner by using phrases and abbreviations as appropriate.
- Document all telephone calls made or received by you that are related to a patient's care.
- Avoid using judgmental language (e.g., "good," "bad," "normal," "abnormal," "appears to be").
- Avoid evaluative statements (e.g., "Patient is uncooperative," "Patient is lazy"); instead, cite specific behaviors or actions that you observed (e.g., "Patient said, 'I hate this place,' and kicked the trash can.").
- State time intervals precisely (e.g., "every 3 hours" instead of "occasionally").
- Do not make relative statements (e.g., "a mass the size of an egg"); instead, be specific (e.g., "3 cm × 5 cm mass").
- Draw pictures when appropriate (e.g., location of scars, bruises, skin lesions).
- Refer to findings by using anatomic landmarks, such as LUQ (left upper quadrant).

Methods of Documentation

- **Narrative charting** is done in a story format that describes the patient's status, interventions, and treatment, as well as the patient's response to treatment.
- **SOAP** is a structured method of narrative charting. SOAP stands for:
  ○ **S**ubjective data (what the patient says)
  ○ **O**bjective data (assessment findings, such as vital signs and laboratory results)
  ○ **A**ssessment and analysis (the conclusion reached on the basis of the data collected)
  ○ **P**lan (actions to be taken to change the status of the patient's problem)
- **PIE** is also a structured method of narrative charting. PIE stands for:
  ○ **P**roblem
  ○ **I**ntervention
  ○ **E**valuation
- **Charting by exception (CBE)** is a method of charting that requires the nurse to document only deviations from preestablished norms.

Documentation based on the nursing process facilitates effective care, as the story of the patient's care can be traced from assessment to the identification of problems, through planning, implementation, and evaluation of nursing care.

NURSING PROCEDURES

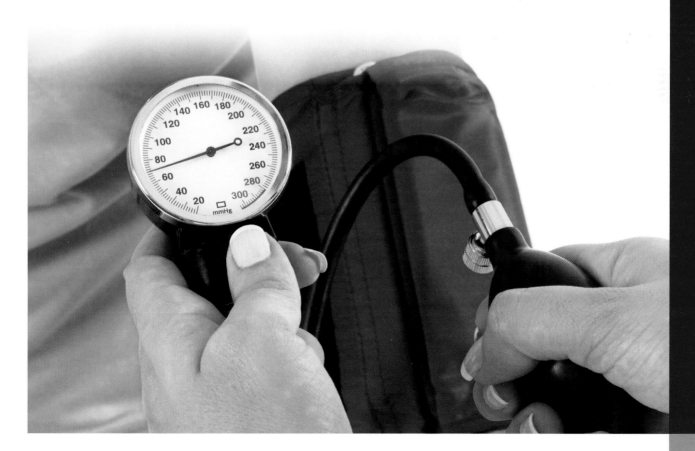

3

Introduction

Procedural skills are an integral part of nursing practice. The ability to perform these skills requires a combination of nursing knowledge, fine motor skills, practice, and patience. This chapter provides step-by-step instructions on how to perform some of the most common nursing procedures, such as starting an intravenous (IV) line, inserting an indwelling catheter, changing an ostomy bag, performing a blood transfusion, and more. Figures are provided when available.

Clean Technique vs. Aseptic Technique

Nursing procedures are performed using clean technique or aseptic technique.

Clean Technique

Clean technique refers to the use of hand hygiene and nonsterile gloves during patient care. It is used to prevent the spread of microorganisms during noninvasive procedures, such as caring for superficial wounds, removing sutures, or giving injections.

Clean Technique Procedure
1. Perform hand hygiene (wash hands, or clean them with an alcohol-based gel or foam if hands are not visibly soiled).
2. Put on gloves.
3. Perform the procedure.
4. Remove gloves.
5. Perform hand hygiene.

Aseptic Technique

Aseptic technique refers to the use of hand hygiene, sterile gloves and other sterile supplies, and antiseptic during procedures. It is used to prevent the spread of microorganisms during invasive procedures, such as urinary catheterization, IV insertion, and sterile dressing changes. Aseptic technique requires a dedicated sterile field.

Aseptic Technique Procedure
1. Perform hand hygiene.
2. Open the sterile package, and use the corners of the paper to create a sterile field.
3. Put on gloves, making sure to not touch the outsides of the gloves.
4. Apply antiseptic to the area to be treated.
5. Perform the procedure.
6. Remove gloves.
7. Perform hand hygiene.

Vital Signs

Measuring vital signs is normally the first procedure done during any patient encounter.
- When measuring vital signs, the examination room should be quiet, warm, and well lit.
- Prior to measuring vital signs, the patient should be given the opportunity to sit or rest in bed for approx. 5 minutes so that the values are not affected by exertion.
- All measurements should be taken while the patient is seated or reclining.

Temperature

Temperature is most often measured using a thermometer that provides a digital reading when the sensor is placed under the patient's tongue. Temperature is measured in degrees, either Fahrenheit (F) or Celsius (C). A normal temperature for an adult is 86.8°F–99.5°F, or 36°C–37.5°C.
- To convert a temperature from Celsius to Fahrenheit: $([°C] \times 1.8) + 32 = [°F]$

- To convert a temperature from Fahrenheit to Celsius: $([°F] - 32) \div 1.8 = [°C]$

Temperature Sites

- **Oral:** Taken with a clinical thermometer placed under the tongue. It can be taken only if the patient is capable of holding the thermometer securely in his or her mouth; this generally excludes small children, as well as people who are weak, vomiting, or overcome by coughing. A normal oral temperature is approx. 98.2°F (36.8°C).
- **Axillary:** Taken with a clinical thermometer placed under the armpit (or axilla). A normal axillary temperature is approx. 97.7°F (36.5°C).
- **Rectal:** Taken with a clinical thermometer placed in the rectum (via the anus). A rectal temperature is considered the method of choice for infants. If not done correctly, this method can be uncomfortable and, in some cases, painful for the patient. A normal rectal temperature is approx. 97.3°F (36.3°C).

Types of Thermometers

- **Clinical (medical) thermometer:** Used for measuring human body temperature, with the tip of the thermometer being inserted into the mouth (oral temperature), under the armpit (axillary temperature), or into the rectum via the anus (rectal temperature). A medical thermometer may be glass or digital.
- **Digital thermometer:** A clinical thermometer that uses a sensor based on thermistors (solid-state electronic devices whose electrical characteristics change with temperature). The reading is recorded within seconds. Some digital thermometers have a red light or other device to indicate when maximum temperature is reached.
- **Mercury thermometer:** An oral thermometer that consists of mercury in a glass tube. Calibrated marks on the tube allow the temperature to be read by the length of the mercury within the tube, which varies according to heat. Mercury is a toxic and hazardous chemical. The U.S. Environmental Protection Agency, the American Academy of Pediatrics, and other organizations warn against using mercury thermometers. If a mercury thermometer breaks, the mercury may be inhaled or absorbed into the skin. In health care settings, mercury thermometers have been replaced by digital thermometers or glass thermometers that use alcohol or Galinstan instead of mercury.
- **Tympanic membrane thermometer:** A thermometer that is placed in the ear; it measures the temperature of the tympanic membrane.
- **Basal thermometer:** Used to take the basal (base) body temperature, or the temperature upon waking. Basal body temperature is the lowest temperature attained by the body during rest (usually during sleep). Compared to daytime temperatures, basal body temperatures are much less affected by environmental factors such as exercise and food intake. This allows small changes in body temperature to be detected, such as those caused by ovulation or changes in thyroid function.

Blood Pressure

Blood pressure (BP) is normally checked using a sphygmomanometer. Readings are reported in millimeters of mercury (mm Hg).

- The size of the BP cuff will affect the accuracy of the readings.
  - If the cuff is too small, the readings will be artificially elevated.
  - If the cuff is too large, the readings will be artificially lowered.
- Normal systolic pressure for an adult is less than 120 mm Hg.
- Normal diastolic pressure for an adult is less than 80 mm Hg.

Types of BP Equipment

- **Sphygmomanometer:** An instrument for measuring arterial BP. It consists of an inflatable cuff that is placed around the upper arm at roughly the same vertical height as the heart and is attached to a mercury or aneroid manometer.
- **Aneroid manometer:** A portable, handheld BP measurement unit consisting of a cuff that is easily applied with one hand, a built-in or attachable stethoscope, a valve

that inflates and deflates the cuff automatically, and an easy-to-read data display screen.

- **Electronic manometer:** An instrument used to digitally measure BP.
- **Mercury manometer:** Considered to be the gold standard for arterial pressure measurement. It measures the height of a column of mercury, giving an absolute result without need for calibration, and consequently is not subject to the errors and drift of calibration that affect other methods. The use of mercury manometers is often required in clinical trials and for the clinical measurement of hypertension in high-risk patients.
- **Oscillometric method of BP measurement:** Includes an electronic pressure sensor transducer fitted in the cuff to detect blood flow. The pressure sensor is a calibrated electronic device with a numerical readout. To maintain accuracy, calibration must be checked periodically, unlike the inherently accurate mercury manometer. In most cases, the cuff is inflated and released by an electrically operated pump and valve, which may be fitted on the upper arm.

Pulse

Pulse can be measured at any place where there is a large artery or by listening to the heart with a stethoscope.

- For the sake of convenience, the radial pulse is the usual site for checking a pulse; palpate the radial pulse using the index and middle finger on the inside of the wrist at the base of the thumb.
- A normal adult pulse is 60–100 beats per minute (at rest).

Respirations

Respirations are measured by counting the number of breaths the patient takes per minute.

- Respirations should be counted for at least 30 seconds; the total number of breaths in a 15-second period (which would then be multiplied by 4) is relatively small, and miscounting could result in large errors.
- Try to count respirations as inconspicuously as possible so that the patient does not consciously alter his or her rate of breathing; this can be done by observing the rise and fall of the patient's hospital gown while you appear to be taking his or her pulse.
- A normal respiratory rate for an adult is 12–20 breaths per minute.

> Respiratory rate can be a reliable indicator of pulmonary dysfunction.

Urine Specimen Collection

The type of urine testing to be done determines the method of urine collection to be used; all urine collection requires the use of universal precautions to prevent the transmission of microorganisms.

Indications

- Disease diagnosis (e.g., urinary tract infection, diabetes, kidney disease)
- Disease monitoring (e.g., diabetes, kidney disease)
- Drug screening
- Pregnancy testing

Contraindications

There are no known contraindications to urine specimen collection.

Equipment Needed

- Gloves
- Specimen container
- Ice (for 24-hour specimen collection)

Routine Urinalysis

A specimen for a routine urinalysis can be collected at any time using a clean container.

1. Ask the patient to void into a specimen cup.
2. After the patient urinates into the specimen container, put on gloves.
3. Seal the container, label it, and place it in a biohazard bag for transport to the laboratory.
4. Send the specimen to the laboratory immediately for testing.
5. Remove gloves and perform hand hygiene.

> Urine specimens need to be submitted to the laboratory immediately to prevent the growth of bacteria or changes in the urine's composition.

24-Hour Urine Specimen

Urine is collected over a 24-hour period and stored in a plastic gallon container that contains a preservative; if the analyte to be studied is light sensitive, a dark plastic container is needed.

1. At the beginning of the collection period, ask the patient to void and discard the first specimen.
2. Ask the patient to save all subsequent urine until the end of the 24-hour period.
3. At the end of the 24-hour period, ask the patient to void one more time.
4. Put on gloves.
5. Seal and label the container.
6. Send the specimen to the laboratory.
7. Remove gloves and perform hand hygiene.

> Throughout the 24-hour period, 24-hour urine specimen collection containers should be refrigerated or kept on ice.

Closed-Drainage System Collection

Closed-drainage system collection is used to collect sterile specimens.

1. Perform hand hygiene and put on gloves.
2. Manipulate the tubing so that urine drains from the tubing into the collection bag.
3. Clamp the tubing below the aspiration port for 10–15 minutes.
4. Cleanse the aspiration port, and insert the needle/syringe to aspirate urine. (This is a sterile procedure.)
5. Transfer the specimen to a sterile container.
6. Seal, label, and transport the sample to the laboratory immediately.
7. Remove gloves and perform hand hygiene.

Clean Specimens

A clean-catch or midstream-voided specimen is done to collect a specimen of urine uncontaminated by skin flora; the first void in the morning is the best time to obtain this specimen.

- Different techniques are used for women, men, and children:
  - Women are instructed to cleanse from the front to the back.
  - Men are instructed to cleanse from the tip of the penis downward.
  - For infants and young children, a sterile collection bag is placed over the perineum or penis and scrotum.
- The procedure is the same as with routine urinalysis except the patient is instructed to cleanse the area and begin voiding into the toilet; after the patient begins voiding, he or she should stop midstream, and then continue voiding into the specimen container.

> Proper collection technique and timely transport of urine specimens to the laboratory will influence the validity of the results.

Blood Specimens (Venipuncture)

Venous Samples

The following sources of variability can lead to inaccuracy:

- **Hemoconcentration:** Reduced plasma volume and increased concentration of blood cells, plasma proteins, and protein-bound constituents
- **Hemolysis:** Breakdown of red blood cells (RBCs) and the release of hemoglobin
- **Contamination with IV fluids:** When blood is drawn from a site above an IV infusion

Indications
- Obtaining routine laboratory values
- Disease diagnosis
- Disease monitoring
- Type and crossmatch

Contraindications
- Cellulitis
- Abscess
- Venous fibrosis
- Hematoma

Equipment Needed
- Sterile needle and syringe
- Vacuum tube holder with a sterile two-sided needle
- Gloves
- Needle
- Tourniquet
- Tubes
- Gauze
- Needle adapter
- Antiseptic pads

> Use a needle gauge appropriate to the size of the vessel to prevent hemolysis.

Routine Venipuncture Procedure
1. Gather equipment.
2. Explain the procedure to the patient.
3. Apply the tourniquet.
   a. The tourniquet should be placed 3–4 inches above the puncture site.
   b. The tourniquet should not be left on longer than 1 minute; a tourniquet left on too long may cause the following:
      i) **Hemoconcentration:** Too many blood elements in plasma
      ii) **Hemolysis:** Destruction of RBCs
      iii) **Petechiae:** Red spots on the skin
   c. Ask patients with difficult veins to make a fist or squeeze a rubber ball after the tourniquet is applied; once blood starts flowing, ask the patient to open his or her fist or stop squeezing the ball, then release the tourniquet.

Common Sites for Venipuncture

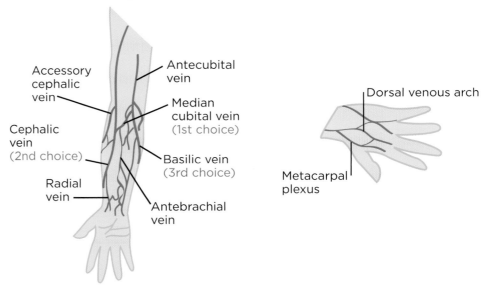

Accessory cephalic vein

Antecubital vein

Median cubital vein (1st choice)

Cephalic vein (2nd choice)

Basilic vein (3rd choice)

Radial vein

Antebrachial vein

Dorsal venous arch

Metacarpal plexus

4. Select the site for the blood draw.
    a. The best veins are usually in the antecubital fossa (inside of the elbow).
    b. If blood is to be drawn from the hand or wrist, you may want to consider using a winged infusion kit (butterfly) with smaller needles.
5. Palpate the vein.
    a. Veins will feel spongy, bouncy, and firm.
6. Clean the site with antiseptic pads.
    a. Clean the area in concentric circles spiraling upward from the puncture site.
    b. Allow to dry before puncturing the skin.
7. Examine the needle for defects.
8. Perform the venipuncture.
    a. Anchor the vein and brace the arm.
    b. Hold the needle with your dominant hand.
    c. Angle the needle 15–30 degrees.
    d. Insert the needle bevel up.
    e. Hold the needle steady.
    f. Keep the needle assembly downward to prevent reflux (backflow).
9. Fill the first tube, and then remove the tourniquet.
    a. To be sure the tourniquet stays on no longer than 1 minute, remove the tourniquet when blood flow has been established.
    b. The tourniquet must be removed prior to needle removal to prevent a hematoma (blood pooling under the skin).
10. If you are drawing more than one tube of blood, change tubes; be sure to hold the needle assembly still in the patient's arm when changing tubes.
11. Remove the last tube before removing the needle to prevent blood from dripping out of the tube.
12. Withdraw the needle.
13. Apply gauze to the puncture area.
14. Press down on the site after the needle has been removed.
    a. Do not bend the arm over the puncture site (this can cause a hematoma).
    b. Apply pressure for up to 2 minutes.
15. Dispose of the needle in the sharps container.
16. Label the tubes properly.
    a. The label should include the patient's name, identification (ID) number, date, and time of draw.
    b. If using computer-generated labels, make sure the correct information is on the label.
17. Deliver the specimen to the laboratory.
18. Remove gloves and perform hand hygiene.

Types of Needles
- **Multisample needles:** A double-ended needle that is used for most blood specimen collections; one tip of the needle pierces the patient's skin, while the other end is inserted into the evacuation tube.
    - Multisample needles have a retractable rubber sleeve that covers the second tip when it is not inserted into the tube.
    - A multisample needle remains in the patient's vein while you exchange one tube for another.
    - The rubber sleeve keeps the blood from leaking onto or into the tube holder while changing tubes.
- **Safety syringe needles:** Patients with small or fragile veins benefit most from the use of a safety syringe needle because the vacuum of the collection tube is likely to cause the vein to collapse; with this type of needle, suction can be applied slowly and gradually.
    - Safety syringe needles come in a variety of sizes, but the most common needle used is a 22-gauge that is 1 inch long.

Blood Collection Tube Additives	
Color	**Additive**
Red	No additive
Lavender	Ethylenediaminetetraacetic acid
Light blue	Sodium citrate
Green	Sodium heparin
Gray	Potassium oxalate
Black	Sodium oxalate

- **Winged infusion kits (a.k.a. butterfly needles):** Winged infusion kits are used for venipuncture on small or fragile veins, such as hand veins and veins in pediatric or elderly patients, and for patients with circulation conditions or problems (e.g., peripheral vascular disease, Raynaud disease).
  - The most common needle size is a 23-gauge (½ inch to ¾ inch long).
  - The needle is held by a plastic butterfly-shaped grip.
  - The needle is connected to flexible latex tubing and, with the proper adapter, can be connected to an evacuation tube.

Needle Adapters

Because most blood collections make use of a multisample needle and an evacuation collection tube, a needle adapter (a.k.a. tube holder) is used to ensure a good connection between them.

- A needle adapter is a translucent plastic cylinder with one small end that accepts the needle, while the other end has a wide opening that accepts the collection tube.
- Needle adapters come in different sizes to fit different tubes.
- To ensure a proper connection between the needle and the tube, adapters have a tube advancement mark indicating how far a tube can be pushed without losing the vacuum.

Arterial Samples
Indications
- To evaluate acid-base balance
- To evaluate gas exchange and oxygenation status

Contraindications
- Hyperthermia
- Immediately after suctioning or respiratory treatments
- Following changes in ventilator settings
- Anticoagulant therapy
- Clotting disorders
- Peripheral vascular disease

Equipment Needed
- Heparinized syringe
- Needle
- Alcohol wipe
- Sterile gauze
- Sterile gloves
- Ice
- Labels

Arterial Puncture Procedure

1. Explain the procedure to the patient.
2. Check radial pulses on both wrists to determine which one to use, and perform Allen test.
3. Shoot most of the heparin from the syringe so that only a small amount remains.
4. Perform hand hygiene.
5. Prepare a sterile field, and put on sterile gloves.
6. Clean the area with alcohol swabs.
7. Turn the bevel of the needle upward, and insert it 5–10 mm distal to the finger directly over the artery; the puncture angle should be approx. 45 degrees toward the direction of the blood flow.
8. Slowly advance the needle with one hand while continuing to palpate the artery with the other hand; stop when you see a flash of arterial blood in the hub of the needle.
9. Fill the syringe.
10. Remove the needle, and press down on the puncture site with gauze.
11. Cap and label the syringe.
12. Put the syringe in the cup of ice until it can be analyzed.
13. Continue to apply pressure to the site until it stops bleeding.
14. Remove gloves and perform hand hygiene.

Wound Care

The procedure for wound care will depend on the type of wound, the type of dressing or skin closures, and whether the wound has a drain. Caring for open wounds requires aseptic technique; caring for superficial wounds requires clean technique.

Skin Care

The following products are used for skin care in nursing:

- **Cleanser:** A skin care product that is used to remove dead skin cells, oil, dirt, and other types of pollutants from the skin surface. Using a cleanser to remove dirt is a better alternative to using bar soap, since bar soap has a high pH (approx. 9–10), whereas the pH of skin cleansers is closer to the skin's natural pH of 5.5.
- **Lotion:** Used for moisturizing skin.
- **Moisture barrier cream:** Provides protection against urine and fecal matter while moisturizing and soothing reddened, irritated skin.
- **Ointment:** Used topically on a variety of body surfaces, including the skin and the mucous membranes of the eye, vagina, anus, and nose. An ointment may or may not be medicated.
- **Protective skin barriers:** A liquid barrier film that dries quickly to form a breathable, transparent, protective film, or "second skin." Designed to protect intact or damaged skin from urine, feces, other bodily fluids or secretions, and tape trauma and friction. Some skin barriers contain calamine; aloe vera; and vitamins A, D, and E to promote healing of fragile or irritated skin. Others contain antimicrobial properties to protect against infection and reduce odor.
- **Skin paste:** A thick, rich paste applied to protect and condition sensitive, excoriated, inflamed skin resulting from contact with caustic diarrhea or enzymatic drainage. Commonly used for severe incontinence.
- **Soap:** Used for cleaning skin.

Dressings

Dressings are used to cover and protect wounds. There are several different types of dressings:

- **Absorptive dressing:** A bulky dressing designed to absorb drainage from a wound.
- **Ace wrap:** Rubber-reinforced cotton for wrapping sprains and strains; available in a variety of sizes, all of which can be laundered and reused.

- **Adhesive bandage:** A bandage consisting of plain absorbent gauze held in place by a plastic or fabric tape coated with adhesive.
- **Antiseptic dressing:** Gauze impregnated with antiseptic material.
- **Compression bandage:** A bandage designed to provide pressure to a particular area (i.e., a pressure dressing) or a bandage that stops the flow of blood from an artery by applying pressure.
- **Drain sponge:** A nonwoven, highly absorptive dressing that has been precut to fit around most drains, tubes, and catheters.
- **Elastoplast:** An elastic adhesive bandage for covering cuts, wounds, or incisions.
- **Foam dressing:** A highly absorbent dressing that allows less-frequent changing of dressings and less maceration of surrounding tissues; used for wounds with heavy exudate (especially after debridement or desloughing, when drainage peaks) and for deep cavity wounds or weeping ulcers.
- **Gauze:** A thin, loosely woven surgical dressing, usually made of bleached cotton cloth.
- **Gauze bandage roll (Kerlix):** A self-adherent and conforming gauze roll bandage that is used to hold dressings in place.
- **Hydrocolloid dressing (DuoDERM):** An opaque dressing used to protect wounds from contamination and to provide a moist, wound-healing environment. Hydrocolloid dressings are biodegradable and nonbreathable and adhere to the skin, so no separate taping is needed.
- **Laparotomy pad, or abdominal (ABD) pad:** Sterile, all-purpose bandage and wound cleaning pad that is flexible, absorbent, and breathable. Made from several layers of gauze folded into a rectangular shape, and used as a sponge for packing off the viscera in abdominal operations. Also used to control bleeding and prevent contamination of large wounds.
- **Montgomery strap:** A 7 × 11–inch breathable strap with reinforced eyelets that are tied together with twill ties. Most commonly used when a wound requires a large, bulky dressing that needs to be changed frequently.
- **Nonadherent dressing (Telfa):** Consists of an absorbent, nonadherent pad with a nonwoven adhesive backing. Used for nondraining and lightly draining wounds, abrasions, lacerations, surgical incisions, skin tears, and IV sites.
- **Nonstick pad:** Sterile gauze pad with a porous membrane that allows fluids to be absorbed without adhering to the wound surface. Used for abrasions and burns.
- **Occlusive dressing:** A dressing that seals a wound from contact with air or bacteria, or a plastic film placed over medication that has been applied to the skin. The dressing enhances absorption of the medication.
- **Petrolatum gauze:** Gauze saturated with petrolatum; used as an occlusive or non-stick dressing.
- **Pressure dressing:** Exerts pressure on a covered area to prevent collection of fluids in underlying tissues. The constant pressure may also control bleeding.
- **Sponge:** A gauze pad used to absorb blood and other fluids; can be used in surgery or as a wound dressing.
- **Tegaderm:** A transparent dressing that can be used to cover and protect wounds and catheter sites. Allows visualization and monitoring of the wound without changing the dressing.
- **Wet dressing:** Dressings that are presaturated with normal saline or medicated solutions; wet dressings aid in the cleaning, drainage, and debridement of a wound.
- **Tape:** A narrow, long strip of fabric or other flexible material that adheres to skin and other materials.

> Some wounds require dressings to add moisture, whereas others need dressings to absorb it.

Skin Closures

A skin closure is any means used to close the open skin of a wound. Skin closures include sutures, staples, and adhesives.
- **Sutures:** Stitches used to hold tissues together. There are two types of sutures:
  - **Absorbable sutures:** Sutures that are broken down in the tissue after a given

period of time (anywhere from 10 days to 8 weeks) and therefore do not need to be removed. Occasionally, absorbable sutures can cause inflammation and be rejected by the body rather than absorbed.
  - ○ **Nonabsorbable sutures:** Sutures that are not metabolized by the body and therefore need to be removed after a given period of time.
- **Skin (surgical) staples:** Specialized staples used in surgery in place of sutures to close skin wounds. Stapling is much faster than suturing by hand, as well as more accurate and consistent.
- **Butterfly stitches:** Thin adhesive strips that can be used to close small wounds. They are applied across the laceration in a manner that pulls the skin on either side of the wound together. They are often used in addition to or in place of sutures for small wounds.
- **Skin (dermal) adhesive (skin glue):** A sterile, liquid glue that holds wound edges together, eliminating the need for sutures. A glued closure produces less scarring and is less prone to infection than a sutured or stapled closure. There is also no residual closure to remove, so follow-up visits for removal are not required.
- **Steri-Strips:** Strips of adhesive-backed paper tape that are placed across an incision or minor cut to keep the edges of a wound together as it heals. May be used in place of sutures because they cause less scarring; also may be applied when sutures are removed to support the incision line.

Drains

A drain is a device that is used for removing fluid from a cavity or wound. Drainage systems are used to prevent infection and skin breakdown. Drainage containers need to be frequently emptied and the fluid measured. There are two common types of wound drainage systems:
- **Open drainage system:** Inserted during surgery; uses gravity to drain fluid onto a dressing. There are two common types of open drainage systems:
  - ○ **Penrose drain:** Consists of a soft rubber tube that is placed in a wound area to prevent the buildup of fluid.
  - ○ **T-tube:** Used following open gallbladder procedures to drain bile. The tube allows bile to drain out of the patient's body into a small pouch, known as a bile bag. Before removing a T-tube, an X-ray should be taken to make sure that the duct has healed and no stones remain.
- **Closed drainage system:** Inserted during surgery; tubing is connected to a portable vacuum unit, which is a collection unit that suctions fluids from the wound site. There are two common types of closed drainage systems:
  - ○ **Spring evacuator drain (Hemovac):** A three-spring evacuator drain container is connected to an internal plastic drainage tube and provides reliable suction for surgical cases with larger amounts of drainage.
  - ○ **Bulb drain, or Jackson-Pratt drain (JP drain):** Consists of a flexible plastic bulb (shaped something like a hand grenade) that connects to an internal plastic drainage tube. Removing the plug and squeezing the bulb removes air, which creates lower air pressure within the drainage tube.

Wound Drainage

There are three types of wound drainage:
- **Serous exudate,** which is primarily serum (the clear portion of blood); appearance is watery and has a low protein count; seen with mild inflammation, such as blister formation after a burn.
- **Purulent exudate,** which is pus; generally occurs with severe inflammation and infection; this type of exudate is thick because of the presence of leukocytes, liquefied dead tissue debris, and bacteria; purulent drainage may vary in color (e.g., yellow, brown, green), depending on the causative organism.
- **Hemorrhagic exudate,** which is primarily RBCs and is caused by capillary damage; this type of exudate is associated with severe inflammation. The color of the exudate reflects whether the bleeding is fresh (bright red) or old (dark red).

Open Wound Care According to Wound Color

Wound Color	Care
Red	Make sure the wound is moist and clean. Cover it, and protect it from trauma. Use a transparent dressing over a gauze dressing moistened with saline solution, or use a hydrogel foam or hydrocolloid dressing.
Yellow	Clean the wound. Remove the yellow layer. Use a moisture-retentive dressing like a hydrogel to cover the wound, or use a moist gauze dressing with or without a debriding enzyme. Consider hydrotherapy.
Black	Debride the wound per orders. Use an enzyme product, conservative sharp debridement, or hydrotherapy. Do not debride noninfected heel ulcers or wounds having inadequate blood supply; keep them dry and clean.

Moisture Scale

Absorb Moisture		Neutral (maintain existing level)		Add Moisture	
Alginates	Foams	Composites	Transparent films	Sheet hydrogels	Amorphous hydrogel
Specialty absorptives	Hydrocolloids	Mini-VAC device	Biologic dressings		Debriding agents
Vacuum-assisted closure (VAC) device	Compression dressings		Collagen dressings		
Gauze			Contact layers		
			Warm-Up therapy system		

Nutrition

Physiologic Basics
- The consumption of nutrients is necessary to support the physiologic activities of digestion, absorption, and metabolism, as well as to maintain homeostasis.
- Nutrients are classified into three groups:
  - **Energy nutrients**, which release energy for maintenance of homeostasis
  - **Organic nutrients**, which build and maintain body tissues and regulate body processes
  - **Inorganic nutrients**, which provide a medium for chemical reactions, transport materials, maintain body temperature, promote bone formation, and conduct nerve impulses

Diet Therapy
- **Nothing by mouth (NPO):** Nothing to eat or drink; this intervention is ordered to rest the gastrointestinal (GI) tract, either prior to surgery or certain diagnostic procedures or when the source of the patient's nutritional problem is unidentified.
- **Clear-liquid diet:** Consists of liquids that have no residue, such as water, apple juice, and gelatin; dairy products are not allowed.
- **Liquid (full-liquid) diet:** Consists of clear liquids and substances that are liquid at room temperature (e.g., ice cream, pudding).
- **Soft diet:** Consists of foods that are soft in texture or that have been mashed, pureed, or liquefied to soften the texture. Promotes mechanical digestion of foods; used for patients with difficulty in chewing or swallowing or with impaired digestion or

absorption; foods to be avoided include nuts, seeds (including tomatoes and berries with seeds), raw fruits and vegetables, fried foods, and whole grains.

- **Low-residue diet:** Consists of reduced fiber and cellulose; prescribed to decrease GI mucosal irritation; foods to be avoided are raw fruits (except bananas), vegetables, seeds, plant fiber, and whole grains; dairy products are limited to 2 servings per day.
- **High-fiber diet:** Consists of foods high in fiber or cellulose; used to increase the forward motion of indigestible wastes through the colon.
- **Diabetic diet:** Used to control blood sugar. Consists of smaller portions spread throughout the day and a variety of whole grains, fruits, and vegetables. The timing and amount of carbohydrates to be consumed is determined by a dietitian. Foods that should be limited are foods that are high in sugar, fatty foods, salt, and alcohol.
- **Sodium-restricted diet:** Used with patients who have excess fluid volume, hypertension, heart failure, myocardial infarction, or renal failure; sodium intake may be restricted as follows:
  - **Mild:** 2000–3000 mg (2–3 g)
  - **Moderate:** 1000 mg (1 g)
  - **Strict:** 500 mg (0.5 g)

Parenteral Nutrition
Parenteral nutrition is given through a route outside the alimentary tract.

- The solution is infused directly into the vein to meet daily nutritional needs.
- Total parenteral nutrition (TPN) consists of an IV solution containing dextrose, amino acids, fats, essential fatty acids, vitamins, and minerals.

Enteral Nutrition
Enteral nutrition is used for patients who have a functional GI tract and will not or cannot eat and therefore are at risk for malnutrition. Various feeding tubes, methods, and formulas are used, depending on the patient's diagnosis and condition.

Feeding Tubes
A feeding tube is a flexible, narrow plastic or rubber tube inserted into some portion of the digestive tract to provide nutrition to patients who cannot obtain nutrition by swallowing. The state of being fed by a feeding tube is called enteral feeding or tube feeding. Placement may be temporary for the treatment of acute conditions or lifelong in the case of chronic disabilities.

Types of Enteral Formulas		
Formula Type	**Brand Names**	**Characteristics**
Standard	Ensure, Isocal, Osmolite	Most common form of enteral nutrition; well tolerated by patients; contains a mixture of protein, polysaccharides, and fat
Concentrated	Ensure Plus, TraumaCal	Has more nutrients and calories and less fluid than the standard solution; used for patients who are on fluid restriction
High protein	Isocal HN, Osmolite HN	Used for patients who need more protein
High fiber	Nutrison Multi Fibre, Ultracal, Sustagen Plus Fibre, Ensure Fibre	Contains additional fiber; used for relief of diarrhea or constipation

A variety of feeding tubes are used in medical practice; they are classified by site of insertion and intended use. Feeding tubes are usually made of polyurethane or silicone. The diameter of a feeding tube is measured in French units (F). Each French unit equals 0.33 mm. Feeding tubes are classified by site of insertion and intended use.

- **Gastrostomy tube (G-tube):** A G-tube is inserted directly into the stomach through a small incision in the abdomen; it is used for long-term enteral nutrition. The most common type is the percutaneous endoscopic gastrostomy (PEG) tube.
  - Advantages:
    - Can be used long term
    - Allows for intermittent feeding
    - Allows for normal gastric emptying time
    - Is not visible to others
    - Makes medication administration easier
    - Less risk of infection
    - Does not irritate esophagus
  - Disadvantages:
    - Requires surgical placement with sedation or local anesthesia
    - Necessitates local skin care
    - May ulcerate gastric mucosa
- **Nasogastric (NG) tube:** An NG tube is passed through the nares, past the pharynx, down the esophagus, and into the stomach. NG tubes are used for patients who are unable to ingest nutrients by mouth. The length of tube required can range from 36 to 45 inches. Placement must be checked before each feeding.
  - Advantages:
    - Smaller tube, so more comfortable
    - Less risk of aspiration and reflux
  - Disadvantages:
    - Placement requires X-ray confirmation.
    - Placement is difficult.
    - The patient's head must remain elevated.
    - Constant infusion is needed because of the osmotic response of the small intestine.
    - Cramping, diarrhea, vomiting, and distension are common.
    - Improper placement can lead to aspiration.
    - Because of alkaline environment, risk of infection is greater.
    - Period of use is limited (4 weeks maximum).
- **Jejunostomy tube (J-tube):** A J-tube is surgically implanted in the upper section of the small intestine called the jejunum, which is just below the stomach. The primary reason for use of the J-tube is to bypass the stomach.
  - Advantages:
    - Tube position is guaranteed.
    - Tube is not visible.
    - There is less risk of reflux and aspiration.
  - Disadvantages:
    - Placement requires general anesthesia.
    - Continuous infusion is required.
    - Cramping, diarrhea, vomiting, and distension are common.
    - May lead to peritonitis.
    - Because of alkaline environment, risk of infection is greater.

Tube feedings are contraindicated in patients with diffuse peritonitis, intestinal obstruction, intractable vomiting, or severe diarrhea.

NG Tube Placement

An NG tube is the only type of feeding tube that is placed by the nurse. All other feeding tubes are placed surgically.

Indications

- Evaluation of the upper GI tract
- Feeding and medication administration
- Intestinal obstruction
- Aspiration of stomach contents

Contraindications

- Esophageal stricture
- Severe facial trauma
- Recent nasal surgery

Equipment Needed

- Nonsterile gloves
- NG tube
- 60 mL irrigation syringe
- Water-soluble lubricant
- Adhesive tape
- Wall suction, suction tubing, and container (if indicated)
- Cup of water with a straw
- Emesis basin
- pH indicator strips

NG Tube Insertion Procedure

1. Assemble the equipment.
2. Explain the procedure to the patient.
3. Place the patient in an upright position.
4. Perform hand hygiene and put on gloves.
5. Measure the tubing from the bridge of the nose to the earlobe, then to the point halfway between the xiphoid and the navel.
6. Lubricate the end of the tube.
7. Gently insert the tube into the nostril.
8. When the tube reaches the pharynx, the patient may begin to gag; have the patient sip the water through the straw and swallow as you continue to pass the tube into the esophagus and down to the stomach.
9. Verify the position of the tube by aspirating a small amount of the gastric contents and conducting a pH test (pH should be less than 6); obtain a chest X-ray if there is any doubt as to proper placement.
10. Secure the tube to the nose with adhesive tape.
11. If indicated, attach the tube to suction.
12. Remove gloves and perform hand hygiene.

> Immediately withdraw the NG tube if the patient shows signs of respiratory distress, if the patient begins bleeding profusely from the nose, or if the tube meets significant resistance.

Managing Problems with Tube Feedings

Complication	Nursing Interventions
Obstruction of tube	• Flush out tube with warm water; replace tube if needed. • Flush out tube with 50 mL of water after every feeding to remove excess formula, which could block the tube.
Constipation	• Provide additional fluids if patient can tolerate them. • Give patient a bulk-forming laxative. • Increase sugar, fruit, or vegetable content of feeding.
Bloating, diarrhea, cramps, or vomiting	• Reduce rate of flow. • Administer metoclopramide to increase motility of GI. • Warm formula to prevent GI distress. • Position patient on right side with head elevated to facilitate gastric emptying for 30 minutes after feeding. • Notify physician.
Aspiration of gastric secretions	• Stop feeding immediately. • Perform tracheal suction of aspirated contents. • Notify physician. • Check placement of tube before feeding to prevent complications.
Electrolyte imbalance	• Monitor serum electrolyte levels. • Notify physician; he or she may want to adjust the content of the formula to correct the deficiency.
Hyperglycemia	• Monitor levels of blood glucose. • Notify physician; he or she may want to adjust the glucose content of the formula. • Give insulin if ordered.
Nasal, oral, or pharyngeal irritation or necrosis	• Provide oral hygiene frequently, and treat cracked lips. • Change tube's position; replace tube if needed.

IV Line Insertion
Indications
- Fluid administration
- Medication administration
- Blood transfusions

Contraindications
- Severe edema at insertion site
- Burns or trauma at insertion site
- Cellulitis at insertion site

Equipment Needed
- Gloves
- 14- to 25-gauge IV catheter
- Tourniquet
- Saline lock
- Alcohol swab
- Transparent dressing
- Tape

IV Line Insertion Procedure

1. Gather the equipment.
2. Explain the procedure to the patient.
3. Apply the tourniquet and choose the insertion site.
4. Perform hand hygiene and put on gloves.
5. Clean the site with an alcohol pad.
6. Stabilize the vein with your nondominant hand.
7. Insert the needle at a 10- to 30-degree angle; reduce the angle as you advance the needle.
8. When you see the "flash back," continue to advance the needle another 1 cm.
9. Hold the catheter in place with your thumb and index finger; pull the needle back 1 cm with your middle finger.
10. Slowly advance the catheter until the hub is against the skin.
11. Remove the tourniquet.
12. Apply the transparent dressing.
13. Occlude the tip of the catheter with your nondominant hand; carefully remove the needle.
14. Attach the saline lock, and flush with saline.
15. Secure with tape.
16. Remove gloves and perform hand hygiene.

Taping a Venous Access Site

Use one of these methods to attach the venous access device to the insertion site with sterile tape.

U Method

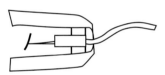

H Method

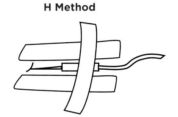

Chevron Method

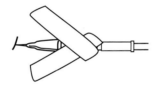

Blood Transfusions

Indications

- Anemia
- Hemorrhage
- Blood loss replacement during surgery
- Illness (e.g., cancer, blood diseases, liver failure)

Contraindications

- Megaloblastic anemia
- Iron deficiency anemia

Equipment Needed

- Gloves
- IV access device
- Normal saline
- Blood administration kit
- Blood or blood component

> Because blood products need to be refrigerated, blood transfusions should be started within 30 minutes after the blood is checked out of the laboratory; if circumstances require a delay, return the blood to the laboratory.

Blood Transfusion Procedure

1. Gather the equipment.
2. Explain the procedure to the patient.
3. Obtain baseline vital signs.
4. Administer pretransfusion medications if applicable.
5. Ask another nurse to verify the patient's identity and blood type with you; compare with the name and blood type on the unit of blood. Make sure the ID number on the unit of blood matches the number on the patient's ID band.
6. Check the expiration date on the unit of blood, and look for any clumping, gas bubbles, or abnormal color.
7. Perform hand hygiene and put on gloves.
8. Open the blood administration packet, and label the tubing.
9. Spike the normal saline bag with one of the spikes on the Y tubing, and prime the tubing; when the tubing is primed, close off the clamp.
10. Spike the blood component bag with the other spike on the Y tubing; prime the tubing with normal saline.
11. Gently invert the unit of blood several times.
12. Hang the normal saline and the unit of blood on an IV pole.
13. Connect the infusion unit to the patient's IV site; prime with normal saline.
14. Start the infusion; adjust the flow as prescribed.
    a. Stay with the patient for the first 15 minutes, checking vital signs every 5 minutes; watch for infusion reactions.
    b. If you see signs of an infusion reaction, stop the infusion immediately and notify the physician.
15. If there are no signs of a reaction, continue with the infusion, checking vital signs according to organizational protocol.
16. After the infusion is complete, disconnect the tubing and discard the used equipment.
17. Remove gloves and perform hand hygiene.

> If the patient appears to be experiencing a transfusion reaction:
> - Stop the transfusion.
> - Assess the patient's condition.
> - Disconnect the IV line from the needle.
> - Alert the physician.

Blood Products	
Blood Component & Volume	**Indications**
Albumin 5% (buffered saline); albumin 5% (salt poor) A small plasma protein made by fractionating pooled plasma **Volume:** 5% = 12.5 g/250 mL; 25% = 12.5 g/50 mL	Hypoproteinemia; loss of volume because of shock from infection, surgery, trauma, or burns
Cryoprecipitate Insoluble portion of plasma recovered from fresh frozen plasma (FFP) **Volume:** Approx. 30 mL (freeze-dried)	Bleeding related to fibrinogen and factor XIII deficiencies
FFP Uncoagulated plasma separated from RBCs and rich in coagulation factors V, VIII, and IX **Volume:** 180–300 mL	Warfarin reversal; thrombotic thrombocytopenic purpura; coagulation factor deficiency
Packed RBCs Same RBC mass as whole blood but with 80% of the plasma removed **Volume:** 250 mL	Symptomatic chronic anemia; sickle cell disease (red cell exchange); symptomatic oxygen-carrying capacity deficiency; inadequate circulating red cell mass
Platelets Platelet sediment from RBCs or plasma **Volume:** 35–50 mL/unit	Prevention of bleeding because of thrombocytopenia; bleeding because of critically decreased circulating or functionally abnormal platelets

Blood Transfusion Reactions

Reaction	Causes	Signs and Symptoms
Transfusion-related lung injury	Antibodies activate granulocytes, causing leakage into lungs	Tachypnea, dyspnea, hypotension, cyanosis, chills, fever, tachycardia
Plasma protein incompatibility	Immunoglobulin A incompatibility	Diarrhea, abdominal pain, dyspnea, fever, chills, flushing, hypotension
Hemolytic	Blood stored improperly; cross-matching done improperly; intradonor incompatibility; RH or ABO incompatibility	Dyspnea, flushed face, fever, chest pain, shaking, chills, hypotension, flank pain, oliguria, hemoglobinuria, bloody oozing at surgical incision or infusion site, burning feeling along vein getting blood, shock, renal failure
Febrile	Bacterial lipopolysaccharides; antileukocyte recipient antibodies directed against donor white blood cells	Fever, headache, chills, flushed face, cough, palpitations, increased pulse rate, chest tightness, flank pain
Bacterial contamination	Organisms that can survive cold temperatures (e.g., *Staphylococcus* and *Pseudomonas*)	Fever, chills, abdominal cramping, vomiting, diarrhea, shock, renal failure
Allergic	Donor blood has allergen; donor blood hypersensitive to certain drugs	Anaphylaxis, nausea, vomiting, fever

Indwelling Catheter Insertion

Indications
- Urinary retention
- Bladder obstruction
- Measuring urine output
- Obtaining uncontaminated urine specimens
- Assessing fluid status during surgery

Contraindications
- Urethral trauma

Equipment Needed
- Nonsterile gloves
- Soap and water
- Washcloth
- Indwelling catheter kit
- Privacy drape

Indwelling Catheter Insertion Procedure

1. Gather the equipment.
2. Explain the procedure to the patient.
3. Provide privacy.
4. Position the patient.
   a. Female: Knees flexed and feet flat on the bed.
   b. Male: Lying flat with knees slightly apart.
5. Drape the patient so that only the perineal area is exposed.
6. Perform hand hygiene and put on nonsterile gloves.
7. Wash the perineal area with soap and water.
8. Remove gloves and perform hand hygiene.
9. Open the catheter kit; use aseptic technique to create a sterile field.
10. Place the pad under the patient, plastic side down.
11. Apply a sterile drape to the perineal area.
12. Put on sterile gloves using aseptic technique.
13. Pour lubricating gel into the tray.
14. Test the balloon with the prefilled syringe; deflate the balloon, and leave the syringe attached.
15. Pour antiseptic solution over the cotton balls.
16. Insert catheter:
    a. Female:
       i) With your nondominant hand, separate the labia and locate the urinary meatus.
       ii) Using your dominant hand, grasp the cotton balls with the forceps; cleanse one side from top to bottom, then the other side, then down the middle. Use only one swipe per cotton ball.
       iii) Using your dominant hand, lubricate the first 1–2 inches of the catheter.
       iv) Insert the catheter into the meatus; when urine begins to flow, advance it another 1 inch.
    b. Male:
       i) Using your nondominant hand, retract the foreskin if present.
       ii) Grasp the shaft of the penis with your nondominant hand.
       iii) Using your dominant hand, grasp the cotton balls with the forceps; cleanse from the center of the meatus to the outside, using a circular motion (one circle per cotton ball).
       iv) Using your dominant hand, lubricate the first 1–2 inches of the catheter.
       v) While holding the penis upright, insert the catheter into the meatus, advancing it to the bifurcation at the Y of the catheter.
17. Inflate the balloon.
18. Connect the drainage bag to the end of the catheter.
19. Tape the catheter to the patient's leg.
20. Hang the drainage bag on the bed rail, below the level of the bladder.
21. Remove gloves and perform hand hygiene.

> If resistance is felt during catheter insertion, rotate the catheter slightly or gently apply pressure; do not force.

Male Catheter Insertion

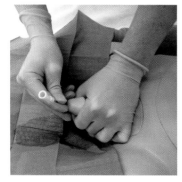

Changing an Ostomy Bag

Equipment Needed

- Gloves
- Pouching system (wafer and pouch)
- Washcloth
- Adhesive remover or alcohol wipes
- Skin care products (if ordered)
- Additional adhesive (if applicable)

Procedure for Changing on Ostomy Bag

1. Gather the equipment.
2. Explain the procedure to the patient.
3. Perform hand hygiene and put on gloves.
4. Place a clean towel under the existing pouch.
5. With your nondominant hand, gently push down on the skin around the existing stoma while using the dominant hand to remove the existing wafer and pouch (pull from the top down); use adhesive remover or alcohol wipes if the existing pouch is difficult to remove.
6. Gently clean around the stoma with lukewarm water (do not use soap); dry with a towel.
7. Inspect the stoma (should be pink or red and moist).
8. Measure the stoma with the existing pattern or with the guide that comes with the kit.
9. Cut the wafer to the appropriate size.
10. Remove the inner backing on the wafer.
11. Apply skin care products if ordered.
12. Apply additional adhesive to the wafer as applicable.
13. Center the wafer over the stoma, and press it into place.
14. Remove the outer backing on the wafer.
15. Remove gloves and perform hand hygiene.

Oxygen Administration

Indications
- Hypoxemia
- Pulmonary hypotension
- Increased heart workload (e.g., acute myocardial infarction, congestive heart failure)

Contraindications
There are no absolute contraindications to oxygen therapy when indications are present.

Equipment Needed
- Oxygen source
- Oxygen delivery device

Oxygen Administration Procedure
1. Gather the equipment.
2. Explain the procedure to the patient.
3. Connect the oxygen delivery device to the oxygen delivery source.
4. Adjust the oxygen flow rate as ordered.
5. Place the oxygen delivery device on the patient.
6. Assess patient comfort.

Oxygen Delivery Devices
- **Nasal cannula:** A device consisting of a plastic tube that fits behind the ears and a set of two prongs that are placed in the nostrils; it is connected to an oxygen source. Oxygen flows from the prongs into the nasal airway. A nasal cannula is the most commonly employed device for low-flow oxygen delivery. It provides supplemental oxygen at flows ranging from 0 to 8 L/min, enabling a maximum of 40% oxygen (O_2) to be delivered. Each liter increases the fraction of inspired oxygen (FiO_2) by 4%.
- **Oxygen mask:** Covers the nose and mouth (oral-nasal mask) or the entire face (full-face mask). It may be made of plastic, silicone, or rubber and is hooked up to an O_2 source. This is a low-flow delivery system.
- **Partial rebreather mask:** An O_2 mask with a reservoir bag. O_2 flow should always be supplied to maintain the reservoir bag at least one-third to one-half full on inspiration. At a flow of 6–10 L/min, the system can provide 40%–70% O_2. It is considered a high-flow delivery system.

- **Nonrebreather mask (NRB):** Similar to the partial rebreather mask, except that it has a series of one-way valves. One valve is placed between the bag and the mask to prevent exhaled air from returning to the bag. There should be a minimum flow of 10 L/min. The delivered FiO_2 of this system can be greater than 70%, depending on the O_2 flow and breathing pattern.
- **Venturi mask, or air-entrainment mask:** Delivers a known O_2 concentration (FiO_2) to patients on controlled O_2 therapy. Venturi masks are considered high-flow O_2 therapy devices. Venturi masks are able to provide total inspiratory flow at a specified FiO_2 to patients. The Venturi mask kits usually include multiple jets in order to set the desired FiO_2.
- **Ambu bag, or bag-valve-mask (BVM):** A handheld device used to provide ventilation to a patient who is not breathing (respiratory arrest) or who is breathing inadequately. An O_2 reservoir bag is attached to a central cylindrical bag, which is attached to a valved mask that administers O_2 at 8–15 breaths per minute. The central bag is squeezed manually to deliver a "breath" to the patient or to assist the patient in breathing by doing some of the work for the lungs.
- **Nebulizer:** A device used to administer medication in the form of a mist inhaled into the lungs. The most common nebulizer is the jet nebulizer, which is also called an atomizer. Jet nebulizers are connected by tubing to a compressed air source that causes air or O_2 to blast at high velocity through a liquid medicine to turn it into an aerosol, which is then inhaled by the patient.

Circulatory Care Techniques & Equipment

- **Cardioversion:** Refers to the conversion of one cardiac rhythm (electrical pattern) to another, almost always from an abnormal to a normal one. This conversion can be accomplished by pharmacologic means (i.e., using medications) or by electrical cardioversion (i.e., using a defibrillator).
  - **Pharmacologic cardioversion:** Involves a process similar to synchronized electrical cardioversion but uses medication instead of an electrical shock to convert the cardiac arrhythmia.
  - **Synchronized electrical cardioversion:** The process by which an abnormally fast heart rate or a cardiac arrhythmia is terminated by the delivery of a therapeutic dose of electric current to the heart at a specific moment in the cardiac cycle.
- **Defibrillator:** A device used to deliver a therapeutic dose of electrical energy to the heart. This depolarizes a critical mass of the heart muscle, terminates the arrhythmia, and allows a normal sinus rhythm to be reestablished by the body's natural pacemaker, the sinoatrial node of the heart. Defibrillators can be external, transvenous, or implanted, depending on the type of device used.
  - **Automated external defibrillator (AED):** A portable electronic device that automatically diagnoses the potentially life-threatening cardiac arrhythmias of ventricular fibrillation and ventricular tachycardia and is able to treat them through defibrillation (i.e., the application of electrical therapy), which stops the arrhythmia, allowing the heart to reestablish an effective rhythm.
  - **Implantable cardioverter-defibrillator (ICD) or automatic internal cardiac defibrillator (AICD):** Constantly monitors the patient's heart rhythm and automatically administers shocks for various life-threatening arrhythmias, according to the device's programming. These are implanted, similarly to pacemakers, and can also perform the pacemaking function.
  - **Manual external defibrillator:** Used in conjunction with (or have built in) electrocardiogram (ECG) readers, which the clinician uses to diagnose heart rhythms. The energy level of the shock delivered will depend on the diagnosis. The clinician will then decide what charge (in joules) to use, based on his or her prior knowledge and experience, and will deliver the shock through paddles or pads on the patient's chest.

- ○ **Manual internal defibrillator:** Virtually identical to the external version, except that the charge is delivered through internal paddles in direct contact with the heart. These are almost exclusively found in surgical areas, where the chest is likely to be open or can be opened quickly by a surgeon.
- **Electrocardiogram (ECG or EKG):** A recording of the electrical activity of the heart over time, usually in a noninvasive method via skin electrodes.
- **Pacemaker:** A device that uses electrical impulses, delivered by electrodes in contact with the heart muscles, to regulate the heartbeat. The primary purpose of a pacemaker is to maintain an adequate heart rate, either because the heart's natural pacemaker is not fast enough or because there is a block in the heart's electrical conduction system.
- **Epicardial (temporary) pacing:** Used during open-heart surgery should the surgical procedure create atrioventricular block. The electrodes are placed in contact with the outer wall of the ventricle (i.e., the epicardium) to maintain satisfactory cardiac output until a temporary transvenous electrode has been inserted.
- **Permanent pacing:** Involves transvenous placement of one or more pacing electrodes within one or more chambers of the heart. The procedure is performed by incision of a suitable vein into which the electrode lead is inserted and passed along the vein and through the valve of the heart until positioned in the chamber. The procedure is facilitated by fluoroscopy, which enables the cardiologist to view the passage of the electrode lead. After satisfactory placement of the electrode is confirmed, the opposite end of the electrode lead is connected to the pacemaker generator.
- **Temporary pacing:** Used to stimulate cardiac contraction until the underlying pathology is corrected or a permanent pacing device is inserted.
- **Transcutaneous pacing (TCP), or external pacing:** Used for the initial stabilization of hemodynamically significant bradycardia of all types. It is an emergency procedure that acts as a bridge until transvenous pacing or other therapies can be applied.
- **Transvenous pacing:** Used as an alternative to transcutaneous pacing. A pacemaker wire is placed into a vein, under sterile conditions, and then passed into either the right atrium or the right ventricle. The pacing wire is then connected to an external pacemaker (outside the body). Transvenous pacing is often used as a bridge to permanent pacemaker placement. It can be kept in place until a permanent pacemaker is implanted or until there is no longer a need for a pacemaker.
- **Telemetry:** A technology that allows the remote measurement and reporting of information. Telemetry is used for patients who are at risk of abnormal heart activity. The patient is outfitted with measuring, recording, and transmitting devices. A data log can be useful in diagnosis of the patient's condition, and an alerting function can notify nurses if the patient is suffering from an acute or dangerous condition.

Products

- **Compression stockings:** Used to support the venous and lymphatic systems of the leg. They offer graduated compression with maximum compression achieved at the ankle and decreasing as you move up the leg. This compression, when combined with the muscle pump effect of the calf, aids in circulating blood and lymph fluid through the legs.
- ○ **Thromboembolic deterrent (TED) antiembolism stockings:** These stockings are designed to prevent blood clots in the recumbent (bedridden) patient. TED stockings have graduated compression to speed blood flow.
- **Sequential compression devices (SCDs), or lymphedema pumps:** Designed to limit the development of deep vein thrombosis and peripheral edema in immobile patients. They consist of an air pump connected to a disposable sleeve by a series of air tubes. The sleeve is placed around the patient's leg. Air is then forced into different parts of the sleeve in sequence, creating pressure around the calves and improving venous return.

Managing Shock

Type	Pathophysiology	Causes	Physical Findings	Treatment
Septic	Functional hypovolemia; chemical mediators activated in response to invading organisms	Any type of bacteria	*Early:* Flushed, pink skin; shallow, rapid respirations; full, rapid, bounding pulse; normal to slightly elevated blood pressure *Late:* Cyanotic, pale skin; shallow, rapid respirations; weak, rapid, thready pulse; hypotension	IV fluids; antimicrobials; oxygen; vasopressors; mechanical ventilation; surgery
Neurogenic	Severe vasodilatation	Spinal cord injury; anesthesia	Bounding pulse; hypotension; bradycardia; warm, pale, dry skin	IV fluids; vasopressors; oxygen
Hypovolemic	Ventricular filling decreased; cardiac output decreased; less venous return to the heart because of lost fluid; metabolic acidosis, tissue anoxia	Acute blood loss; burns; dehydration	Shallow, rapid respirations; cool, clammy, pale skin; thready, rapid pulse; orthostatic vital signs; decreased sensorium; urine output <20 mL/hr mean arterial pressure <60 mm Hg (adults)	Fluid and blood replacement; lying flat; vasopressors
Cardiogenic	Myocardial ischemia; sympathetic compensation; cardiac output decreased; left ventricular dysfunction	Myocardial infarction; myocarditis; myocardial ischemia; acute mitral or aortic insufficiency; ventricular septal defect; ventricular aneurysm; papillary muscle dysfunction	Cold, clammy, pale skin; thready, rapid pulse; shallow, rapid respirations; gallop rhythm, faint heart sounds; mean arterial pressure <60 mm Hg (adults)	IV fluids; inotropics; vasopressors; defibrillation or cardioversion; temporary pacemaker; analgesics; sedatives; oxygen
Anaphylactic	Edema; fluid shifts, bronchospasms, blood vessel dilation	Allergic reaction to antigens	Cool, pale skin; rash; swelling of the face, eyes, or tongue; respiratory distress	IV fluids; oxygen; epinephrine; antihistamines; steroids

NURSING
CHEMISTRY

4

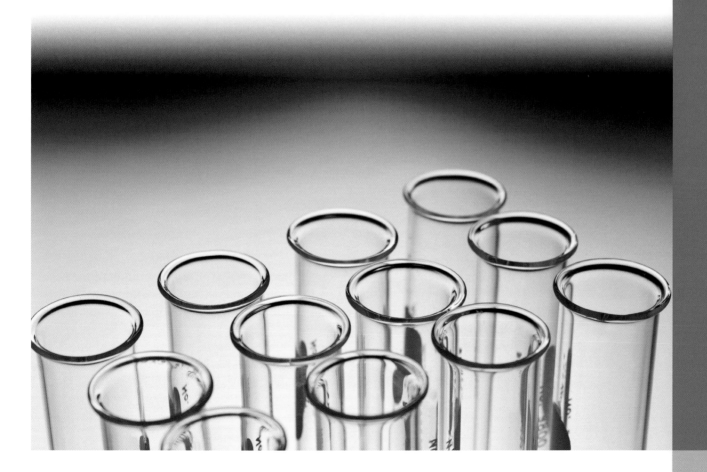

Introduction

Chemistry is the science that explains how materials behave, whether in a process as simple as the evaporation of water or one as complex as the replication of DNA in the nucleus of a living cell. Chemistry helps us understand how substances react with other materials, as well as how external conditions influence the things we see around us. In nursing, you are exposed to most aspects of chemistry, from the fundamentals of general chemistry to the advanced features of biochemistry that help in the diagnosis and treatment of diseases. At times, you may feel like a scientist as you explore, for example, the impact of diet on health, as our diet is the chemical input that keeps our bodies working properly. The mathematics of chemistry comes into play, for example, when you administer oxygen to a patient with lung dysfunction or monitor the dose of a pain reliever. Every disease and medical treatment has as its basis the chemistry of the human body. Understanding chemistry provides an essential set of knowledge that will make you a more effective nurse, and it can often provide explanations for why we do the things we do in the medical field.

Science & Measurement

Science is the experimental study of nature. A scientist uses observed data to guide the experimental process to test hypotheses, refine theories, and develop scientific laws in a process called the **scientific method**.

A scientific **hypothesis** is an attempt to explain observations scientifically. A scientific **theory** is a predictive hypothesis supported by many experiments. Scientific **laws** bring together phenomena having common causes and explanations.

Chemistry is the study of matter and the changes that matter undergoes. **Matter** is the material part of the universe and is composed of pure substances and mixtures. A **pure substance** has a fixed composition, while a **mixture** is a combination of substances of variable composition.

Elements are the fundamental building blocks for all matter, as an element cannot be decomposed into a simpler substance by chemical or physical means. Elements chemically combine to form **compounds** with a fixed chemical composition; compounds can be chemically broken down into elements. **Chemical reactions** alter the chemical makeup of substances. In contrast, **physical processes** change only the form or phase of a substance and are easily reversed. The highest-energy processes are **nuclear reactions**, that change the nucleus of an atom.

Scientific data are used to describe phenomena or properties of matter. Data have numerical values and, in most cases, descriptive units. If no unit is given, one is often assumed. The **unit** is a quantity adopted as a standard for a given type of data. The **English system** includes common nonstandard units, the **metric system** is based on a consistent set of units, and **SI units** (International System) make use of the metric system and are used in scientific work. The metric system provides the decimal-based units used in chemistry. The standard metric units are:

- **Time**, in seconds (s)
- **Mass**, in grams (g)
- **Length**, in meters (m)
- **Volume**, in liters (L)

A **unit prefix** is used to denote the decimal fraction or power of 10 multiple of the base unit. The resulting unit is a shorthand way to account for a wide range of numerical values (e.g., 1000 g becomes 1 kg; 0.001 m becomes 1 mm). Some of the common experimental phenomena encountered in chemistry include:

- **Temperature**, or relative "hotness," measured in °C (Celsius) or K (Kelvin). The Fahrenheit scale (°F) is the English unit often used. Normal body temperature is 98.6°F, or 37°C. The **Temperature Scales** figure (p. 81) provides a visual comparison of the three scales.
- **Mass**, or the quantity of matter (given in grams) determined experimentally using a scientific balance.

➕ ❗ Understanding units is important to good health therapy. Even dosages have units: 1/day? 3/day? Grams, milligrams, or kilograms? Misreading dosage units can have tragic results, as many drugs become toxic in high concentrations.

Common Unit Prefixes	
Prefix (abbreviation)	**Meaning**
micro- (μ)	10^{-6}
milli- (m)	10^{-3}
centi- (c)	10^{-2}
kilo- (k)	10^{3}
mega- (M)	10^{6}
giga- (G)	10^{9}
See chapter 5, **Medical Math**, for more metric prefixes.	

Temperature Scales

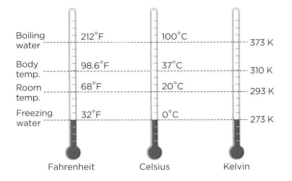

	Fahrenheit	Celsius	Kelvin
Boiling water	212°F	100°C	373 K
Body temp.	98.6°F	37°C	310 K
Room temp.	68°F	20°C	293 K
Freezing water	32°F	0°C	273 K

- **Volume**, or the space occupied by matter. Liquid volume is measured using a calibrated graduated cylinder or syringe. For a solid, measure the dimensions and use a geometry formula for the specific shape to calculate the volume.
- **Pressure**, or the force per unit of area exerted by a gas on the walls of a container or by a liquid pumped through a pipe. Blood pressure measures the pressure of the blood in the body's blood vessels.
- The **mole**, or Avogadro's number of atoms or molecules. It is used for chemical calculations that describe compounds and chemical reactions.
- The **density**, or mass per unit of volume, of an object or sample of gas. The common units are g/mL or g/cm^3.
- **Specific gravity**, or the density relative to the density of pure water at 4°C. Specific gravity has no units.
- **Concentration**, or the quantity of a substance in a volume of solution. Examples include vinegar, saline reagents, and blood. Common units for denoting the amount of dissolved materials are molarity (moles per liter) and g/L.

Example

A packet of saline solution has a mass of 55.0 g and a volume of 50.0 mL. Therefore, the density of the solution is 55.0 g/50 mL, or 1.1 g/mL.

When working with data and units, the units often must be changed to fit the needs of the scientist. A **conversion factor** is an equivalence statement (i.e., a ratio or an equation) used to convert from one set of units to another. The **factor-label method** is the technique used to convert units from one system to another (e.g., from grams to kilograms).

Example
A box of hospital gloves weighs 5000 g. What is the mass in kg?

The conversion factor is 1 kg = 1000 g, so multiply by 1 kg/1000 g to convert grams to kilograms:

5000 g × 1 kg/1000 g = 5.0 kg. The old unit (g) is canceled, leaving the new unit (kg).

➕ ❗ You may encounter different temperature units, so check equipment scales and readouts. You may see °C or °F, so be aware of the differences. Water freezes at 32°F, or 0°C. Hot water and fevers are a bit over 100°F, or 37°C. If you get mixed up, there could be dire consequences!

A **conversion equation** is used to convert between the Fahrenheit and Celsius temperature scales. The key equations are as follows:

- To convert a temperature from Celsius to Fahrenheit: $([°C] \times 1.8) + 32 = [°F]$
- To convert a temperature from Fahrenheit to Celsius: $([°F] - 32) \div 1.8 = [°C]$

Example
Body temperature is 98.6°F. What is normal body temperature using a Celsius thermometer?

We use the equation $[°C] = ([°F] - 32) \div 1.8$; therefore, body temperature

$[°C] = (98.6°F - 32) \div 1.8 = 66.6 \div 1.8 = 37°C$.

Data should be analyzed for reliability. An experimental measurement is never exact—it includes a limited number of digits because of the uncertainty of the measuring device. The number of **significant figures** establishes the degree to which you can trust data.

➕ A measurement of 5.0 g on a triple-beam balance has an uncertainty of 0.1 g. The same measurement using an electronic balance gives 5.000 grams, with an uncertainty of 0.001 grams.

Fundamental Constants
- **Gas constant for energy calculations:** $R = 8.314$ J mole^{-1} K^{-1}
- **Gas constant for gas property calculations:** $R = 0.082$ L atm mole^{-1} K^{-1}
- **Avogadro's number:** $N_A = 6.022 \times 10^{23}$ mole^{-1}
- **Boltzmann constant:** $k = R/N_A = 1.381 \times 10^{-23}$ J molecule^{-1} K^{-1}
- **Elementary charge of the electron, e:** 1.602×10^{-19} C
- **Faraday's constant, $\mathcal{F}$:** Charge of one mole (N_A) of electrons
- **Mass of a proton, m_p:** 1.673×10^{-27} kg
- **Mass of a neutron, m_n:** 1.675×10^{-27} kg
- **Mass of an electron, m_e:** 9.110×10^{-31} kg
- **Planck's constant, h:** 6.626×10^{-34} J • s
- **Speed of light in a vacuum, c:** 2.9979×10^8 m • s^{-1}

Atomic Structure & the Periodic Table

All matter is composed of atoms. An **atom** is the smallest unit of matter that retains elemental properties. The **nucleus**, the dense center of positive charge in the atom, contains **neutrons** (uncharged nuclear particles) and **protons** (positively charged nuclear particles). These particles have about the same mass. The **electrons** are the negative particles outside the nucleus; they are less massive than protons or neutrons. The **electron configuration** is used to tally the number and type of electrons for a given atom. The **valence electrons** are the electrons in the outermost shell of an atom that determine the chemical properties of the element.

Elements are defined by their **atomic number (Z)**, which is the number of protons in the nucleus. The **mass number (A)** is the sum of protons and neutrons. The **atomic**

mass is the total mass of the atom in atomic mass units (amu). Elements often have several **isotopes**, which are two forms of the same element that have the same Z values but different A values (i.e., the number of neutrons is different, but the number of protons is the same). The term **radioisotope** refers to an isotope that emits radioactivity. Such isotopes are used in a number of medical applications.

Because most elements have more than one isotope, the mass of the elements in a compound is described using the **atomic weight**, which is the element's average atomic mass accounting for the different isotopes found in natural samples.

The **periodic table** (*see* appendix C) is a tabular depiction of the elements organized by atomic number, with chemically similar elements in the same column. A **period** is a horizontal row of elements in the periodic table, whereas a **group** (a.k.a. family) is a vertical column of elements in the periodic table.

Did you ever wonder why it is called the "periodic" table? Elements in the same column of the table have the same number of valence electrons, which gives them similar chemical behavior. **Periodicity** is the term used to describe predictable trends in atomic properties tied to an atom's column location in the table. In terms of the general properties of elements in the table, **metals** are located on the left side of the periodic table and **non-metals** on the right side of the periodic table. **Metalloids** form a "staircase" boundary between metals and nonmetals because they can exhibit both metallic and nonmetallic properties, depending on what they react with.

Some groups of elements have specific names. The **alkali metals** form group 1; they are very reactive metals. The **alkaline earth metals** form group 2; they are also reactive metals, but not as reactive as the alkali metals. The **transition metals** form a large part of the table, groups 3–12; transition metals display varied chemistry, with cations exhibiting a number of possible valences. The **halides** form group 17, which are very reactive nonmetals. Finally, we find the **noble, or inert, gases** in group 18, named for the fact that they are nonreactive elements.

In most cases, we find elements in chemical compounds or as dissociated ions in solutions. An **ion** is a charged particle formed by a molecule or atom when it loses or gains one or more electrons. An **anion** is a negative ion formed by electron gain relative to the neutral atom or molecule. A **cation** is a positive ion formed by electron loss relative to the neutral atom or molecule.

The chemical behavior of elements is driven by the energy of atoms and ions. Energy is not a random property. **Quantum mechanical principles** predict the energies of electrons in atoms. Atoms with filled outermost electron shells are the most stable. The *most* stable elements are the noble gases because each has a filled outer valence shell. This also helps explain the chemical properties of elements. An element that is one electron short or one electron in excess of the configuration of a noble gas is *very* reactive. Chemical reactions occur when atoms exchange electrons to match the electron configurations of noble gases. Metals have more electrons than the nearest noble gas, so they tend to lose electrons, becoming cations. Nonmetals have fewer electrons than the nearest noble gas, so they tend to gain electrons, becoming anions.

Compounds: Bonds & Formulas

A **chemical formula** is a depiction of a compound using elemental symbols and numerical subscripts. The compound's name is often a unique description of a compound, covering the same information as its formula. **Nomenclature** is the term used to describe a formal system for chemical names. The force that holds atoms together in a material is called a **chemical bond**. A **molecule** is formed by two or more bonded atoms.

A **covalent bond** is a bond formed with bonding electrons: Two atoms share one pair of electrons in a **single bond** (e.g., H–H, diatomic hydrogen or H_2). For a **double bond**, two atoms share two pairs of electrons (e.g., O=O, diatomic oxygen or O_2). In the strongest bond, a **triple bond**, two atoms share three pairs of electrons (e.g., N≡N, diatomic nitrogen or N_2).

Radioactive materials are the source of X-rays in computed tomography (CT) scans. Radioactive iodine is used to treat thyroid conditions. Positron-emitting isotopes are used in positron emission tomography (PET) scans.

Oxygen (for respiration therapy), chlorine (used in disinfectants), and helium and argon (inert gases) are all elemental gases used in medicine.

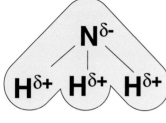

Dipole Moment

$N^{\delta-}$
$H^{\delta+}$ $H^{\delta+}$ $H^{\delta+}$

Ammonia

Lewis Structure

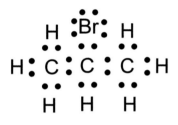

H :Br: H

H:C:C:C:H
  H   H   H

⊕ Many common plastics, paints, and glues are made of various polymers. Plastic materials in the hospital are made of polyethylene, which is a long carbon chain consisting of thousands of atoms forming monomers of ethylene, or C_2H_4.

In symmetrical molecules, the atoms equally share the bonding electrons. In an ionic bond, atoms are held together by electrostatic attractive forces resulting from electron transfer (e.g., sodium chloride [NaCl], or table salt, formed from sodium cations and chloride anions). Most bonds tend to have both ionic and covalent character and are called **polar covalent bonds**. Electrons in a polar covalent bond are not equally shared by the two atoms. Polar covalent molecules have a permanent electric **dipole moment**, which is produced by an asymmetrical electron density in a bond, giving rise to a partial negative charge at one end of a bond or molecule. Thus, polar covalent molecules are often called **dipolar molecules**.

Bonding Principles

Chemical bonding is explained by a number of principles. **Electronegativity** is the tendency of an atom in a molecule to attract shared electrons. This describes the process of atoms interacting with other atoms to form chemical bonds. The **octet rule** helps explain molecular stability: a bonded atom is most stable when it is surrounded by eight valence electrons. Atoms in stable molecules "look" like rare gas atoms. It is important to note, however, that hydrogen accommodates only two electrons, and sulfur (and larger atoms) can accommodate more than eight electrons and, therefore, more than four bonds. These are considered exceptions to the octet rule, but they are consistent with the rare gas guideline, since helium has two valence electrons and larger atoms have up to 18 electrons in the valence shell.

Describing Bonding

A **Lewis structure** is a visual depiction of molecule showing bonds and valence electrons for each atom. This does not describe the geometry, just the bonds. A **lone pair** is an electron pair *not* involved in bonding; it does affect the geometry and molecular electronic features.

Molecular Properties

The properties of a molecule are derived from the bonding in the molecule, as well as its interactions with other molecules. Some molecules, such as gaseous oxygen, are diatomic—that is, they contain two atoms. Other molecules contain thousands of atoms. **Polymers** are chain molecules formed by chemically linking small molecules, called **monomers**. Many cellular chemicals are polymers: Starch (a carbohydrate) is a sugar polymer. Proteins are polymers of amino acids. DNA and RNA, which are nucleic acids, are polymers of nucleotides. Fats contain fatty acids, which contain polymer chains of carbon atoms. Biochemical polymers use monomers with reactive –OH and –NH groups, and thus cellular metabolism uses many polymer-making and polymer-breaking reactions.

The complex chemistry of the human body is largely caused by the variations in polar character found in biomaterials. A **hydrophilic** material is a polar molecule that is attracted to water; dipole-dipole interactions or hydrogen bonding enhances the solubility of these materials in water. Conversely, **hydrophobic** substances are nonpolar molecules that repel water and are therefore less water soluble.

Biochemical and organic materials often have both features in one molecule. Fatty acids have a polar head and a nonpolar tail, sugars have carbon backbones with polar –OH groups, and amino acids consist of a polar amine and acid part combined with a variety of nonpolar organic groups.

Common Types of Compounds

- The key feature of **organic compounds** is their carbon backbone. Examples include methane, ethanol, glucose, and benzene. Added chemical groups alter the properties of the compound, which helps to explain why there are millions of possible organic compounds.
- **Inorganic materials** are all the nonorganic substances, covering the chemical properties of the other 90 natural elements.
- Water and inorganic salts, in addition to proteins, fats, carbohydrates, and vitamins (organic compounds), are important within the chemistry of living cells.
- **Elemental gases** are the simplest compounds. Examples include hydrogen (H_2), nitrogen (N_2), chlorine (Cl_2), and oxygen (O_2).

- **Acids** commonly encountered include hydrochloric acid (a digestive acid found in the stomach), acetic acid (vinegar), nitric acid (found in acid rain), and phosphoric acid (a component of DNA and RNA).
- Common **bases** include sodium hydroxide (used in degreasers and sink drain cleaners), sodium bicarbonate (baking soda), ammonium hydroxide (used in window cleaners and kitchen sprays), and amines (organic bases found in DNA and RNA).
- **Ionic salts** may be water soluble (e.g., table salt [NaCl] and washing soda [sodium carbonate]) or insoluble (e.g., magnesium oxide and calcium carbonate) minerals. In some cases, the ions can interact with water, giving acidic or basic solutions.
- **Small molecules** are some of the most important chemicals encountered: carbon dioxide (CO_2), ammonia (NH_3), and water (H_2O).

Types of Organic Compounds

Type of Compound	Examples
Alkane	CH_4
Alkene	>C=C<
Aromatic ring	$-C_6H_5$
Alcohol	R–OH
Ether	R–O–R'
Aldehyde	$\overset{\displaystyle O}{\overset{\|}{R-C-H}}$
Ketone	$\overset{\displaystyle O}{\overset{\|}{R-C-R'}}$
Carboxylic acid	$\overset{\displaystyle O}{\overset{\|}{R-C-OH}}$
Ester	$\overset{\displaystyle O}{\overset{\|}{R-C-OR'}}$
Halide	R–Cl, R–Br
Amine	N–RR'R"
Amide	$\overset{\displaystyle O}{\overset{\|}{R-C-NRR'}}$

Typical Behavior of C, N & O

Atom	Number of Valence Electrons	Typical Behavior	Single Bond Example	Double Bond Example	Triple Bond Example
Carbon (C)	4	4 bonds	–C–C– alkane	>C=C< alkene	–C≡C– alkynes
Nitrogen (N)	5	3 bonds, 1 lone pair; 4 bonds for cation	>N– ammonia	R=N–	–C≡N cyanide
Oxygen (O)	6	2 bonds, 2 lone pairs	–O– water	>C=O carbonic acid	Not observed

Reactions: Calculations & Equations

Chemical reactions convert one material into another material. A **chemical equation** is used to tally the details of the reaction. An equation has the general form Reactants → Products. The **product** is the reaction result and is placed on the right side of the equation. The **reactant** is the starting material and is placed on the left side of the equation. For example:

$$O_2 \text{ [g]} + C \text{ [s]} \rightarrow CO_2 \text{ [g]}$$

A **balanced equation** accounts for the conservation of mass, charge, and specific elements. Balancing gives a correct assessment of how much material reacts and how much product is obtained from the reaction. To balance an equation, use the following steps:
1. Count the atoms of each element.
2. Determine which atoms are balanced and which are not.
3. Change coefficients to balance each element.
4. Balance one atom at a time, using coefficients.
5. Balance pure elements last.
6. Check your work; is it balanced?

Examples of Reactions & Processes

- **Decomposition** is the breakdown of a substance into component elements or simpler compounds.
- **Double replacement** occurs by mixing two solutions, allowing the ions to form new compounds.
- **Acid-base processes** include dissociation, the use of buffers, and neutralization.
- **Oxidation-reduction reactions** involve atoms in compounds exchanging electrons.
- **Dehydration** is the loss of water (in either a chemical or a physical process).
- **Hydrogenation** adds hydrogen to an organic compound.
- **Ionic reactions**, **dissociation**, **hydration**, and **hydrolysis** are all reactions that involve water.

Typical evidence of a reaction is the generation of heat or flame, the production of a gas, a color change, or the formation of a precipitate.

Complete Reactions & Equilibrium

A reaction that goes to completion converts all reactants to products. For a process exhibiting **equilibrium**, the reaction does not go to completion; reactants and products coexist in equilibrium. Equilibrium is quantified using a constant, K_{eq}, called the **equilibrium constant**. K_{eq} is calculated from product and reactant concentrations at equilibrium; its magnitude denotes which direction is dominant: a large K_{eq} means products are more prevalent, and a small K_{eq} means reactants are more prevalent.

Chemical Calculations

Atomic masses vary from element to element, so the mass of a molecule depends on the elements in the compound. Because the number of atoms in a typical sample of material is not practical for routine use, a counting unit called the **mole** is used in chemical calculations. This allows balanced equations to be used to calculate masses of products and reactants, as in the following equations:

$$1 \text{ mole } + 1 \text{ mole } \rightarrow 1 \text{ mole}$$

$$C + O_2 \rightarrow CO_2$$

$$12 \text{ g } + 32 \text{ g } \rightarrow 44 \text{ g}$$

The **mole** is defined as Avogadro's number of particles (6.022×10^{23} particles). **Formula weight** is the mass of a formula unit of a compound relative to a standard atomic mass (the carbon-12 isotope). **Molar mass** is the mass in grams of one mole of a substance, regardless of whether it is an element, molecule, or solid material. To calculate the molar mass, add all atomic weights of the elements in the compound multiplied by formula coefficients.

Theoretical yield is the predicted mass of the product using a balanced equation, the reactant mass, and the molar masses of products and reactants. The **limiting reagent** is the first depleted reagent in a reaction; it is present in the smallest molar quantity as defined by the balanced equation.

Energy & Kinetics

Thermodynamics

Thermodynamics describes the heat and work associated with a physical or chemical process and therefore whether a reaction will occur and if heat is absorbed or released. Thermodynamics introduces three key terms: enthalpy, entropy, and free energy.

The **change in enthalpy (ΔH)** for a process is the heat released or absorbed at constant pressure (i.e., normal laboratory conditions). An **exothermic** process has a negative ΔH; heat is released to the surroundings, making the reaction vessel feel hot (e.g., gas condensing to liquid, respiration, combustion of a fuel). An **endothermic** process has a positive ΔH; heat is absorbed from the surroundings, making the vessel feel cold (e.g., evaporation of liquid to form gas, melting of ice).

The **change in entropy (ΔS)** for a process measures the change in system disorder. Gases have more entropy or disorder than liquids or solids. A value of ΔS greater than zero denotes an increase in entropy. A common example is the evaporation of water. A value of ΔS less than 0 denotes a decrease in entropy, which would apply to the condensation of water vapor.

The **change in free energy (ΔG)** for a process shows whether a specified reaction is spontaneous; that is, whether it will occur for the given conditions. This is the most important practical issue to address with the thermodynamics of a reaction. An **exogenic** process has a negative ΔG; it is spontaneous. An **endogenic** process has a positive ΔG; it is not spontaneous. A process at equilibrium has $\Delta G = 0$. The magnitude of ΔG reflects the degree of spontaneity or lack of spontaneity. For example, the combustion of fuels on oxygen has a large negative ΔG.

In most cases cellular chemistry involves multistep reactions. **Hess's law** states that the thermodynamic properties of a combination of reactions are obtained by adding the respective ΔG, ΔH, and ΔS of the reactions. Enthalpy, entropy, and free energy are related by the equation:

$$\Delta G = \Delta H - T\Delta S$$

As this shows, exothermic reactions with a positive ΔS tend to be spontaneous. Endothermic reactions need help from ΔS and a high temperature to be spontaneous. Note that T is always positive; it is the absolute temperature in Kelvin.

Equilibrium can also be defined in terms of thermodynamic variables. A large equilibrium constant is associated with a large and negative ΔG. The change in free energy is related to the equilibrium constant by the following equation:

$$\Delta G = -RT\ln K_{eq},$$

where R is the ideal gas constant, T is the absolute temperature in Kelvin, and K_{eq} is the equilibrium constant.

Kinetics

Kinetics answers a second key question about a chemical reaction: How fast does the reaction go? Does it take a few seconds or many years to get a product? The speed of a

➕ Respiration releases heat to the body, keeping the body warmer than its surroundings and matching the needs of catalyzed cellular processes.

➕ Sweating is endothermic, serving to release heat from the body. An alcohol bath cools the skin as the isopropyl alcohol evaporates.

➕ Cellular respiration is exogenic; it produces excess heat and free energy to drive other endogenic reactions in the body. Otherwise, the body could not synthesize the thousands of chemicals required for life.

➕ The body's metabolism is an example of Hess's law, as it has many coupled exothermic and endothermic reactions. The net result is a stable temperature that supports all of the body's living cells.

reaction also provides insight into the way the reaction occurs, called the **mechanism**, which identifies the simple chemical steps that together form the overall reaction.

The **rate of a reaction** depends on the concentrations of the reactants. The mathematical form of the behavior tells us how the reaction occurs. To illustrate this, consider a reaction $A + B \rightarrow C$. For a **first-order** reaction, the rate depends on the concentration of a single reagent, which may be either:

$$\text{Rate} = k[A] \text{ or } \text{Rate} = k[B]$$

For a **second-order** reaction, the rate depends on the product of two reagent concentrations, which may be either:

$$\text{Rate} = k[A][B], \text{Rate} = k[A]^2, \text{ or } \text{Rate} = k[B]^2$$

A **rate constant (k)** is used to characterize each reaction rate equation. A larger k is associated with a faster reaction. The order of the reaction reflects the nature of the **rate-determining step**, which is the highest-energy step of the reaction. The magnitude of this energy barrier is called the **activation energy, E_a**. This barrier exists because bonds must be broken for the reaction to happen; this requires the addition of energy. This is the crucial part of the mechanism that controls the overall rate of the reaction and nature of the product.

The activation energy governs the rate and controls the formation of products. Any change to the activation energy alters the reaction rate. If this energy barrier increases, the reaction is slower. Conversely, if the barrier is lowered using a **catalyst**, the reaction becomes faster. In addition, increasing the temperature increases the reaction rate and lowering the temperature decreases the rate.

States of Matter

There are three states of matter: gas, liquid, and solid. A **gas** is fluid that fills a container, a **liquid** is a fluid that takes the shape of a container, and a **solid** has a defined size and shape. The standard variables used to describe phase behavior are pressure (P) in atmospheres (atm), volume (V) in liters, number of moles (n), and temperature (T) in Kelvin, the absolute scale. Solids are found at low temperature and high pressure. Gases are found at high temperature and low pressure.

States of Matter

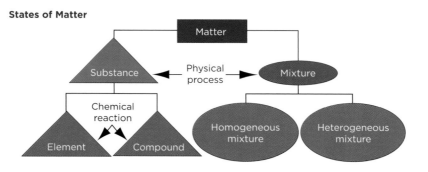

A **barometer** is used to measure the pressure of gas. A number of units are used for pressure: atm, mm Hg (millimeters of mercury), in Hg (inches of mercury), or psi (pounds per square inch). These are related as follows:

$$1 \text{ atm} = 760 \text{ mm Hg} = 14.696 \text{ psi} = 29.92 \text{ in Hg}$$

The **volume** of a gas or liquid is measured in L or mL using a calibrated container. The volume of a solid is calculated from measured size dimensions, usually in m^3 or cm^3. A **thermometer** is used to measure temperature in °C or °F. **Standard temperature and pressure (STP)** is 273 K and 1 atm (760 mm Hg). Liquids contained in a pressurized system are measured using these pressure units as well.

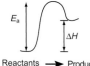

+ Fever produces an elevated body temperature, increasing the rate of cellular reactions. Hypothermia has the opposite effect: as the body temperature drops, crucial reactions become slower. Both processes can lead to cellular damage or death.

Reaction Energy

Endothermic

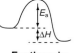

Exothermic

+ An **enzyme** is a biochemical catalyst, a specific protein that catalyzes one specific reaction in the body. Our bodies contain thousands of reactions, each with a matching enzyme that works at peak efficiency at 98.6°F.

Enzyme Catalyst

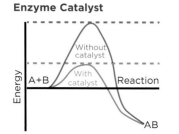

+ Blood pressure is measured in units of mm Hg, similarly to air pressure. The blood pressure ratio is systolic-to-diastolic (the maximum-to-minimum) pressure exerted on blood vessels. If the pressure is too high, vessels can be damaged, leading to stroke; if it is too low, fluid builds up in the lungs and other body tissues. Both extremes harm the body.

The **normal boiling point (T_b)** for a compound is the temperature at which the liquid changes to gas at standard pressure of 1 atm. The **melting point (T_m)** is the temperature at which the solid changes to liquid at standard pressure of 1 atm. **Evaporation** is the conversion of a liquid to gas when the temperature is less than the boiling point. All liquids exhibit a characteristic vapor pressure, increasing to 1 atm at the boiling point. **Condensation** converts a gas to a liquid. A **phase diagram** denoting boiling points, melting points, and vapor pressure for the material is often used as a graphical depiction of the phase behavior.

✚ When administering oxygen gas to a patient, you will need to monitor the pressure or gas flow using a dial setting, so be aware of the pressure unit; is it atm, mm Hg, psi, or in Hg?

Gas Laws

Gases are the easiest phase to describe using scientific laws to calculate properties under various experimental conditions of temperature, pressure, and volume.

Avogadro's law states that gas volume is directly proportional to n (the number of moles of gas) at constant pressure and temperature (e.g., double n, and V doubles). **Boyle's law** states that gas volume varies inversely with pressure at constant temperature and fixed moles of gas (e.g., double P, and V is halved). **Charles' law** states that gas volume is directly proportional to temperature at constant pressure and fixed moles of gas (e.g., triple T in Kelvin, and V is tripled). It is important to remember that for all gas laws, T is in Kelvin.

Phase Relationships

SOLID

sublime   melt T_m

T_b

GAS   boil   LIQUID

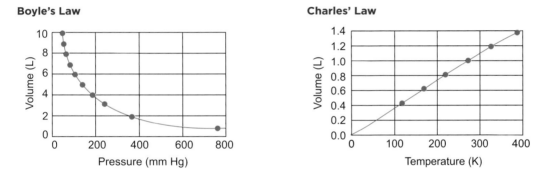

Avogadro's, Boyle's, and Charles' laws can be combined to give the **ideal gas law**:

$$PV = nRT$$

The creation of a single equation requires the introduction of a constant, R, called the **ideal gas constant**.

$$R = 0.082 \ \frac{\text{L atm}}{\text{mol K}}$$

These units match the most common units for P (in atm), V (in liters), and n (in moles).

The ideal gas law is accurate at low pressure and high temperature, meaning it works for common gases such as oxygen and nitrogen at room temperature. It is important to note that this model omits molecular properties and intermolecular forces. So at low temperature and high pressure, it fails to describe gas liquefaction. Other, more complex equations, such as the van der Waals gas equation, form the basis of more realistic models and therefore address the shortcomings of the ideal gas law.

In many cases in everyday life we work with mixtures of gases. **Dalton's law** states that the total pressure for a gas mixture is the sum of partial pressures, which is the pressure exerted by each component. The most common example of a mixture of gases is the Earth's atmosphere, composed of approx. 80% nitrogen and 20% oxygen, with minor amounts of argon, water vapor, and residual components such as CO_2 and air pollutants. Because CO_2 plays a role in insulating the Earth from heat loss, much of the discussion of climate change focuses on the amount of CO_2 in the atmosphere.

✚ Inhaled air contains oxygen that is absorbed by the bloodstream in the lungs and carried to the cells in the body's tissues for use in respiration. Exhaled air contains less oxygen and more CO_2, a product of cellular oxidation of carbon-containing dietary proteins, carbohydrates, and fats.

Intermolecular Forces

All atoms and molecules interact with surrounding atoms or molecules. In some cases, these interactions are strong, as seen in ionic solids bonded together by strong electrostatic forces or atoms in molecules held together by chemical bonds. The more general interactions are the weaker intermolecular forces that are observed as molecules or atoms interact with neighbors in liquids or gases. **Dipole-dipole interactions** are attractive forces between polar molecules. The **hydrogen bond** is a special type of dipole-dipole interaction arising from the attraction between the H atom of –OH or –NH and another atom with unshared electrons (often O, N, or S). The **London force** is a weak attraction caused by short-lived dipoles arising from electronic motion in atoms or symmetrical molecules.

The term **van der Waals force** is often used to describe the dipole-dipole and London forces that cause gases to liquefy at low temperatures and influence real gas pressure-volume behavior. London forces apply to gases such as oxygen, argon, and neon, as well as to all molecules.

Dipole molecules are attracted to one another by dipole-dipole interactions. Polar covalent bonds give rise to molecules with dipole moments if the molecule is asymmetrical. Nonpolar molecules and monatomic gases interact only through London forces.

Water & Hydrogen Bonding

Understanding the chemical and physical properties of water requires a clear understanding of hydrogen bonding. This strong intermolecular force gives liquid water a loose structure and helps explain a number of water's properties. Water has a high boiling point and low freezing point relative to molecules of comparable size. Water's low vapor pressure arises from the stability of liquid water and its surface molecules.

Sugar, table salt, and alcohol are soluble in water because of the interactions of water molecules with these materials, and thus water is often called the "universal solvent." Hydrogen bonding allows water to be stable on our planet's surface and therefore allows life to exist. Any search for extraterrestrial life starts with finding liquid water.

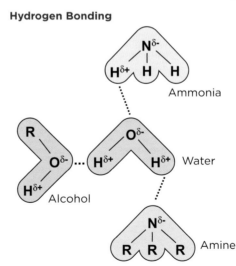

Hydrogen Bonding

Ammonia

Alcohol

Water

Amine

➕ Our body is mostly water. The stability of water as a liquid helps stabilize cellular processes and allows for the variety of chemistry arising from the thousands of compounds found in the body.

Solutions & Mixtures

We encounter mixtures of materials much more often than pure elements and individual compounds. A **solution** is a uniform physical mixture of solids, liquids, or gases. The **solute** is the minor component (e.g., dissolved salt in the ocean). The **solvent** is the major component (e.g., liquid water in seawater). A solution may contain one or many solutes and can be described with the following general equation:

$$\text{Solution} = \text{Solute [s]} + \text{Solvent}$$

A **colloid** is a mixture of larger particles that scatter light. For example, a cloud is made of water droplets mixed with air. In the human body, blood is made of cells and other components in water. An **emulsion** is a colloid of interacting liquid phases. For example, soap works by forming an emulsion of grease in water; otherwise, the water alone will not dissolve the grease or dirt. A **suspension** is a nonequilibrium mixture; the particles will settle to the bottom of the container over time.

Solubility, or the "solubility limit," is the amount of a substance that will dissolve in a given volume of solvent at a specified temperature. A **saturated solution** contains the maximum dissolved solute. A **supersaturated solution** is an unstable mixture that is concentrated beyond its saturation point.

Henry's law governs the solubility of gases in water or any liquid. According to the law, the amount of dissolved gas is proportional to gas pressure. This is why high altitudes put stress on the body: there is less oxygen in the air, so less gets drawn into the lung tissue.

We often use the term *insoluble* to describe a solute that is less than 1% soluble, although this can vary with application. A general rule for solutions is that "like dissolves like"—that is, materials with similar properties will mix. This is especially true for gases; all gases mix because in this phase the atoms and molecules exhibit weak interactions. This is why any gas will mix with the air, as will evaporated molecules of volatile liquids, such as alcohols and ethers.

Liquid solutions require favorable interactions between the solutes and the solvent. A polar solvent dissolves polar solutes. For example, water dissolves hydrochloric acid (HCl). Nonpolar solvents dissolve nonpolar solutes. The organic solvents benzene and hexane readily mix. Hydrogen bonding also serves to promote solvation, as seen with water and alcohol mixtures.

Solids in water exhibit varied behavior. Many mineral silicates and oxides are insoluble in water, providing material for continents on planet Earth. Otherwise everything would dissolve in the oceans. Ionic salts have varied solubility. Most nonpolar organic solids are not very soluble. Lard, an animal fat, is not soluble in water. Table salt, NaCl, is a soluble salt.

Expressing Solution Concentration

Concentration is the proportion of solute in a solution. A number of units are used to quantify concentration. Three common examples are:

- **Molarity (M):** Moles of solute/L of solution
- **Weight/volume percent [% (W/V)]:** g of solute/mL of solution × 100%
- **Weight/weight percent [% (W/W)]:** g of solute/g of solution × 100%

The amount of a solute is measured in terms of mass or moles of solute; the amount of a solution is measured in volume or mass of solution. The following are examples of these units:

- **1 M:** 1 mole of solute in 1 L of solution
- **1% (W/V):** 1 g of solute in 100 mL of solution
- **1% (W/W):** 1 g of solute in 100 g of solution

Very dilute solutions have concentration given in **parts per million (ppm)** of solute. A 1 ppm solution contains 1 mg of solute in 1 kg of solution. For water, 1 kg = 1 L. This is used as a convenience to avoid potential confusion by working with a solution unit of 0.00001 M or 0.0000005% (W/V).

Molecular & Electrolyte Solutes

All solutes do not behave in the same way; some remain as molecules, while others break into ions. An **electrolyte** dissolves in water to produce ions and conducts an electrical current. Common examples are acids, bases, and soluble salts. The electrolyte is strong if it fully dissociates (e.g., HCl, sodium hydroxide [NaOH], NaCl) and weak if it dissociates only partially. A weak electrolyte always has a significant amount of the molecular form present. Weak acids, such as acetic acid, and weak bases, such as NH_3, are examples of weak electrolytes.

The amount of oxygen that dissolves in the bloodstream and passes through lung tissue is proportional to the oxygen pressure in the air. To get more oxygen into the bloodstream, more oxygen must be inhaled. This is the basis for hyperbaric chambers and the use of oxygen therapy to assist patients with breathing problems.

Blood tests check for the amount of lipid in the sample. Some fats are essential to the body and dissolve in the blood. Undesirable fats tend to be less soluble and form solid deposits in the blood vessels. The term **LDL** (low-density lipoprotein) cholesterol describes the less-soluble fats; **HDL** (high-density lipoprotein) cholesterol, the healthier component, describes the more soluble ones.

Physiological saline is 0.9% (W/V) NaCl. All intravenous (IV) solutions use this as the starting material, and then you add glucose, morphine, or other medicines as needed.

Proper muscle and nervous system function depends on the sodium-to-potassium ratio in the body. This is why dehydration presents a health risk because the electrolytes cease to work properly.

To keep track of this behavior, we focus on the amount of dissolved ions, not the total amount of solute. The term *equivalent of an electrolyte* is used to denote the strength of the electrolyte by giving the number of grams corresponding to Avogadro's number of electrical charges.

Membrane Phenomena

A **membrane** is a layer of material that limits the flow of solvent or solute between two solutions. The cell membrane plays this role in living cells, controlling the flow of water and essential chemicals into and out of the cell.

Osmosis is the net flow of a solvent across a semipermeable membrane in response to a concentration gradient. Water can flow into or out of the cell depending on which side of the membrane has a higher concentration of solute.

A **hypertonic solution** outside the cell is more concentrated than the cellular fluids; as a result, water is forced from the cell through the membrane, potentially resulting in the shrinkage of red blood cells (**crenation**). Conversely, a **hypotonic solution** is more dilute than cellular fluids. Osmotic pressure draws water into the cell, which may force the cell to rupture (**cytolysis**). Under **isotonic conditions**, the concentration and osmotic pressure are balanced inside and outside of the cell.

Solutions

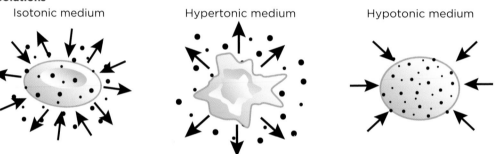

Isotonic medium   Hypertonic medium   Hypotonic medium

Working with Solutions

The two most common types of solution problems are dilutions and the determination of the total amount of solute. When performing solution calculations, pay attention to the units of mass, moles, and volume.

In some cases, you will need to interconvert moles and mass. This is calculated using the molar mass of the solute. The two conversions are:

- Moles to mass conversion: Mass = Moles × Molar Mass

- Mass to moles conversion: Moles = $\dfrac{\text{Mass}}{\text{Molar Mass}}$

The total amount of solute in a solution is determined by multiplying the concentration by the solution volume or mass, as illustrated in the following equations (always make sure that the units match):

Amount of Solute = Concentration × Volume

For molarity, M × Volume of Solution = Moles of Solute

For % (W/V) units, % (W/V) × Volume of Solution = Mass of Solute

Amount of Solute = Concentration × Mass of Solution

For % (W/W) units, % (W/W) × Mass of Solution = Mass of Solute

Solution dilutions require the addition of a solvent to produce a solution with a new lower concentration. The key is to figure out how much solvent to add to obtain the desired concentration. Dilution calculations are governed by the following equation:

$$C_1 \times V_1 = C_2 \times V_2$$

This calculation uses four variables, with any three used to calculate the fourth term:

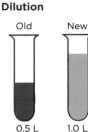

Dilution

C_1 = old concentration

C_2 = new concentration

V_1 = old volume or mass

V_2 = new volume or mass

Radioactivity

Radioactivity is the nuclear process by which atoms emit high-energy particles or rays from the nucleus. Nuclear reactions are much more energetic than chemical reactions or physical processes, since the nuclear makeup is changed. **Background radiation** is the radiation that emanates from radioactive elements, such as uranium and radium, found in the Earth's crust. **Natural radioactivity** denotes the spontaneous decay of a nucleus to produce high-energy particles or rays. **Artificial radioactivity** accompanies the forced conversion of a stable nucleus to an unstable nucleus in a nuclear reactor or particle collider.

Common Types of Radiation

An **alpha (α) particle** is composed of two protons and two neutrons, the same composition as the helium nucleus, and has a +2 charge. A **beta (β) particle** is an electron formed by the neutron-proton conversion in the nucleus of an unstable atom; β particles have a −1 charge. A **gamma (γ) ray** is a high-energy photon released as a nucleus undergoes change; because it is uncharged, it easily penetrates matter. A **positron (β⁺)** has the mass of an electron, but with a +1 charge. A **neutron (n)** is a neutral nuclear particle emitted from the nucleus. All forms of radiation are energetic enough to penetrate materials, including tissue, and therefore present a health risk. An α particle is slow moving and easily absorbed by air. A β particle is smaller and faster; it penetrates air but is absorbed by most solids. γ rays are the most penetrating and therefore dangerous, since they easily pass through most materials; they are stopped only by thick layers of dense metals like lead. Radioactive samples must be stored in lead containers to limit exposure to these harmful emissions.

Nuclear Reactions

Nuclear equations must be balanced with respect to charge and mass. However, you must track changes from one element to another in these reactions. The **nuclide symbol** is used to denote element and isotope mass (e.g., $^{198}_{79}$Au or Au-198). This allows you to keep track of essential isotopic data. The following are examples of nuclear reactions:

α decay: Ra-224 → Ra-222 + α

β decay: Th-234 → Pa-234 + β

γ + β decay: I-131 → Xe-131 + γ + β

Radioactive emissions are characterized by the decay **half-life**, which is the length of time for one-half of the sample to decay. Note, however, that the half-life is *not* the time required for the material to totally decay to a harmless material. Even after several half-lives, a small portion of the isotope is still emitting radiation. **Radiocarbon dating** is used to estimate an artifact's age by determining the isotopic ratios of C-14 and C-12 in an archeological sample.

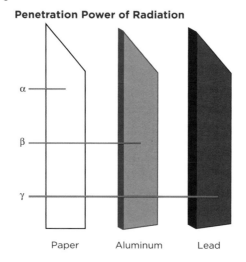

Penetration Power of Radiation

α

β

γ

Paper   Aluminum   Lead

Dealing with Radioactive Emissions

Ionizing radiation is a radioactive emission that causes ion formation when the emission is absorbed by another atom or molecule. This raises safety issues in any facility that uses radioactive isotopes. Nuclear technologies require shielding and regular monitoring of exposure to these emissions. The health effects from exposure to radioactive emissions are cumulative.

Measurements of Radiation Intensity

A number of units are used to describe radioactive exposure. The **curie** is the quantity of radioactive material that produces 3.7×10^{10} disintegrations per second. The term **rad** stands for radiation absorbed dose; 1 rad corresponds to 2.4×10^{-3} calories per kilogram of tissue. **RBE** (short for relative biologic effect of radiation) is used to describe how different materials interact with radiation.

The term **rem** stands for roentgen equivalent in man; the product of rad and RBE, rem describes the net radiation damage to the body. A more general unit, the **roentgen**, tracks the ionization caused by the radiation. One roentgen produces 2.1×10^9 ions in 1 cm^3 of air at 0°C and 1 atm. The lethal impact of radiation is quantified using the measure **LD_{50}**, which is the dose fatal for 50% of the exposed population within 30 days. So, like half-life, this measure of risk must be understood as a standard measure for laboratory work, not simply for safety.

Nuclear Medicine

Radiation is used for various diagnostics and therapeutic modalities:
- Diagnostic scans use radiation that passes through the body, providing a diagnostic picture of how the body absorbs the particles or X-rays.
- Cancer treatments use high-energy particles to destroy dysfunctional cells in the body.
- Tracer techniques use diagnostic radioisotopes (e.g., I-131 is used for the thyroid).
- Radiography is a routine tool for imaging the body's hard tissue; a radioactive isotope is often the X-ray source.
- A PET scan is positron emission tomography.
- A computerized tomography (CT) scan provides a three-dimensional picture of the body.

Radiation detectors allow the measurement of radiation exposure. Geiger counters detect ionizing radiation using a meter and speaker to warn of exposure. Film badges use photographic film sensitive to radioactive emissions; this is an important safety tool for anyone working with radioactive isotopes or associated technology.

Synthetic radioactive isotopes are prepared using cyclotrons, nuclear reactors, and other particle accelerators. Neutron bombardment is used to produce radioactive gold: $n + $ Au-197 $\rightarrow$ Au-198. Proton bombardment converts zinc to gallium: $p + $ Zn-66 $\rightarrow$ Ga-67. A nuclear reactor uses uranium fission to generate a beam of neutrons.

Acids & Bases

Acids and bases are some of the most common chemical reagents. We find them in the kitchen, the chemical industry, and pharmaceutical manufacturing, and they are key players in biological chemistry.

An **Arrhenius acid** is any material that produces the hydronium cation, H_3O^+, in water. An **Arrhenius base** yields the hydroxide anion, OH^-. A **Brønsted-Lowry acid** is a proton donor; a **Brønsted-Lowry base** is a proton acceptor. A **Lewis acid** is an electron-pair acceptor; a **Lewis base** is an electron-pair donor. The Lewis system gives a more general definition that applies to organic compounds and nonaqueous solutions.

Amphiprotic materials behave either as an acid or a base, depending on the reaction conditions. An important example in the body is the amino acids that react to form proteins. **Polyprotic** and **polybasic** chemicals have two or more reactive groups.

A strong acid or strong base exhibits full dissociation into ions, depleting the molecular form. A weak acid or weak base partially dissociates, establishing an equilibrium of molecular and ionic components. **Le Chatelier's principle** describes the shift in equilibrium that follows the addition of an acid, base, or other reagent to a solution.

A **buffer** is a material that resists changes in pH with the addition of an acid or base. The most common buffers are solutions that contain either a weak acid and its salt or a weak base and its salt. Buffer capacity measures the ability of a solution to resist large changes in pH.

> ➕ Blood is buffered at a pH of approx. 7.4 by carbonic acid and bicarbonate; **acidosis** is a harmfully low pH, whereas **alkalosis** is a harmfully high pH.

Conjugate Acid-Base Pairs

The **conjugate acid** of a base is formed by adding one proton to the base. The **conjugate base** of an acid is formed by the removal of one proton from the acid. These conjugate acid-base pairs allow one to understand acid-base equilibrium and buffers, as in the following examples:

> ➕ All IV fluids and topical eyedrops are buffered to prevent a shift in the pH of bodily fluids.

$$\text{Acid HCl} + H_2O \leftrightarrow H_3O^+ + \text{Conjugate Base Cl}^-$$

$$\text{Base NH}_3 + H_2O \leftrightarrow \text{Conjugate Acid NH}_4^+ + OH^-$$

Water in Acid-Base Chemistry

Acid-base chemistry is closely tied to the fact that water can dissociate into ions. Water self-ionizes in any solution or as a pure liquid to give OH^- and H_3O^+, forming a weak equilibrium as described in the following equation:

$$2H_2O \leftrightarrow H_3O^+ + OH^-$$

The equilibrium constant is defined as $K_w = [H_3O^+][OH^-] = 1.0 \times 10^{-14}$ at 25°C. H_3O^+ is formed from the protonation of the water molecule. Conversely, OH^- is formed from the deprotonation of a water molecule.

Acid-Base Reactions

In the neutralization reaction, an acid fully reacts with a base, yielding a salt solution:

$$Acid + Base \rightarrow Water + Salt$$

$$HCl + NaOH \rightarrow H_2O + NaCl$$

A **titration** is an experimental procedure for analyzing acid or base samples. The amount of acid needed to neutralize an unknown base is used to calculate the base's concentration. In a similar manner, the amount of base added to neutralize an acid sample is used to quantify the acid sample. These procedures use a burette to add the variable reagent and a chemical indicator or electronic pH meter to identify the neutralization point.

pH Scale

The pH scale is a numerical representation of acidity, where $pH = -\log[H^+]$, with the concentration in molarity. The scale ranges from 0 to 14. A **neutral solution** has a pH of 7. A **basic solution** has a pH greater than 7, with a strong base in the 12–14 range and a weak base in the 8–10 range. An **acidic solution** has a pH less than 7, with a strong acid in the 0–2 range and a weak acid in the 4–6 range. The pH scale provides a simple way to describe acidic *and* basic solutions without having to deal with molarity.

The pH Scale

Strong Acid	Weak Acid		Weak Base	Strong Base
		Neutral		
0 1 2	3 4 5	6 7 8	9 10 11	12 13 14
		H_2O		
HCl, HNO$_3$	H_2CO_3		NH$_3$	NaOH
H$_2$SO$_4$	HAc		Ca(OH)$_2$	KOH
		NaCl		
	NH$_4^+$ Salts		Ac$^-$ or CO$_3^{2-}$ Salts	

Examples of Bases

The mineral strong bases are formed from reactions of alkali metals and alkaline earth metals with water. Common examples are potassium hydroxide (KOH) and NaOH. This explains why the term **alkali** is used to denote these mineral bases and aqueous bases in general. Organic bases tend to be weak and often are derived from NH_3. Examples of weak bases include ammonium hydroxide (NH_4OH), amines, purines, and pyrimidines.

Examples of Acids

The mineral strong acids include HCl, nitric acid (HNO_3), sulfuric acid (H_2SO_4), and phosphoric acid (H_3PO_4). The oxyacids are formed from the reaction of oxides with water. Organic acids tend to be weak and are often derivatives of carbonic acid. (Fatty acids are one class of organic acid.) The most common weak organic acid is acetic acid, found in vinegar.

Natural rain is slightly acidic (pH = 5.2) because of the formation of carbonic acid ($H_2O + CO_2 \rightarrow$ carbonic acid). Soil and aquatic pH must be 5–8 for most animals and plants to survive. Acid rain denotes the presence of sulfuric and nitric acids formed from oxide pollutants in rainwater. Acid rain has a pH less than 5 and destroys life in lakes and harms plants.

Organic Chemistry

Organic chemistry is the chemistry of carbon compounds. Biochemistry is the subset of organic chemistry that deals with the chemicals specific to living organisms. The simplest organic compounds are the **hydrocarbons**, carbon chains bonded with hydrogen

➕ RNA and DNA are characterized by the sequence of nitrogenous bases along their polymer strands.

➕ The stomach contains hydrochloric acid, a strong acid that assists with digestion. If this acid were present elsewhere in the body, it would destroy proteins and cells.

➕ Many water-soluble vitamins are acids. DNA and RNA are nucleic acids. Fatty acids are the dietary fats essential to a balanced diet.

accounting for the rest of the bonded positions on each carbon atom (octet rule). There are an unlimited number of possible organic compounds, a testament to the varied chemistry exhibited by carbon. As we add more types of bonding and other elements, we construct the various classes of organic compounds.

Organic Names & Formulas

The molecular formula gives the atoms and the number of each type of atom; it does not provide information on molecular structure. The **structural formula** is a visual depiction that shows atoms and exhibits all bonds as lines. The **line formula** hides H atoms, with lines used to denote chains of bonded carbon atoms.

IUPAC nomenclature refers to naming standards established by the International Union of Pure and Applied Chemistry. When naming a compound, the **parent compound** is the longest carbon chain containing the functional group. A **functional group** (a.k.a. substituent) is an atom (or group of bonded atoms) that imparts specific properties to a molecule; the chemical name must denote the functional group and its position in the parent compound. Unfortunately, many compounds also have common names that have no connection with IUPAC names.

Carbon chains are named based on how many carbon atoms are in the chain. Each length has a characteristic prefix (*see* **Carbon-Chain Prefixes** table). The number of various substituents is also defined using prefixes, much as in naming salts and inorganic compounds. For example, carbon monoxide and carbon dioxide are distinct compounds, as denoted by the *mono-* and *di-* prefixes (*see* **Substituent Prefixes** figure).

Carbon-Chain Prefixes			
Number of Carbon Atoms	Prefix	Number of Carbon Atoms	Prefix
1	meth-	11	undec-
2	eth-	12	dodec-
3	prop-	13	tridec-
4	but-	14	tetradec-
5	pent-	15	pentadec-
6	hex-	16	hexadec-
7	hept-	17	heptadec-
8	oct-	18	octadec-
9	non-	19	nonadec-
10	dec-	20	eicos-

Substituent Prefixes

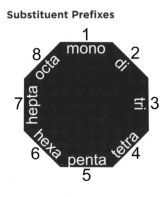

Hydrocarbons

Hydrocarbons are composed of only two elements: carbon and hydrogen. The two classes are called **aliphatic** and **aromatic**. Aromatic hydrocarbons are derivatives of benzene. Aliphatic hydrocarbons are alkanes, alkenes, and alkynes.

Isomers are chemical compounds with the same formula but different structural features. The terms **cis** and **trans** describe the different spatial arrangement of groups on opposite sides of a double bond in alkenes. Groups attached to a ring, as well as carbon rings with a flexible structure, are also described with these terms. **Geometric isomers** differ in the placement of substituents on a double bond or ring. In a cycloalkane or cycloalkene, the carbon backbone forms a ring structure. Many important biologic molecules adopt cyclic structures.

An **unsaturated hydrocarbon** contains at least one multiple (i.e., double or triple) bond. A **substituted hydrocarbon** has one or more hydrogen atoms replaced by another group. Each substitution position creates a unique compound, as does the number of substitutes.

An **alkane** is a saturated hydrocarbon that follows the general formula C_nH_{2n+2}. An **alkyl group** is formed by removing an H atom from an alkane. For example, a methyl group, $-CH_3$, is formed by removing one H atom from methane. **Alkyl halides** substitute halogen atoms for H atoms on an alkane. The term **saturated hydrocarbon** is often used to describe an alkane, as it is saturated with as many bonded H atoms as possible. Alkanes contain only carbon single bonds along the carbon chain. The covalent nature of the bonding in alkanes makes these materials nonpolar, and as a result most alkanes are not soluble in water. The boiling point of an alkane increases with the mass or length of the chain; larger molecules are heavier and interact more with other molecules, making it harder to evaporate the material. For example, methane is a gas at room temperature, whereas hexane is liquid.

Alkane (Propane)

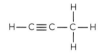

Alkane Nomenclature

The IUPAC naming scheme for an alkane uses the carbon fragment name and adds *-ane*. For example, for methane (CH_4), *meth-* denotes the fragment and *-ane* denotes it is an alkane.

Alkenes are hydrocarbons with one or more carbon-carbon double bonds. These are called unsaturated and have the general formula C_nH_{2n}. The same term comes into play with dietary fats. The most common alkene in practical use is ethylene and its derivatives, which are used to manufacture polyethylene and other commercial plastics.

Alkene (Cis-2-Butene)

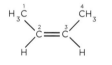

Alkene Nomenclature

The IUPAC naming scheme for an alkene uses the carbon fragment name and adds *-ene*. Examples include:
- $H_2C=CH_2$ (ethene)
- $H_2C=CH_2CH_2CH_2CH_2$ (1-hexene, based on the carbon number that locates the double bond + *hex-* + *-ene*)

Alkene (Trans-2-Butene)

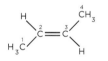

Alkynes are hydrocarbons with one or more carbon-carbon triple bonds; these are also unsaturated, with the general formula C_nH_{2n-2}. Triple bonds are the strongest carbon bonds and are not very common in cellular chemistry. The most common alkyne is acetylene, a gas used as a fuel for welders' torches.

Alkyne (Propyne)

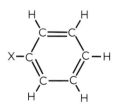

Alkyne Nomenclature

The IUPAC naming scheme for an alkyne uses the carbon fragment name and adds *-yne*. Examples include:
- $HC\equiv CH$ (ethyne, a.k.a. acetylene)
- $HC\equiv CCH_3$ (propyne)

Substituted Aromatic

Benzene (and substituted benzene compounds) is **aromatic**: the molecule is stabilized because of the delocalization of electrons in the carbon ring. Benzene has all H atoms on the ring. Replacing the H with other groups yields a series of compounds, such as toluene ($-CH_3$), phenol ($-OH$), aniline ($-NH_2$), benzoic acid ($-COOH$), chlorobenzene ($-Cl$), nitrobenzene ($-NO_2$), and anisole ($-OCH_3$). Heterocyclic aromatic compounds have one or more noncarbon atoms in the aromatic ring.

Hydrocarbon reactions allow you to add functional groups and convert alkanes to alkenes to alkynes, as well as reverse these processes. The following are common examples of hydrocarbon reactions:

- **Addition:** The addition of a molecule to an alkene double bond or an alkyne triple bond

- **Halogenation:** The replacement of a carbon-hydrogen bond of a hydrocarbon with a carbon-halogen bond:

Chlorine [g] + Alkane → Chloroalkane

- **Hydration:** The addition of water (as H and OH) to a molecule:

Water + Alkene → Alcohol

- **Dehydration:** The loss of water (as H and OH) from a molecule:

Alcohol → Water + Alkene

- **Hydrogenation:** The addition of hydrogen (H_2) to a double or a triple bond:

H_2 + Alkene → Alkane (e.g., $H_2 + C_2H_4 \rightarrow C_2H_6$)

H_2 + Alkyne → Alkene (e.g., $H_2 + C_2H_2 \rightarrow C_2H_4$)

- **Hydrohalogenation:** The addition of a hydrohalogen, such as HCl, to an unsaturated bond as H and Cl

Markovnikov's rule predicts products for unsymmetrical alkenes; the addition of hydrogen atoms to the carbon leads to more bonded hydrogen atoms.

Alcohols, Ethers & Thiols

Alcohols

Alcohols are organic compounds that contain **hydroxyl** (–OH) groups attached to an alkyl group. The hydroxyl group imparts polar character to an alcohol and makes it water soluble. Alcohols and their cousins, the sugars—molecules that contain several hydroxyl groups—play key roles in biochemistry because of their solubility in water. Without the hydroxyl group, these materials would not dissolve in cellular fluids.

Phenol (ArOH) is an aromatic alcohol. In some reactions, the hydrogen of the hydroxyl group dissociates, making phenol a weak organic acid. A **diol** is a di-alcohol, that is, with two –OH groups. **Glycerol** is a tri-alcohol, a three-carbon molecule with an –OH group on each carbon atom; glycerol is a key part of the triglyceride fat molecule. Sugar is a carbohydrate with multiple –OH groups.

Alcohols form three categories, or degrees, depending on the nature of the carbon bonded to the hydroxyl group: primary, secondary, or tertiary. A primary carbon is bonded to another carbon and three hydrogen atoms. A secondary carbon is bonded to two carbon atoms and two hydrogen atoms. A tertiary carbon is bonded to three carbon atoms and one hydrogen atom. The classes of alcohols form by replacing one of the hydrogen atoms with an –OH group. Methanol has a single carbon bonded to three hydrogen atoms with the –OH group replacing the carbon atom.

Glycerol

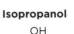

Isopropanol

T-butanol

Alcohol Degrees	
Degree	**Examples**
Primary (1°) alcohol RCH_2OH	$CH_3–CH_2–OH$ (ethanol); $CH_3–OH$ (methanol)
Secondary (2°) alcohol $R_2CH–OH$	Isopropanol $(CH_3)_2CH–OH$
Tertiary (3°) alcohol $R_3C–OH$	T-butanol $(CH_3)_3C–OH$

Alcohols & Hydrogen Bonding

The polar –OH group on an alcohol molecule interacts favorably with water and promotes dissolution. In contrast, the nonpolar R group, an alkyl fragment, inhibits dissolution in water. In terms of overall solubility, an alcohol with a large R group is less soluble. The addition of –OH groups enhances solubility; therefore, glycerol and sugar, which have multiple –OH groups, are very soluble in water. In terms of physical properties, alcohols remain solid or liquid at higher temperatures than comparable alkanes and ethers. This is another example of hydrogen bonding's stabilizing a phase.

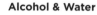

Alcohol & Water

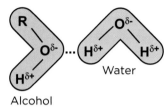

Alcohol
Water

⊕ ! Common Alcohols

- **Methanol** (methyl alcohol, wood alcohol) is a common solvent. It is extremely toxic if ingested and extremely flammable.
- **Ethanol** (ethyl alcohol, grain alcohol) is a solvent and disinfectant. It is produced by fermentation of sugars by yeast.
- **2-propanol** (isopropyl alcohol, rubbing alcohol) is commonly used as a disinfectant and solvent.
- **1,2-ethanediol** (ethylene glycol) is a component in antifreeze.
- **1,2,3-propanetriol** (glycerol) is a component of triglycerides, dietary fats in the body.

Alcohols undergo a number of chemical reactions, which center on the –OH group and the attached carbon atom:

- The **oxidation** of an alcohol corresponds to the gain of oxygen or loss of hydrogen; in practice, an alcohol is oxidized to an aldehyde or ketone; third-degree alcohols are nonreactive. Further oxidation of the aldehyde can produce a carboxylic acid. Fermentation of natural sugars produces ethanol. With aging, the ethanol is converted to vinegar.
- The **reduction** of a carbonyl compound (aldehyde or ketone) produces an alcohol, corresponding to the loss of oxygen or gain of hydrogen.
- **Dehydration** is the removal of water. As a physical process, this refers to simply removing liquid water. However, it also refers to a chemical reaction that results in the removal of a water molecule, usually a hydrogen atom and –OH group from adjacent atoms. Dehydration converts an alcohol to an alkene. As the reaction occurs, two possible alkenes may be obtained as products, and the nature of the alkene product is governed by **Zaitsev's rule**, which states that the favored product has fewer hydrogen atoms on the C=C group. Therefore, the alkene with more R groups is the dominant product.

⊕ In biological chemistry, oxidation is the gain of O and the loss of H, whereas reduction is the loss of O and the gain of H. **Redox** reactions are important in the metabolic pathways that harvest energy from the oxidation of dietary fuels; enzymes, called *oxidoreductases*, catalyze these reactions. Coenzymes serve as H acceptors and donors. Note that if one material is oxidized, something else must be reduced to account for the electronic changes.

Ethers

Ethers are formed by two alkyl or aryl groups attached to an oxygen atom. The formula will be ROR, ArOR, or ArOAr. Ethers are structurally related to alcohols; however, they are less polar than alcohols and less water soluble and have lower boiling points. This is because of the presence of a second organic R group attached to the oxygen atom.

! Ethers are chemically inert but *very* flammable, presenting safety risks. Even worse, they can form explosive peroxide compounds if stored at room temperature.

Ether Nomenclature
Ethers are named by denoting the two R groups, followed by *ether*. Diethyl ether has two ethyl groups bridged by an O atom (i.e., $CH_3CH_2OCH_2CH_3$).

⊕ Diethyl ether is the first general anesthetic that works by interfering with nerve impulses, creating analgesia, a state of lessened pain perception. Current anesthetics are the safer, less-flammable halogenated ethers.

Ethers are synthesized by the reaction of two alcohols:

$$ROH + R'OH \rightarrow ROR' + H_2O$$

Select the alcohols that have functional groups that exhibit the properties desired in the ether.

Thiols

If we substitute a sulfur atom for the oxygen atom in an alcohol, we produce a **thiol**. The thiol group is –SH; thiols are similar to alcohols in structure and reactivity.

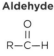
The amino acid cysteine has a thiol group; proteins containing cysteine may form disulfide bonds.

Aldehydes & Ketones

Aldehydes and ketones share a common feature: the **carbonyl** functional group. For an **aldehyde**, the carbonyl group is bonded to a hydrogen atom *and* to a hydrogen or alkyl or aryl group. With a **ketone**, the carbonyl group is bonded to two alkyl or aryl groups. The key chemical feature of the carbonyl group is the electron-rich carbon-oxygen double bond (>C=O). The most common ketone is acetone.

Because these compounds contain the polar carbonyl group, aldehydes and ketones hydrogen bond with water; the positive end of the water molecule interacts with the oxygen lone pairs, and the negative end of the water molecule interacts with the positive charge on the carbon of the carbonyl group. The carbonyl group is polar, but the organic R groups weaken dipole interactions. Aldehydes and ketones with larger R groups are not very soluble in water. Water solubility decreases as the sizes of the R groups increase. Acetone, the ketone formed with two methyl groups, is very soluble in water.

Aldehyde

$$\underset{\underset{R-C-H}{\overset{\overset{O}{\|}}{}}}{}$$

Ketone

$$\underset{\underset{R-C-R'}{\overset{\overset{O}{\|}}{}}}{}$$

Aldehyde Nomenclature

An aldehyde is named with the alkyl group, adding the suffix *-al*. Examples include:
- HCOH (methanal, a.k.a. formaldehyde)
- $HCOCH_3$ (ethanal, a.k.a. acetaldehyde)

Ketone Nomenclature

Ketones are named with the alkyl group that describes the carbon chain plus a number denoting the position of the C=O and the suffix *-one*. Examples include CH_3COCH_3 (propanone, a.k.a. acetone). A non-IUPAC naming scheme names a ketone by denoting the two alkyl groups + *ketone*. Using this system, acetone is called *dimethyl ketone*.

Reactions of aldehydes and ketones primarily involve changes in the carbonyl group to increase oxygen or increase hydrogen composition: oxidation or reduction.

- **Hydrogenation** is an example of reduction; hydrogen is added to the double bond of the carbonyl group.
- Alcohols can be **oxidized** to aldehydes or ketones, and aldehydes can be oxidized to carboxylic acids (in each case, the product molecule has relatively more oxygen and less hydrogen than the reactant molecule):

Oxidize 1° Alcohol → Aldehyde

Oxidize 2° Alcohol → Ketone

Oxidize Aldehyde → Carboxylic acid

Ketones and aldehydes can undergo reduction, producing an alcohol:

H_2 + Ketone or Aldehyde → Alcohol

Carboxylic Acids & Their Derivatives

The key chemical feature of carboxylic acids is the acidic **carboxyl** group, –COOH. The hydrogen atom can dissociate, forming weak acid solutions. Carboxylic acids have the general formula RCOOH. **Fatty acids**, important in biochemistry, have long-chain alkene or alkane groups attached to the carboxyl group (e.g., stearic acid).

Carboxylic Acid

$$\underset{\underset{R-C-OH}{\overset{\overset{O}{\|}}{}}}{}$$

Hydrogen bonding influences the physical properties and solubility of carboxylic acids in water. The acid part, the carboxyl group, is polar and can ionize. The organic part is the nonpolar R group. The carboxyl group interacts favorably with water, while the organic chain tends to diminish solubility. The dissociation of a carboxylic acid looks like a typical weak acid:

$$RCOOH \rightarrow RCOO^- + H^+$$

Acid dissociation enhances the solubility of the acid in water, since the ions are stabilized by interactions with water. Carboxylic acids with small organic groups (e.g., acetic acid) tend to be water soluble. Compounds with large R groups (e.g., longer chains from fatty acids) tend to be less soluble. Carboxylic acids tend to have elevated boiling points and freezing points compared with alkanes, aldehydes, ketones, and alcohols. The polar carboxyl group interacts with other like molecules, just as it does with water, through hydrogen bonding.

Chemical Derivatives of Carboxylic Acid

An **ester** is formed by the reaction of a carboxylic acid and an alcohol (catalyzed by an acid or a base). The general formula for an ester is RCOOR′. The R group comes from the acid, and the R′ group comes from the component alcohol. A **phosphoester** is the product of the reaction between phosphoric acid and an alcohol. A **thioester** (RCOSR) looks like an ester, but a sulfur atom replaces the oxygen atom in the compound. Thioesters are produced by the reaction of thiols and carboxylic acids: R′SH + RCOOH.

 Cellular enzymes catalyze thioester formation. **Coenzyme A** is a thiol that participates in cellular metabolic reactions; it is an acyl group activator, whose action results in the formation of a thioester, **acetyl-coenzyme A** (acetyl-CoA), which is part of the citric acid cycle. Coenzyme A helps to oxidize fatty acids to produce adenosine 5′-triphosphate (ATP).

Carboxylic Acid Nomenclature

Using IUPAC conventions, carboxylic acid names are formed with the name of the parent compound + *-oic* + *acid*. Examples include:
- CH_3COOH (ethanoic acid, a.k.a. acetic acid)
- $HCOOH$ (methanoic acid, a.k.a. formic acid)
- C_6H_6COOH (benzoic acid)
- $CH_3(CH_2)_{16}COOH$ (octadecanoic acid, a.k.a. stearic acid)

Ester Nomenclature

Using IUPAC conventions, ester names are formed with the name of the ester R′ group plus the name of the acidic part + *-oate*. The R′ group comes from the alcohol that was used to make the ester.
- $CH_3CO_2CH_2CH_3$ (ethyl ethanoate, a.k.a. ethyl acetate)
- $C_6H_5CO_2CH_2CH_3$ (ethyl benzoate)

Stearic Acid

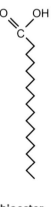

Thioester

$$\underset{R'-S-C-R}{\overset{O}{\underset{\|}{}}}$$

Ester
$$\underset{R-C-OR'}{\overset{O}{\underset{\|}{}}}$$

Reactions of carboxylic acids take advantage of the acidic carboxylic group. These are weak organic acids that react with bases. Esters dissociate to produce carboxylic acids. Phosphoesters are produced by the reaction of acidic phosphate with alcohols. Reactions include:

- **Dissociation** in water of carboxylic acid:

$$RCOOH + H_2O \rightarrow RCOO^- + H_3O^+$$

- **Acid-base neutralization reactions:**

$$RCOOH + NaOH \rightarrow H_2O + RCOO^- Na^+$$

- **Hydrolysis** of esters, often acid or base catalyzed:

$$Ester + H_2O \rightarrow Alcohol + RCOOH$$

Phosphoesters, which have the general formula $ROPO(OH)_2$, are formed by the reaction of phosphoric acid and an alcohol or sugar (i.e., any group with a reactive –OH). The acidic phosphate group can react with two groups, forming a polymer chain. Phosphoesters of monosaccharides include ATP, adenosine diphosphate (ADP), and adenosine monophosphate (AMP), the cell's energy storage compounds.

> ### Saponification & Soap
> **Saponification** is soap synthesis (i.e., base-catalyzed ester hydrolysis), and a **soap** is an alkali metal fatty acid salt. The polar COO hydrogen bonds with water, and the nonpolar R group mixes with oily dirt. Soap works by forming an emulsion of soap, grease, and water.

➕ ATP is the cell's energy currency. It consists of adenine bonded to a phosphoester of the sugar ribose. ATP is a source of energy for the cell, using the exothermic hydrolysis of the phosphate group.

➕ Phosphoesters in the cell include ATP and related compounds.

Nitrogen-Based Organic Molecules: Amines & Amides

A number of important biologic chemicals have nitrogen as a key chemical component. The **amines** are organic derivatives of NH_3 in which one or more hydrogen atoms are replaced by organic groups. Amines are weak organic bases because the lone pair on the nitrogen atom can be protonated, resulting in the formation of the hydroxide anion. One particularly important kind of amine is the amino acid, which combines amine with carboxylic acid functionality. An amine has the general formula RNH_2 (a first-degree amine), R_2NH (a second-degree amine), or R_3N (a third-degree amine), depending on how much substitution occurs on NH_3 molecules. The R groups on amines can be alkyl or aryl groups or hydrogen atoms.

Phosphoric Acid

```
        OH
        |
  O = P — OH
        |
        OH
```

Phosphoester

```
        O
        ||
  R—O—P—OH
        |
        OH
```

> ### Amine Nomenclature
> For IUPAC names, name the R groups of the amine and specify how they are attached to the nitrogen atom, followed by -*amine*. Examples include:
> • $N(CH_3)_3$ (N-N-dimethylmethaneamine, a.k.a. trimethylamine)
> • $H_2N–C_6H_5$ (benzeneamine, a.k.a. aniline)
> Note that common names simply list the R groups followed by *amine*, unless a compound is commonly known by another name.

Amines can also form **quaternary ammonium salts (QASs)** by reactions with acids. These amine salts have the general formula $R_4N^+A^-$. A^- is the anion from the acid used in the neutralization. The quaternary ammonium salt is analogous to the ammonium cation formed in water: water dissociates, losing a proton to form a hydroxide anion; the NH_3 gains a proton to form an ammonium cation:

$$NH_3 + H_2O \leftrightarrow NH_4^+ + OH^-$$

Other reactions of amines include:
• **Dissociation** into a QAS and an anion:

$$CH_3NH_2 + H_2O \leftrightarrow CH_3NH_3^+ + OH^-$$

• **Neutralization** with acid:

$$NH_3 + HCl \leftrightarrow NH_4^+ + Cl^-$$

$$CH_3CH_2NH_2 + HCl \leftrightarrow CH_3CH_2NH_3^+ + Cl^-$$

➕ QASs are commonly used as antiseptics and detergents, as the nitrogen end of the molecule is polar, whereas the R group is nonpolar. Because they have a weak acid feature, they have a mild antiseptic action, such as that in mouthwashes.

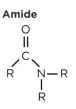

Amide

O
‖
C
R   N—R
    |
    R

Amino Acid

COOH
|
H₂N—C—H
|
R

Zwitterion

COO⁻
|
H₃N⁺—C—H
|
R

➕ Proteins are amino acid polymers.

➕ Carbohydrates have a key dietary role: they are oxidized in the cell for energy. One component in blood analysis is the amount of glucose in the sample, which reflects the health of the body's glucose consumption.

Amides, the other important nitrogen-containing compounds, are formed by the reaction of carboxylic acid and an amine. This produces the amide bond, formed when the carbonyl carbon of a carboxylic acid molecule bonds to the amino nitrogen of an amine molecule.

Amino acids are compounds with an amine group and a carboxylic acid group. This allows an amino acid to react as an acid or a base depending on which end of the molecule is involved. Amino acids are the monomers that form protein polymers in living cells. Peptide bonds are the amide bonds between two amino acids in a peptide chain. The distinct features of an amino acid depend on the organic R group; because of this, amino acids are not named using the IUPAC system. For example, if the R group is a hydrogen atom, then the amino acid is called *glycine*. The presence of a methyl group produces alanine. Amino acids can also ionize through proton exchange to form **zwitterions**, which are neutrally charged molecules that contain positive and negative charges at different locations in the molecule that are unlike dipole charges.

> ### Amide Nomenclature
> Both common and IUPAC names are derived from the names of corresponding carboxylic acids. Remove the *-ic* acid ending of the common name or the *-oic* acid ending of the IUPAC name of the carboxylic acid, and replace it with *-amide*. For example, CH_3CONH_2 is called *ethanamide* (from ethanoic acid) but is commonly called *acetamide* (from acetic acid).

Biochemistry

Carbohydrates

Carbohydrates are truly "hydrates," as water is reflected in the chemical formula, appearing as hydrogen atoms and –OH groups on the carbon backbone. Carbohydrates are often called *sugars*. In the body, dietary carbohydrates are broken down into simple sugars and metabolized to release energy; they also provide chemical building blocks for making other biochemicals the body needs. A **monosaccharide** is a single unit of carbohydrate. Sugars are very soluble in water, as the numerous polar –OH groups bond with the hydrogen in water. Sugars can adopt a cyclic form or a linear form. Examples of sugars include glucose, fructose, lactose, ribose, and deoxyribose. **Polysaccharides** are polymers of monosaccharides. Important examples include cellulose, starch (amylose), and glycogen. Reactions include:

- Polymer synthesis:

$$\text{Monosaccharide} \rightarrow \text{Disaccharide or Polymers}$$

- **Dehydration** (the removal of water), as well as its reverse, hydrolysis:

$$\text{Sugar} + \text{Sugar} \leftrightarrow \text{Disaccharide (e.g., sucrose)} + H_2O$$

Carbohydrates also react with phosphoric acid groups to form phosphoesters.

Glucose

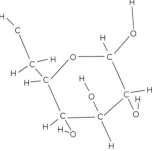

Amylose

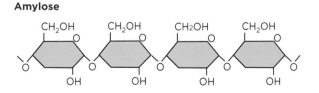

Peptides, Proteins & Enzymes

Amino acids are the building blocks of peptides and proteins. The **peptide bond** is the amide bond (C–N) between two amino acids. Peptides vary from a few units long to many thousands. A **dipeptide** is formed by the reaction of two amino acids: the –NH$_2$ group of one amino acid reacts with the –COOH group of another amino acid. The peptide bond connects the nitrogen atom and the –CO group.

Dipeptide

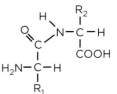

Proteins are polymers of amino acids and are also called polypeptides. Proteins select from 20 different amino acids, giving infinite variety to protein structures. The protein is defined by the **primary structure**, the amino acid sequence, as well as more subtle **secondary and tertiary structures** of the polymer. Proteins have some of the most complex structures and specific chemical reactivity of any known molecules.

Protein

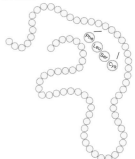

In the cell, many proteins function as **enzymes** for biochemical reactions. Most cellular reactions require a specific enzyme and are fine-tuned for body temperature. The name of the enzyme is based on the reaction or substrate, with the ending -*ase*. For example, the enzyme for digesting lactose is called *lactase*. The enzyme for lipid hydrolysis is called *lipase*.

Nucleic Acids

Nucleic acids are the materials in the cell that direct reproduction and protein synthesis. A **nucleic acid** is a polymer of units called *nucleotides*. **Nucleotides** consist of a base, a sugar, and an acid phosphate. The sugars are either deoxyribose (in DNA, or **deoxyribonucleic acid**) or ribose (in RNA, or **ribonucleic acid**). The bases can be grouped into pyrimidines (cytosine, uracil, and thymine) and purines (adenine and guanine).

Ribose

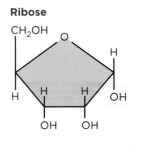

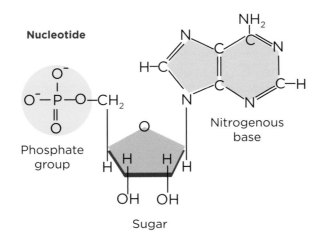

DNA Characteristics

- A double helix polymer forms as base pairs line up to form the "rungs" of the ladder.
- **Chargaff's rule** states that adenine goes with thymine and cytosine goes with guanine.
- The sequence of base pairs in DNA is used by RNA to code for proteins.
- DNA is located in the nucleus and is the genetic code for the cell and organism. Replication of DNA allows cells to reproduce.

RNA Characteristics

- RNA is a single-stranded polymer.
- RNA carries out protein synthesis; several types of RNA coordinate this process.
- RNA is defined by the sequence of bases along the strand.

DNA Replication

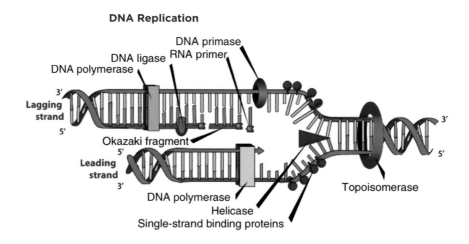

Lipids & Membranes

Lipids, also called **fats**, are the hydrophobic compounds in the cell, which have limited water solubility. These materials play key roles in metabolism, as well as the formation of cell membranes and many important hormones. Examples of lipids include **fatty acids**, which are weak organic acids with the general structure RCOOH, where the R group is a long carbon chain. The nature of the acid depends on the R group. For a **saturated fat**, the R group is an alkyl group. **Unsaturated fats** contain an R group with an alkene character, having at least one C=C linkage. A **polyunsaturated fat** has two or more C=C linkages.

Fatty acids in the body are stored as **triglycerides**, formed from three fatty acids and a glycerol molecule. **Phospholipids** are formed from an acid-phosphate group and a lipid, such as triglyceride fatty acid, and are key materials for cell membranes. Other important lipids are the **steroids**, cholesterol, fat-soluble vitamins, and hormones. These complex molecules often have very complex chemical structures; steroids, for example, have a fused cyclic molecular structure. Lanosterol exhibits the type of structure characteristic of this class of lipids.

Example of Triglyceride

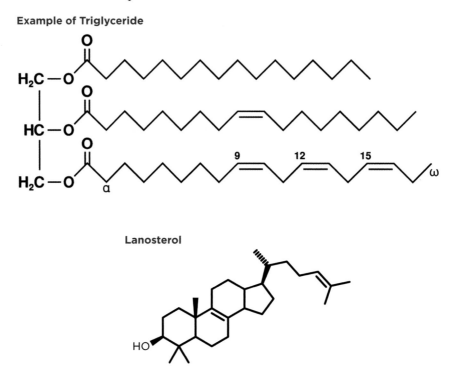

Lanosterol

MEDICAL MATH

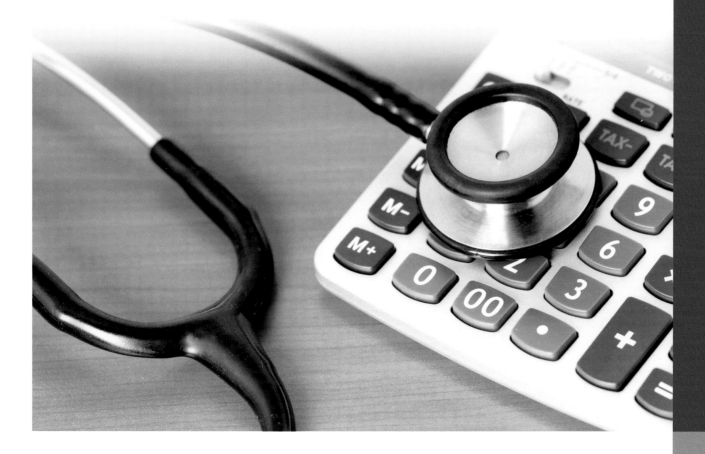

Introduction

Before you begin to study nursing pharmacology, you need to have a good understanding of medical math. This chapter provides an overview of the metric and apothecary systems, including abbreviations, conversion formulas, and equivalent measures. It also includes reimbursement calculations, coding measurements, and health care operating indices.

Basics

Metric Prefixes

Equivalents

mega-	1,000,000
kilo-	1000
hecto-	100
deka-/deca-	10
deci- (one-tenth)	1/10 (0.1)
centi- (one-hundredth)	1/100 (0.01)
milli- (one-thousandth)	1/1000 (0.001)
micro- (one-millionth)	1/1,000,000 (0.000001)

Abbreviations

M	mega-
k	kilo-
h	hecto-
da	deka-/deca-
d	deci-
c	centi-
m	milli-
mc	micro-

Length

Equivalents

1 mm	0.1 cm
1 mm	0.039 in
1 cm	10 mm
1 cm	0.39 in
10 mm	1 cm
10 mm	0.39 in
2.54 cm	1 in
2.5 cm	25.4 mm
1 ft	12 in
1 yard	3 ft
1 m	1000 mm
1 m	100 cm
1 m	1.09 yards
1 m	3.28 ft
1 dm	3.94 in
1 dam	32.81 ft
1 km	0.62 mile
1 km	3280.08 ft

Abbreviations

mm	millimeter
cm	centimeter
dm	decimeter
dam	dekameter
m	meter
in	inch
ft	foot/feet

Conversion Formulas

cm = in × 2.54
in = cm × 0.394

Examples

cm	in
51	20
56	22
61	24
66	26
71	28
76	30
81	32
86	34
91	36
97	38
102	40
107	42
117	46
122	48
127	50
132	52
137	54
142	56
147	58

Area

Equivalents

1 square centimeter (cm^2) = 100 square millimeters (mm^2)

1 cubic decimeter = 1000 cubic centimeters (cm^3)

1 cubic meter (m^3) = 1000 cubic decimeters

Abbreviations

cc	cubic centimeter

Weight

Equivalents

1 gr	64.79 mg
20 gr	1 scruple
60 gr	2.19 dr
16 dr	1 oz
1 g	15.432 gr
1 g	1000 mg
1 g	0.035 oz
1 g	1 mL
10 g	1 dekagram
1 dekagram	0.35 oz
100 g	1 hectogram
1 hectogram	3.53 oz
1 mg	1000 mcg
1 mg	0.001 g
1 centigram	0.15 gr
1 centigram	0.01 g
1 decigram	0.1 g
1 decigram	1.54 gr
1 kg	1 L of water
1 kg	2.2 lb
1 kg	1000 g
1 oz	28.35 g; 16 dr
1 Tbsp	4 dr
1 Tbsp	3 tsp
1 lb	16 oz
1 lb	0.45 kg

Abbreviations

dr	dram
g	gram
gr	grain
kg	kilogram
L	liter
lb	pound
mcg	microgram
mg	milligram
mL	milliliter
oz	ounce
Tbsp	tablespoon
tsp	teaspoon

Conversion Formulas

$kg = lb \times 0.454$
$lb = kg \times 2.205$

Examples

Pounds (lb)	Kilograms (kg)
10	4.5
25	11.4
50	22.7
75	34.1
95	43.1
100	45.4
125	56.8
150	68.1
175	79.5
200	90.8

Fluids

Equivalents

15 gtt	1 mL
1 mL	0.001 L
1000 mL	1 L
1 cL	0.01 L
1 dL	0.1 L
1 dL	100 mL
1 daL	10 L
1 hL	100 L
1 kL	1000 L
1 cup	8 oz
1 cup	236.5 mL
1 pt	16 oz
1 pt	473 mL
1 pt	2 cups
1 pt	16 fl oz
1 qt	32 oz
1 qt	2 pt
1 qt	0.946 L
1 qt	4 cups
4 qt	1 gal
4 qt	16 cups
1 gal	3785 mL
1 gal	3.785 L
1 gal	4 qt
1 glass	8 oz
1 teacup	6 oz
1 gtt	1 minim
1 gtt	0.06 mL
1 fl dr	3.96 mL
1 fl dr	60 minims
1 fl oz	8 fl dr
1 fl oz	6 tsp
1 fl oz	2 Tbsp
1 fl oz	29.57 mL
1 dr	$27\frac{11}{32}$ gr
1 oz	16 dr
1 oz	2 Tbsp
1 oz	6 tsp
1 tsp	60 gtt
1 tsp	$1\frac{1}{3}$ fl dr
1 tsp	5 mL
1 Tbsp	3 tsp
1 Tbsp	4 fl dr
1 Tbsp	½ oz
1 Tbsp	15 mL
1 mL	0.27 fl dr
1 mL	16.23 minims

Abbreviations

cL	centiliter
daL	dekaliter
dL	deciliter
fl dr	fluid dram
fl oz	fluid ounce
gal	gallon
gtt	drop
hL	hectoliter
kL	kiloliter
pt	pint
qt	quart
Tbsp	tablespoon
tsp	teaspoon

Temperature

Equivalents

0°C	32°F (freezing water)
35°C	95°F
37°C	98.6°F
100°C	212°F (boiling water)

Abbreviations

°C	degrees Celsius (centigrade)
°F	degrees Fahrenheit

Conversion Formulas

Celsius to Fahrenheit:

$$([°C] \times 1.8) + 32 = [°F]$$

Fahrenheit to Celsius:

$$([°F] - 32) \div 1.8 = [°C]$$

Examples

°F	°C
97.0	36.1
98.0	36.7
98.6	37.0
99.0	37.2
100.0	37.8
103.0	39.4
104.0	40.0
105.0	40.6
106.0	41.1
107.0	41.7

Hot & Cold Application Temperatures		
Description	**°F**	**°C**
Very hot	105–115	41–46
Hot	98–105	37–41
Warm	93–98	34–37
Tepid	80–93	26–34
Cool	65–80	18–26
Cold	50–65	10–18

Measurement Systems

Household System

The household system is based on measuring devices found in the home; it is commonly used for cooking. The household system is considered the least accurate of the systems because the size of the devices may vary greatly. Popular unit measurements include drops, teaspoons, tablespoons, ounces, cups, pints, quarts, and gallons.

Household Measurements & Liquid Volume Equivalents

60 drops	1 tsp
3 tsp	1 Tbsp
2 Tbsp	1 oz
8 oz	1 cup
2 cups	1 pt
2 pt	1 qt
4 qt	1 gal

Apothecary System

The apothecary system is an old system of pharmaceutical measure that is becoming less common because its measures are approximate.

- Basic unit of weight: grain (gr)
- Basic units of volume: minim (m); dram (dr); ounce (oz)
- Uses lowercase roman numerals, with the unit abbreviation before the number (e.g., 7 drams = dr vii)

Equivalents

16.23 minims	1 mL
1 fl dr	3.697 mL
1 fl oz	29.57 mL
1 pt	500 mL
1 qt	1.05 L
1 qt	1000 mL
1 gr	64.79 mg
15.432 gr	1 g
1 drap	3.888 g
60 gr	1 drap
480 gr	1 ozap
31 g	1 ozap
12 ozap	1 lbap

Abbreviations

b.i.d., BID	twice a day
drap	dram apothecary
h.s., HS	at bedtime (or hour of sleep)
lbap	pound apothecary
o.d.	once a day
ozap	ounce apothecary
p.c.	after meals
po	by mouth
q	every
q.a.m.	every morning
q.d.	every day
q.h.	every hour
q.2.h.	every 2 hours
q.h.s.	every night
q.i.d.	4 times a day
q.o.d.	every other day
ss	one-half
tab	tablet
Tbsp	tablespoon
t.i.d.	3 times a day
tsp	teaspoon

Metric System

The metric system is the most common measurement system in the world and in medicine because it is based on the decimal system and is easy to use.

- Basic unit of length: meter (m)
- Basic unit of weight: gram (g)
- Basic unit of volume: liter (L)

Common Equivalents

1 kg	2.2 lb	—
30 mL	1 oz	—
240 mL	8 oz	1 cup
5 mL	1 tsp	—
15 mL	3 tsp	1 Tbsp

Conversion between Systems

Metric	Apothecary	Household
64.79 mg	1 gr	—
1 g	15 gr	—
1 kg	—	2.2 lb
0.45 kg	—	1 lb
5 mL	—	1 tsp
15 mL	1/2 oz	1 Tbsp
29.57 mL	—	1 fl oz
30 mL	1 oz	2 Tbsp
473.176 mL	—	1 pt
946.35 mL	—	1 qt
1000 mL	—	33.8 oz
1 cm	—	0.4 in
2.5 cm	—	1 in

Laboratory Measures

Abbreviations

cm	centimeter		mL	milliliter
cm³	cubic centimeter		mm	millimeter
dL	deciliter		mm Hg	millimeters of mercury
fl oz	fluid ounce		oz	ounce
g	gram		pt	pint
L	liter		QNS	quantity not sufficient
lb	pound		qt	quart
m	meter		U	unit
mg	milligram		wt	weight

Roman Numerals

I (i)	1	VIII (viii)	8
II (ii)	2	IX (ix)	9
III (iii)	3	X (x)	10
IV (iv)	4	L (l)	50
V (v)	5	C (c)	100
VI (vi)	6	D (d)	500
VII (vii)	7	M (m)	1000

Reimbursement Calculators

Resource-Based Relative Value Scale (RBRVS)
(Physician Work + Practice Expense + Malpractice Insurance Costs) × Conversion Factor = Payment × Geographic Adjustment Factor

Medicare Physician Fee Schedule
- **Participating (PAR) physician reimbursement**
  - (Allowed Amount × 80%) − (Patient 20% Co-pay) = Total Reimbursement
- **Non-PAR physician reimbursement**
  - [(Allowed Amount × 80%) × 95%] − (Patient 20% Co-pay) = Total Reimbursement from Medicare
- **Non-PAR limiting charge**
  - Allowed Amount × 115% = Limiting Charge
- **Ambulance fee schedule (Medicare)**
  - (Reasonable Fee × Allowed Percentage) + (Schedule Rate × Phase-in Percentage) = Medicare Payment Amount
  - Seven categories of ambulance services (land and water):
    – Basic life support
    – Basic life support, emergency
    – Advanced life support, level 1
    – Advanced life support, level 1 emergency
    – Advanced life support, level 2
    – Specialty care transport
    – Paramedic intercept
  - Air service ambulance services include:
    – Fixed-wing air ambulance (airplane)
    – Rotary-wing air ambulance (helicopter)

Health Care Operating Indicators

- **Average length of stay (ALOS)**
  - Total Number of Patient Days/Total Number of Discharges and Deaths
- **Inpatient occupancy rate**
  - (Total Number of Inpatient Days/Total Number of Inpatient Beds) × 100
- **Outpatient revenue as a percentage of total patient revenue**
  - Total Outpatient Revenue $/Total Patient Revenue $
- **Average daily inpatient census**
  - Total Number of Inpatient Service Days/Total Number of Days
- **Death rate (gross death rate)**
  - (Total Number of Inpatient Deaths/Total Number of Discharges and Deaths) × 100

- **Net death rate**
  - [(Total Number of Inpatient Deaths – Deaths <48 Hours)/(Total Number of Discharges – Deaths <48 Hours)] × 100
- **Newborn (NB) death rate**
  - (Total Number of NB Deaths/Total Number of NB Discharges and Deaths) × 100
- **Maternal death rate (hospital inpatient)**
  - (Total Number of Direct Maternal Deaths/Total Number of Maternal Discharges and Deaths) × 100
- **Gross autopsy rate**
  - (Total Inpatient Autopsies/Total Number of Inpatient Deaths) × 100
- **Hospital infection rate**
  - (Total Number of Nosocomial Infections/Total Number of Discharges and Deaths) × 100
- **Postoperative infection rate**
  - (Number of Infections in Clean Surgical Cases/Total Number of Surgical Operations) × 100
- **Consultation rate**
  - (Total Number of Patients Receiving Consultations/Total Number of Discharges and Deaths) × 100
- **Community-based birth and infant death rates**
  - (Number of Live Births for a Given Community/Estimated Population of That Community) × 100
- **Incidence rate of disease**
  - (Total Number of New Cases of a Specific Disease/Total Population at Risk) × 100
- **Prevalence rate of disease**
  - (All New and Preexisting Cases of a Specific Disease/Total Population) × 100
- **Balance sheet**
  - Liabilities + Capital = Assets

Calculating Risk

- **Attributable risk:** The part of the incidence of a disease in the exposed population that is caused by the exposure
  - Attributable Risk = Incidence in the Exposed – Incidence in the Nonexposed
  - Attributable Risk Percentage = (Attributable Risk/Incidence in the Exposed) × 100%
- **Population attributable risk:** The part of the incidence of a disease in a population (both exposed and nonexposed) that is caused by exposure
  - Population Attributable Risk = Incidence in the Total Population – Incidence in the Nonexposed
  - Population Attributable Risk Percentage = (Population Attributable Risk/Incidence in the Total Population) × 100%
- **Relative risk:** The relationship between the incidence of a disease in the exposed population and that in the nonexposed population
  - Relative Risk = Incidence in the Exposed/Incidence in the Nonexposed

Coding Measurements

Burns

Use the following tables to calculate the percentage of the body affected.

Infants	
Head and neck	18%
Arm, right	9%
Arm, left	9%
Torso, front	18%
Torso, back	18%
Leg, right	13.5%
Leg, left	13.5%
Genitals	1%

Adults (Rule of Nines)	
Head and neck	9%
Chest	9%
Arm, right	9%
Arm, left	9%
Abdomen	9%
Upper back	9%
Lower back, buttocks	9%
Leg, right, front	9%
Leg, right, back	9%
Leg, left, front	9%
Leg, left, back	9%
Genitals	1%

Children	
Head	10%
Neck	2%
Torso	26%
Arm, upper, front, right	2%
Arm, upper, back, right	2%
Arm, lower, front, right	1.5%
Arm, lower, back, right	1.5%
Hand, front, right	1.25%
Hand, back, right	1.25%
Arm, upper, front, left	2%
Arm, upper, back, left	2%
Arm, lower, front, left	1.5%
Arm, lower, back, left	1.5%
Hand, front, left	1.25%
Hand, back, left	1.25%
Buttocks, right	2.5%
Buttocks, left	2.5%
Leg, upper, front, right	4%
Leg, upper, back, right	4%
Leg, lower, front, right	3.5%
Leg, lower, back, right	3.5%
Foot, front, right	1.75%
Foot, back, right	1.75%
Leg, upper, front, left	4%
Leg, upper, back, left	4%
Leg, lower, front, left	3.5%
Leg, lower, back, left	3.5%
Foot, front, left	1.75%
Foot, back, left	1.75%
Genitals	1%

Note: Variations occur because of the growth factor, and percentages change as the child grows; therefore, these percentages are only averages, especially for legs.

Burn Patient Fluid Retention (Parkland Formula)

4 × Weight in Kilograms × % BSA Burned = Total Fluid Volume to Be Infused, where BSA = body surface area. Give half in the first 8 hours. Give the other half in the next 16 hours.

Degrees of Burns

- **First degree:** Redness of the epidermis (skin)
- **Second degree:** Blisters on the skin; involvement of the epidermis and dermis layers
- **Third degree:** Destruction of all layers of the skin, with possible involvement of the subcutaneous fat, muscle, and bone
- **Necrosis:** The death of the tissue

Excision of Lesions

Widest Measurement of Lesion + (Margin × 2) = Coded Size

Laceration Repair

Code the total of all lacerations on the same coded anatomical site.

Wound Repair

Add together the length of all wounds in the same code grouping for one code.

PHARMACOLOGY

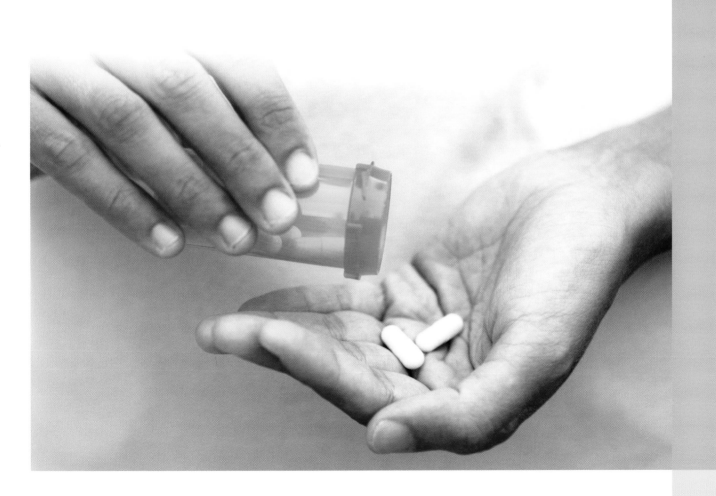

Introduction

Most medications, at least in the inpatient setting, are administered by nurses. Because medications can have serious side effects and patients can develop adverse reactions that can significantly impact morbidity and mortality, it is imperative that nurses have a good understanding of pharmacology.

This chapter includes information about pharmacology and the nursing process, as well as drug names, pharmacology basics, and considerations across the life span. Also included in this chapter is a brief description of many of the major drug classes that are important to nursing pharmacology. For each drug class, one prototype drug is discussed and examined for indications, contraindications, side effects, potential risks, routes of administration, and so forth. As a nurse, you should always seek out detailed information about the individual medications you are administering, as a prototype description cannot be assumed to provide comprehensive information on other drugs in the same class.

Pharmacology & the Nursing Process

Assessment
- Gather the data necessary to evaluate therapeutic effects.
- Gather the data necessary to evaluate adverse reactions.
- Judge if the patient is capable of self-administration.
- Assess any potential risk factors.

Analysis & Diagnosis
- Determine if the prescribed therapeutic plan is appropriate.
- Identify possible drug interactions, adverse reactions, and health problems.

Planning
- Compose a care plan, including nursing interventions and expected outcomes.

Implementation
- Administer the drug.
- Educate the patient about the drug.
- Enact measures that will enhance the drug's effectiveness and minimize adverse reactions.

Evaluation
- Determine the presence or absence of the desired therapeutic response or of adverse reactions.
- Identify if the patient followed the regimen prescribed and is satisfied with treatment.

Pharmacology Basics

- **Pharmacokinetics:** The study of the actions of drugs as they move through the body
  - **Absorption:** Affected by administration route, formulation, patient stress level, stomach contents, and blood flow; may also be affected by other medications
  - **Distribution:** Affected by solubility, protein activity, and blood flow
  - **Metabolism:** Affected by diseases, environment, age, and genetics; may also be affected by other medications
  - **Excretion:** Through kidneys, skin, intestines, lungs, or exocrine glands
- **Pharmacodynamics:** The study of the mechanisms of drug action within the body and of how drugs produce their effects in the body
- **Pharmacotherapeutics:** The study of drugs used to prevent, treat, or diagnose disease

Drug Names
- **Chemical name:** The scientific name, which describes the atomic and molecular structure of a drug
- **Generic name:** The nonproprietary name, often an abbreviation of the chemical name
- **Brand name:** The trade name selected by the pharmaceutical company that makes the drug

Educating Patients

When educating patients about their medications, make sure you include the following:
- Name of the medication and what it is for
- How much to take and when
- How to take the medication
- What to do in the event of a missed dose
- Expected therapeutic response
- Duration of treatment
- How to store the drug
- Major and minor side effects
- Important possible interactions
- Whom to call with questions
- What to do in an emergency

Considerations across the Life Span

Pregnant & Breast-Feeding Women
- Renal excretion rate and hepatic metabolism are accelerated; consider higher doses.
- Intestinal excretion rate is decreased, which leads to a longer absorption time; consider lower doses.
- Assume that all drugs can enter the fetus via the placenta.
- Consult U.S. Food and Drug Administration risk categories for every drug before administration.
- Weeks 3–8 present the greatest risk of drug-induced malformation of the fetus.
- After delivery, doses should be taken directly after breast-feeding to ensure minimal drug concentration in the breast milk for the next feeding.

Pediatric Patients
- Assume increased drug sensitivity because of immature organ system.
- Infants have irregular gastric patterns; absorption rates may vary.
- Infants and young children have thin skin, which may lead to rapid topical drug absorption.
- An infant's blood-brain barrier is not fully developed, which may lead to increased sensitivity to central nervous system (CNS) drugs and risk of toxicity.
- Neonates absorb intramuscular (IM) drugs slower than adults; infants absorb IM drugs faster.
- Infants have reduced protein-binding ability, which can lead to high free concentrations of drugs.
- The liver and kidneys are not fully developed until after 1 year of age; assume reduced hepatic and renal metabolism in infants.
- In children older than 1 year of age, the drug metabolism rate is higher than that in adults.

- Children may have unique side effects from certain drugs, including suppressed growth.
- General rule for dosing adjustment:

$$\frac{\text{Body Surface of Child} \times \text{Adult Dose}}{1.73 \text{ m}^2} = \text{Approximate Dose for Child}$$

Geriatric Patients
- Assume increased drug sensitivity because of deterioration of organ systems.
- Reactions vary greatly based on the individual patient's condition.
- Rate of absorption is generally slowed, which could lead to a delayed therapeutic response.
- Hepatic metabolism rate is likely slowed, which could lead to an extended therapeutic response.
- Renal excretion is likely slowed, which could lead to an accumulation of the drug in the body and an increased risk of adverse effects.
- Determine creatinine clearance prior to drug administration to assess renal function.
- Nonadherence to the prescribed regimen is a common problem; longer or more extensive patient education may be required.
- Polypharmacy can be an issue with elderly patients; anticipate, assess, and manage drug interactions carefully.

Drug Interactions

- **Additive:** Two drugs with similar therapeutic effects have a combined effect that is the sum of their individual effects.
- **Antagonistic:** Two drugs that, when taken together, lead to decreased effectiveness of both.
- **Potentiation:** One drug's potency is enhanced when combined with another.
- **Absorption:** One drug affects the absorption rate of another.
- **Metabolism:** One drug affects the metabolism of another; if metabolism is inhibited, this can cause toxicity.

Adverse Reactions
- Caused by patient sensitivity:
  - Allergic or anaphylactic reaction
  - Idiosyncratic response
- Caused by dose:
  - Secondary or side effects
  - Hypersusceptibility
  - Iatrogenic effects
  - Overdose

Drugs Affecting the Peripheral Nervous System

Anticholinergics
Prototype: Atropine
Other examples: Scopolamine, ipratropium, propantheline, oxybutynin
- **Action:** Acts at muscarinic receptors to competitively block acetylcholine action in the peripheral nervous system
- **Indications:** Spastic conditions, bradycardia, eye disorders, bronchospasm, peptic ulcers, gastrointestinal (GI) disorders, muscarinic poisoning, overactive bladder, motion sickness, vertigo

- **Contraindications:** Myasthenia gravis, narrow-angle glaucoma, tachycardia, severe hemorrhage, hypersensitivity
- **Use with caution in patients with:** GI obstruction risk; urinary tract disorders; chronic cardiac, pulmonary, hepatic, or renal disorder
- **Major interactions:** Tricyclic antidepressants, antihistamines, phenothiazine antipsychotics
- **Administration options:** <u>Oral</u>, intravenous (IV), IM, subcutaneous (subcut), topical (ocular, transdermal patch)
- **Notes for patient education:**
  - **Side effects:** Can cause blurred vision, dry mouth, elevated heart rate, constipation, intraocular pressure, and anhidrosis.
  - Can cause dizziness or drowsiness.
  - Take 30–60 minutes before meals if taking for GI problems.
  - Eat high-fiber foods and drink plenty of fluid to avoid constipation.
  - Stop taking the drug and call the doctor immediately if any of the following occur: rash, inability to urinate, confusion, disorientation, hallucinations, and behavioral changes.

> When more than one administration route can be used, the preferred route is underlined.

Schedules of Controlled Substances

Schedule Class	Characteristics	Examples
Schedule I	High abuse potential; not legal; no acceptable medical use; no prescriptions available	Heroin, lysergic acid diethylamide (LSD), marijuana, methaqualone
Schedule II	High abuse potential and severe dependence liability; current, accepted medical use; prescription drug–signed, not stamped prescription; 30-day supply, no refills	Cocaine, codeine, methamphetamines, oxycodone, fentanyl, methadone
Schedule III	Less abuse potential; low to moderate physical dependence; high psychological dependence; by prescription only, expires within 6 months; maximum 5 refills on one script	Vicodin, products containing not more than 90 mg of codeine per dosage unit (Tylenol with Codeine), anabolic steroids
Schedule IV	Less abuse potential than schedule III drugs; accepted medical use; limited physical and psychological dependence; written or verbal prescription, expires within 6 months; maximum 5 refills on one script	Alprazolam (Xanax), clonazepam (Klonopin), diazepam (Valium), lorazepam (Ativan), temazepam (Restoril)
Schedule V	Limited abuse potential; accepted medical use; small amounts of narcotics used as antitussives (cough medicine) or antidiarrheals; may not need a prescription but must be recorded as a transaction	Cough preparations containing not more than 200 mg of codeine per 100 mL or per 100 g (Robitussin AC, Phenergan with Codeine)

Alpha-Adrenergic Antagonists (Alpha-Blockers)

Prototype: Prazosin
Other examples: Doxazosin, terazosin, alfuzosin, phentolamine
- **Action:** Interferes with alpha-adrenergic receptors on blood vessels
  - **Nonselective:** Inhibits alpha-1 and alpha-2 receptors
  - **Selective:** Inhibits alpha-1 receptors only
- **Indications:** Hypertension, pheochromocytoma, vascular disorders (Raynaud disease), benign prostatic hyperplasia
- **Contraindications:** Hypersensitivity
- **Use with caution in patients with:** Postural hypotension, hepatic disorders
- **Major interactions:** Diuretics, beta-blockers, antihypertensives, propranolol, clonidine
- **Administration options:** <u>Oral</u>, IV (phentolamine only), IM (phentolamine only)
- **Notes for patient education:**
  - **Side effects:** Can cause hypotension, tachycardia, nasal congestion, breathing difficulties, flushing, edema, angina, dry mouth, dizziness, sexual dysfunction, anxiety, insomnia, and diarrhea or constipation.
  - Can cause dizziness or fainting; avoid moving or standing suddenly.
  - Avoid excessive heat.

Beta-Adrenergic Antagonists (Beta-Blockers)

Prototype: Propranolol
Other examples: Metoprolol, timolol, carvedilol, bisoprolol, betaxolol
- **Action:** Interferes with beta-adrenergic receptors on blood vessels
  - **Nonselective:** Inhibits beta-1 and beta-2 receptors
  - **Selective:** Inhibits beta-1 receptors only
- **Indications:** Angina pectoris, cardiac dysrhythmias, hypertension, heart failure, myocardial infarction, migraine, anxiety, open-angle glaucoma
- **Contraindications:** Cardiogenic shock, sinus bradycardia, and partial AV block; asthma, COPD (nonselective beta-blockers)
- **Use with caution in patients with:** Congestive heart failure (compensated), lung disease, hepatic disease, diabetes
- **Major interactions:** Calcium channel blockers, antacids, barbiturates, insulin, anti-inflammatory drugs, rifampin, theophylline, clonidine
- **Administration options:** <u>Oral</u>, IV
- **Notes for patient education:**
  - **Side effects:** Can cause bradycardia, hypotension, atrioventricular (AV) block, bronchospasm, rash, nausea, vomiting, anorexia, fever, sore throat, and diarrhea or constipation.
  - Talk to your doctor before stopping this medication; discontinuing suddenly may result in tachycardia and dysrhythmias.
  - Avoid alcohol.

Antidepressants

Note: Monoamine oxidase inhibitors (MAOIs), bupropion, and other drugs are also indicated for seizure disorders and have varied therapeutic information; the information in this section is applicable only to tricyclic antidepressants and selective serotonin reuptake inhibitors (SSRIs), the two most commonly prescribed classes of drugs for depression.

Tricyclic Antidepressants

Prototype: Imipramine
Other examples: Doxepin, amitriptyline, clomipramine, desipramine
- **Action:** Inhibits the reuptake of the neurotransmitters serotonin and norepinephrine

- **Indications:** Major depression, bipolar disorder, enuresis, chronic pain
- **Contraindications:** Narrow-angle glaucoma, hypersensitivity
- **Use with caution in patients with:** History of cardiovascular disease, seizure disorders, enlarged prostate, diabetes
- **Major interactions:** MAOIs, sympathomimetics, anticholinergics, CNS depressants
- **Administration options:** <u>Oral</u>, IM (imipramine only)
- **Notes for patient education:**
  - **Side effects:** Can cause sedation, orthostatic hypotension, dry mouth, sensitivity to light, blurred vision, urinary dysfunction, tachycardia, constipation, jaundice, sweating, seizures, and hypomanic episodes.
  - Imipramine can cause suicidal thoughts, particularly in young people.
  - Do not take within 14 days of taking MAOIs.
  - Do not take if you have recently had a heart attack.
  - Call your doctor if you experience any of the following:
    - Mood or behavior changes
    - Anxiety or panic attacks
    - Difficulty sleeping
    - Irritability
    - Suicidal thoughts

SSRI Antidepressants

Prototype: Fluoxetine
Other examples: Citalopram, paroxetine, escitalopram, sertraline

- **Action:** Inhibits the reuptake of the neurotransmitter serotonin
- **Indications:** Major depression, eating disorders, panic disorder, premenstrual dysphoric disorder, alcoholism
- **Contraindications:** Current use of an MAOI, thioridazine, or pimozide; hypersensitivity
- **Use with caution in patients with:** Diabetes, seizure disorders, renal or hepatic dysfunction, history of suicidal ideation
- **Major interactions:** MAOIs, tricyclic antidepressants, lithium, warfarin
- **Administration options:** Oral
- **Notes for patient education:**
  - **Side effects:** Can cause nausea, nervousness, insomnia, sexual dysfunction, anxiety, weight gain, rash, and bruxism.
  - Fluoxetine can cause suicidal thoughts, particularly in young people.
  - Do not take within 14 days of taking MAOIs.
  - Tell your doctor if you become pregnant while taking fluoxetine.
  - Call your doctor if you experience any of the following:
    - Mood or behavior changes
    - Anxiety or panic attacks
    - Difficulty sleeping
    - Irritability
    - Suicidal thoughts

Antipsychotics

Atypical Antipsychotics

Prototype: Clozapine
Other examples: Risperidone, ziprasidone, olanzapine, aripiprazole, quetiapine

- **Action:** Primarily inhibits 5-hydroxytryptamine 2 (5-HT_2, serotonin) receptors; secondarily inhibits dopamine 2 (D_2), norepinephrine, histamine, and acetylcholine receptors
- **Indications:** Schizophrenia, acute bipolar mania
- **Contraindications:** CNS depression, uncontrolled epilepsy, granulocytopenia, bone marrow suppression, hypersensitivity

- **Use with caution in patients with:** Angle-closure glaucoma; enlarged prostate; renal, cardiovascular, or hepatic disorder; seizure disorder; diabetes; malnourishment
- **Major interactions:** Drugs that suppress bone marrow function
- **Administration options:** <u>Oral</u>, IM
- **Notes for patient education:**
  - **Side effects:** Can cause dry mouth, weight gain, nausea, vomiting, tachycardia, hypertension, dizziness, sedation, vision problems, sweating, rash, and hyperglycemia.
  - Clozapine can increase your risk of infection; wash hands frequently and avoid crowds.
  - Do not take if you have any of the following:
    - Dementia
    - Untreated or uncontrolled epilepsy
    - A bone marrow disorder
    - Paralytic ileus or intestinal blockage
  - Do not take with other drugs that may increase your risk of infection (e.g., chemotherapy).
  - Call your doctor if you experience flu-like symptoms (e.g., fever, chills, cough, sore throat).

Typical Antipsychotics
Prototype: Chlorpromazine
Other examples: Thioridazine, fluphenazine, haloperidol, pimozide, perphenazine
- **Action:** Inhibits dopamine, histamine, norepinephrine, and acetylcholine receptors
  - **Low potency:** Lower dose necessary; higher incidence of sedation, orthostatic hypotension, anticholinergic effects, QT prolongation; low incidence of extra-pyramidal effects
  - **Medium potency:** Medium dose necessary; moderate incidence of sedation, extrapyramidal effects; low incidence of orthostatic hypotension, anticholinergic effects, QT prolongation
  - **High potency:** High dose necessary; high incidence of extrapyramidal effects; low or moderate incidence of sedation, orthostatic hypotension, anticholinergic effects, QT prolongation
- **Indications:** Schizophrenia, bipolar disorder, Tourette syndrome
- **Contraindications:** Angle-closure glaucoma, hepatic or cardiovascular disease, bone marrow depression, current use of pimozide, hypersensitivity
- **Use with caution in patients with:** Diabetes, seizure disorder, respiratory disease, hyperplasia of the prostate, CNS tumor, intestinal obstruction
- **Major interactions:** Anticholinergics, CNS depressants, direct dopamine receptor agonists, levodopa
- **Administration options:** <u>Oral</u>, IM
- **Notes for patient education:**
  - **Side effects:** Can cause dry mouth, sedation, orthostatic hypotension, sensitivity to light, constipation, tachycardia, blurred vision, breast growth, and menstrual irregularities.
  - Do not use if you have any of the following:
    - Dementia
    - Brain damage
    - Bone marrow depression
  - Avoid alcohol.
  - Call your doctor immediately and stop taking the medication if you experience any of the following:
    - Twitching
    - Uncontrollable movements of the eyes, lips, tongue, face, or limbs

Neurologic & Neuromuscular Drugs

Antiparkinsonians

Prototype: Levodopa

Other examples: Ropinirole, bromocriptine, pramipexole

Note: Anticholinergics, MAOIs, and other drug classes are also indicated for seizure disorders and have varied therapeutic information; the information here refers only to dopamine agonists, the most commonly prescribed class of drugs for parkinsonism.

- **Action:** Balances dopamine levels in the brain
- **Indications:** Parkinson disease, parkinsonism **Contraindications:** Melanoma (past or present)
- **Use with caution in patients with:** Heart disease
- **Major interactions:** Anticholinergic drugs, MAOIs, typical antipsychotics
- **Administration options:** Oral
- **Notes for patient education:**
  - **Side effects:** Can cause nausea, vomiting, hypotension, dyskinesia, confusion, anorexia, and arrhythmias.
  - May cause urine and sweat to be dark in color.
  - May cause drowsiness; avoid alcohol and use caution when driving.
  - Do not take within 14 days of taking MAOIs.
  - Call your doctor immediately if you experience any of the following:
    - Nausea or vomiting
    - Uncontrollable movements of the eyes, lips, tongue, face, or limbs
    - Irregular heartbeat
    - Mood changes

Anticonvulsants

Prototype: Phenytoin

Other examples: Ethotoin, fosphenytoin

Note: Barbiturates, benzodiazepines, and other drug classes are also indicated for seizure disorders and have varied therapeutic information; the information here refers only to hydantoins, the most commonly prescribed class of drugs for seizure disorders.

- **Action:** Blocks sodium entry into overactive neurons in the brain
- **Indications:** Complex partial and tonic-clonic seizure disorders, cardiac dysrhythmias
- **Contraindications:** Hypersensitivity
- **Use with caution in patients with:** Cardiac, hepatic, renal, or respiratory diseases
- **Major interactions:** Corticosteroids, warfarin, oral contraceptives, phenobarbital, carbamazepine, barbiturates
- **Administration options:** Oral, IM, IV
- **Notes for patient education:**
  - **Side effects:** Can cause nystagmus, drowsiness, dizziness, hypotension, dysrhythmias, rash, headache, nausea, abdominal pain, anorexia, and irritability.
  - Phenytoin can cause suicidal thoughts, particularly in young people.
  - Tell your doctor if you become pregnant while taking phenytoin.
  - Avoid alcohol.
  - Call your doctor if you experience any of the following:
    - Mood or behavior changes
    - Anxiety or panic attacks
    - Difficulty sleeping
    - Irritability
    - Suicidal thoughts

Sedative & Antianxiety Drugs

Prototype: Alprazolam

Other examples: Diazepam, zolpidem, eszopiclone

- **Action:** Acts on gamma-aminobutyric acid (GABA) receptors, depressing the CNS
- **Indications:** Panic disorders, anxiety disorders, insomnia, muscle spasms, alcohol withdrawal, adjunct to anesthesia
- **Contraindications:** CNS depression
- **Use with caution in patients with:** Renal, hepatic, or pulmonary impairment; history of drug abuse or dependence or of suicidal thoughts
- **Major interactions:** CNS depressants (barbiturates, opioids)
- **Administration options:** <u>Oral</u>, IV
- **Notes for patient education:**
  - **Side effects:** Can cause lightheadedness, concentration problems, respiratory depression, anterograde amnesia, dry mouth, ataxia, nausea, and vomiting.
  - In some cases, alprazolam can cause reverse effects (insomnia, excitability) in patients with anxiety disorders.
  - Avoid alcohol and other CNS depressants.
  - Do not stop treatment suddenly; sudden withdrawal can cause seizures.
  - Alprazolam can become habit-forming; it is intended for short-term use only.

Drugs Affecting the Respiratory System

Corticosteroids (Inhaled)

Prototype: Fluticasone

Other examples: Budesonide, beclomethasone dipropionate, mometasone furoate

- **Action:** Acts on inflammatory cells and mediators to decrease inflammation and swelling
- **Indications:** Asthma
- **Contraindications:** Acute asthma attack, hypersensitivity
- **Use with caution in patients with:** Glaucoma; diabetes; untreated, active infections; hepatic disorder; systemic corticosteroid therapy
- **Administration options:** Inhalation
- **Notes for patient education:**
  - **Side effects:** Can cause irritation or candidiasis of the mouth, hoarseness, upper respiratory tract infection, and cough.
  - Fluticasone is intended for asthma maintenance; do not use it during an asthma attack.
  - Avoid smoking and environmental respiratory irritants.
  - Rinse mouth following administration to help prevent mouth irritation or infection.
  - Call your doctor if you experience any of the following:
    - Hives
    - Difficulty breathing
    - Facial swelling
    - Blurred vision
    - Exposure to chickenpox or measles

Bronchodilators

Prototype: Albuterol

Other examples: Salmeterol, formoterol, epinephrine, levalbuterol

- **Action:** Stimulates beta-2-adrenergic receptors in lung muscles
- **Indications:** Asthma, chronic obstructive pulmonary disease (COPD)
- **Contraindications:** Uncontrolled cardiac arrhythmias, hypersensitivity

- **Use with caution in patients with:** Hyperthyroidism, diabetes, cardiovascular disease
- **Administration options:** Inhalation
- **Notes for patient education:**
  - **Side effects:** Can cause dry mouth, tachycardia, tremors, angina, and bronchospasm.
  - Keep the inhaler with you at all times, and shake it well before using.
  - Use only the amount prescribed.
  - Avoid smoking and environmental respiratory irritants.

Drugs Affecting the Cardiovascular System

Antiarrhythmics

Prototype: Quinidine
Other examples: Lidocaine, procainamide, disopyramide, moricizine
Note: Beta-blockers (class II agents), potassium channel blockers (class II agents), and calcium channel blockers (class IV agents) are also indicated for arrhythmias and have varied therapeutic information; the information here refers only to sodium channel blockers (class I agents), the most commonly prescribed class of drugs for arrhythmias.

- **Action:** Blocks sodium channels, reducing conduction of impulses to the heart
- **Indications:** Arrhythmias (tachycardia, atrial flutter, atrial fibrillation)
- **Contraindications:** Myasthenia gravis, conduction defects, hypersensitivity
- **Use with caution in patients with:** Bradycardia, renal or hepatic disease, congestive heart failure, hyperkalemia, hypomagnesemia
- **Major interactions:** Digoxin, phenytoin, phenobarbital, warfarin
- **Administration options:** <u>Oral</u>, IV
- **Notes for patient education:**
  - **Side effects:** Can cause vertigo, diarrhea, tinnitus, nausea, vomiting, headache, abdominal cramps, loss of appetite, confusion, blurred vision, light sensitivity, and rash.
  - Call your doctor if you experience any of the following:
    - Vomiting
    - Diarrhea
    - Ringing in the ears or hearing loss
    - Dizziness
    - Vision changes
    - Eye pain
    - Skin changes (yellowing skin or bruising)
    - Dark urine
    - Difficulty breathing
    - New irregular heartbeat or worsening of current condition

Inotropics

Prototype: Digoxin

- **Action:** Elevates calcium levels at cell membranes of the heart, increasing strength of heart contractions
- **Indications:** Heart failure, arrhythmias (tachycardia, atrial fibrillation, atrial flutter)
- **Contraindications:** AV block, uncontrolled ventricular arrhythmias, constrictive pericarditis, idiopathic hypertrophic subaortic stenosis, hypersensitivity
- **Use with caution in patients with:** Hypothyroidism, hypokalemia, hypercalcemia, hypomagnesemia, use of diuretics
- **Major interactions:** Diuretics, sympathomimetics, angiotensin-converting enzyme (ACE) inhibitors, verapamil, quinidine
- **Administration options:** <u>Oral</u>, IV

- **Notes for patient education:**
  - **Side effects:** Can cause fatigue, nausea, vomiting, anorexia, blurred or disturbed vision, bradycardia, and electrocardiogram (ECG) changes.
  - Take with a full glass of water; drink plenty of fluids throughout the day.
  - Avoid becoming overheated.
  - Do not stop taking digoxin without consulting your doctor.
  - Call your doctor if you develop signs of toxicity:
    - Diarrhea
    - Abdominal pain
    - Nausea
    - Vomiting
    - Irritability
    - Headache
    - Confusion
    - Insomnia
    - Depression
    - Vision changes

Anticoagulants

Prototype: Heparin
Other examples: Warfarin (Coumadin)

- **Action:** Encourages antithrombin activity, which inactivates clotting factors
- **Indications:** Unstable angina, pulmonary embolism, deep vein thrombosis, post–myocardial infarction, evolving stroke, disseminated intravascular coagulation, open-heart surgery
- **Contraindications:** Ulcer disease, recent surgery or bleeding, coagulation disorder, malignancy, history of heparin-related thrombocytopenia
- **Use with caution in patients with:** Epidural analgesia, potential bleeding
- **Major interactions:** Antiplatelet drugs
- **Administration options:** <u>Subcut</u>, IV, oral (warfarin only)
- **Notes for patient education:**
  - **Side effects:** Can cause bleeding and excessive bruising.
  - Do not take aspirin, ibuprofen, or naproxen without consulting your doctor.
  - Call your doctor if you develop any of the following:
    - Bruising
    - Red or black stool
    - Dark or discolored urine
    - Unusual bleeding (e.g., nosebleeds, bleeding from the mouth)
  - To prevent bleeding, use electric razors and soft toothbrushes.

Antihypertensives

Diuretics

Prototype: Hydrochlorothiazide (HCTZ)
Other examples: Benzthiazide, cyclothiazide, bumetanide, amiloride

- **Action:** Instigates arteriolar vasodilation, lowering blood volume and resistance in the arteries
  - **Thiazide diuretics:** Maintenance treatment for chronic hypertension
  - **Loop (high-ceiling) diuretics:** Produce stronger effect than thiazides
  - **Potassium-sparing diuretics:** Produce weaker effect than thiazides but do not significantly reduce potassium levels
- **Indications:** Edema, hypertension, renal disorders, cirrhosis
- **Contraindications:** Anuria, hypersensitivity
- **Use with caution in patients with:** Hepatic or renal disorders

- **Major interactions:** Digoxin, lithium, nonsteroidal anti-inflammatory drugs (NSAIDs), ototoxic agents, other antihypertensives
- **Administration options:** <u>Oral</u>, IV
- **Notes for patient education:**
  - **Side effects:** Can cause dehydration, dizziness, drowsiness, cramping, nausea, vomiting, weakness, hyponatremia, hypocalcemia, hypokalemia, hypotension, and photosensitivity.
  - Avoid alcohol.
  - Avoid becoming overheated.
  - Avoid abrupt movements to prevent dizziness.

> Weight and potassium levels should be monitored during HCTZ treatment.

ACE Inhibitors

Prototype: Captopril

Other examples: Benazepril, lisinopril, enalapril, quinapril, ramipril

- **Action:** Blocks ACEs, preventing angiotensin II (which constricts blood vessels) from forming
- **Indications:** Hypertension, managing congestive heart failure, managing myocardial infarction, nephropathy, renal disorders, sodium or water retention
- **Contraindications:** Angioedema with past ACE inhibitor use, hypersensitivity
- **Use with caution in patients with:** Renal or hepatic disorders, diuretic use, hypovolemia, hyponatremia, recent surgery or anesthesia, African American ancestry, history of angioedema
- **Major interactions:** Diuretics, NSAIDs, lithium, other antihypertensives
- **Administration options:** Oral
- **Notes for patient education:**
  - **Side effects:** Can cause cough, dizziness, drowsiness, taste changes, hypotension, weakness, headache, insomnia, vertigo, nausea, and vomiting.
  - Avoid alcohol.
  - Avoid abrupt movements to prevent dizziness.
  - Do not take captopril if you are pregnant.

Endocrine Drugs

Insulin

- **Insulin types:** Insulin lispro, insulin aspart, insulin glulisine, regular insulin, NPH insulin, insulin detemir, insulin glargine
- **Action:** Instigates glucose uptake and glycogen synthesis
  - **Rapid-acting:** Lasts 1–5 hours; use immediately with meals; combined with a longer-acting type
  - **Short-acting:** Lasts 2–8 hours; use within 30–60 minutes of meals
  - **Immediate-acting:** Lasts 3–12 hours; half-day or overnight use; combined with a rapid- or short-acting type
  - **Long-acting:** Lasts 20–36 hours; full-day use; combined with a rapid- or short-acting type
  - **Premixed:** Taken twice a day, prior to meals
- **Indications:** Diabetes mellitus (types 1 and 2), diabetic ketoacidosis
- **Contraindications:** Hypoglycemia, hypersensitivity
- **Use with caution in patients with:** Hepatic or renal disorders, infection
- **Major interactions:** Beta-blockers, sulfonylureas, meglitinides, thiazide diuretics, sympathomimetics, glucocorticoids
- **Administration options:** <u>Subcut</u> (regular insulin options also include IV, IM, inhalation)

- **Notes for patient education:**
  - **Side effects:** Can cause redness or swelling at the injection site, rash, shortness of breath, dizziness, blurred vision, difficulty breathing, sweating, and racing heartbeat.
  - Check blood sugar regularly as instructed by your doctor.
  - Some types of insulin must be refrigerated; check the labels for storage information.
  - Use a different injection site each time you take your insulin.
  - Do not reuse needles.
  - Hypoglycemia may occur with overdose, insufficient food intake, diarrhea, vomiting, exercise, alcohol consumption, or stress; ask your doctor what you should do if you have symptoms of hypoglycemia:
    – Headache
    – Hunger
    – Weakness
    – Sweating
    – Tremor
    – Irritability
    – Difficulty concentrating
  - Call your doctor immediately if you develop symptoms of hyperglycemia:
    – Extreme thirst or hunger
    – Frequent urination
    – Weakness
    – Blurred vision
    – Dry mouth
    – Nausea and vomiting
    – Shortness of breath
    – Breath that smells fruity
    – Decreased level of consciousness

Oral Antidiabetics

Prototype: Glyburide
Other examples: Tolbutamide, chlorpropamide, glipizide

- **Action:** Acts on the pancreas to stimulate insulin production
  - **First generation:** Tolbutamide, chlorpropamide; requires higher dosage
  - **Second generation:** Glyburide, glipizide; requires lower dosage
- **Indications:** Diabetes mellitus (type 2 only)
- **Contraindications:** Type 1 diabetes, ketoacidosis, diabetic coma, current use of bosentan, hypersensitivity
- **Use with caution in patients with:** Renal or hepatic disorders; limited pituitary or adrenal function; recent infection, surgery, or trauma
- **Major interactions:** Beta-blockers, NSAIDs, sulfonamide antibiotics, cimetidine, ranitidine, insulin
- **Administration options:** Oral
- **Notes for patient education:**
  - **Side effects:** Can cause nausea, photosensitivity, dizziness, drowsiness, diarrhea, cramps, headache, increased appetite, heartburn, and vomiting.
  - Check blood sugar regularly as instructed by your doctor.
  - Hypoglycemia may occur with overdose, insufficient food intake, diarrhea, vomiting, exercise, alcohol consumption, or stress; ask your doctor what you should do if you have symptoms of hypoglycemia:
    – Headache
    – Hunger

- Weakness
- Sweating
- Tremor
- Irritability
- Difficulty concentrating
- Call your doctor immediately if you develop symptoms of hyperglycemia:
  - Extreme thirst or hunger
  - Frequent urination
  - Weakness
  - Blurred vision
  - Dry mouth
  - Nausea and vomiting
  - Shortness of breath
  - Breath that smells fruity
  - Decreased level of consciousness

Hypothyroidism

Prototype: Levothyroxine
Other examples: Liothyronine, liotrix, thyroid (desiccated)

- **Action:** As a synthetic hormone, mimics the actions of the natural hormone thyroxine
- **Indications:** Hypothyroidism or thyroid replacement therapy, cretinism, myxedema coma, euthyroid goiters, thyroid cancer
- **Contraindications:** Recent myocardial infarction, hyperthyroidism, hypersensitivity
- **Use with caution in patients with:** Renal insufficiency, cardiovascular disease, adrenocortical disorders
- **Major interactions:** Warfarin, catecholamines, phenytoin, carbamazepine, phenobarbital, sucralfate, cholestyramine, colestipol, antacids, iron and calcium supplements
- **Administration options:** <u>Oral</u>, IV
- **Notes for patient education:**
  - **Side effects:** Can cause sweating, diarrhea, abdominal cramping, heart palpitations, elevated heart rate, angina, elevated blood pressure, increased appetite, weight loss, and arrhythmia.
  - Take dose in the morning to avoid insomnia.
  - Take with a full glass of water.
  - Take on an empty stomach.
  - Treatment is typically lifelong; do not discontinue treatment when symptoms improve.
  - Call your doctor if you experience any of the following:
    - Fast or irregular heartbeat
    - Tremor
    - Nervousness
    - Headache
    - Insomnia
    - Sweating
    - Chest pain

> Because of adverse cardiovascular effects, levothyroxine should be used cautiously in patients with heart disorders.

GI Drugs

Antiulcers

Prototype: Cimetidine
Other examples: Nizatidine, famotidine, ranitidine
Note: Proton-pump inhibitors are also indicated for ulcers and have different therapeutic information; the information here refers only to histamine 2 (H_2) antagonists, the most commonly prescribed class of drugs for ulcers.

- **Action:** Inhibits H_2 receptors to reduce the secretion of gastric acid
- **Indications:** Gastric ulcer, duodenal ulcer, gastroesophageal reflux disease (GERD), acid indigestion, heartburn, Zollinger-Ellison syndrome, aspiration pneumonitis
- **Contraindications:** Hypersensitivity
- **Use with caution in patients with:** Renal disorders, hepatic disorders, porphyria
- **Major interactions:** Antacids, phenytoin, theophylline, warfarin, lidocaine
- **Administration options:** Oral, IV, IM
- **Notes for patient education:**
  - **Side effects:** Can cause headache, dizziness, nausea, constipation, rash, and drowsiness; can cause breast swelling or tenderness in men.
  - May increase risk of contracting pneumonia.
  - Take with a full glass of water.
  - Avoid alcohol.
  - Avoid aspirin, ibuprofen, and naproxen.
  - Avoid cigarette smoke.

Antidiarrheals

Prototype: Loperamide
Other examples: Octreotide, bismuth subsalicylate, polycarbophil
- **Action:** Stimulates opioid receptors during digestion, slowing motility and rate of transit in intestines
- **Indications:** Diarrhea
- **Contraindications:** Unidentified abdominal pain, hypersensitivity, bloody or infectious diarrhea
- **Use with caution in patients with:** Hepatic disorders
- **Major interactions:** CNS depressants
- **Administration options:** Oral
- **Notes for patient education:**
  - **Side effects:** Can cause vomiting, dry mouth, abdominal cramping, constipation, nausea, tachycardia, drowsiness, and CNS depression.
  - Do not take if you have black or bloody stools or diarrhea caused by antibiotic use.
  - Take with a full glass of water.
  - Drink plenty of water throughout the day.

Laxatives

Prototype: Psyllium
Other examples: Methylcellulose, docusate sodium, bisacodyl, magnesium hydroxide
- **Action:** Encourages intestinal motility; hydrates stool to soften it
  - **Bulk-forming:** Psyllium, methylcellulose; acts like dietary fiber to cause fecal matter to expand and soften
  - **Surfactant:** Docusate sodium; takes several days to soften stool
  - **Osmotic:** Magnesium hydroxide; salts cause stool to expand and soften
  - **Stimulant:** Bisacodyl; stimulates intestines, secretes electrolytes into lumen of intestines
- **Indications:** Constipation, irritable bowel syndrome, diverticulitis
- **Contraindications:** Unidentified abdominal pain, vomiting, nausea; hypersensitivity
- **Use with caution in patients with:** Dietary restrictions
- **Administration options:** Oral (dissolved powder, liquid, tablet, capsule), suppository (bisacodyl only)
- **Notes for patient education:**
  - **Side effects:** Can cause feeling of fullness, flatulence, intestinal impaction or obstruction, and diarrhea.
  - Mix powder with 8 oz water or juice; drink plenty of fluids throughout the day.

- o Do not inhale powder when mixing; can cause an allergic reaction.
- o May suppress appetite if taken before a meal.
- o Eat a high-fiber diet.

Antiemetics

Prototype: Ondansetron

Other examples: Dolasetron, aprepitant, dronabinol, prochlorperazine

Note: Corticosteroids, anticholinergics, dopamine antagonists, and other drug classes are also indicated for nausea and have different therapeutic information; the information here refers only to serotonin antagonists, the preferred class of drugs for chemotherapy-associated and postoperative nausea.

- **Action:** Inhibits the serotonin activity in the brain that induces vomiting
- **Indications:** Nausea or vomiting caused by anesthesia, chemotherapy, or radiation; postoperative nausea
- **Contraindications:** Phenylketonuria (for oral tablets), hypersensitivity
- **Use with caution in patients with:** Hepatic impairment, abdominal surgery
- **Major interactions:** CNS depressants, tricyclic antidepressants, antiparkinsonians, phenothiazines, anticholinergics
- **Administration options:** <u>Oral</u>, IV
- **Notes for patient education:**
  - o **Side effects:** Can cause headache, diarrhea, dizziness, dry mouth, insomnia, restlessness, problems urinating, impotence, weakness, and agitation.
  - o Avoid alcohol.
  - o Contact your doctor if you experience any of the following:
    - – Slow heart rate
    - – Difficulty breathing
    - – Anxiety or agitation
    - – Shaking
    - – Dizziness
    - – Decreased urination

Antiallergy, Anti-Inflammatory & Immunosuppressant Drugs

Antihistamines

Prototype: Diphenhydramine

Other examples: Promethazine, phenindamine, azelastine, cetirizine, loratadine

- **Action:** Prevents histamine activity by binding with histamine 1 (H_1) receptor sites
- **Indications:** Allergic reactions, motion sickness, rhinitis, insomnia
- **Contraindications:** Angle-closure glaucoma, hypersensitivity
- **Use with caution in patients with:** Hyperthyroidism, cardiovascular disease, pyloric obstruction, prostatic hypertrophy, hepatic disease
- **Major interactions:** CNS depressants
- **Administration options:** <u>Oral</u>, nasal, IV, IM
- **Notes for patient education:**
  - o **Side effects:** Can cause sedation, dizziness, incoordination, dry mouth, hypo- or hypertension, elevated heart rate, loss of appetite, vomiting, nausea, and diarrhea or constipation.
  - o Can cause drowsiness; use caution when driving.
  - o Take with food to reduce adverse GI effects.
  - o Avoid alcohol and other CNS depressants.

Diphenhydramine should be used cautiously in patients with heart conditions, asthma, or COPD.

Corticosteroids (Systemic)

Prototype: Prednisone

Other examples: Cortisone, hydrocortisone, methylprednisolone, dexamethasone

- **Action:** Suppresses inflammatory response by inhibiting chemical reactions leading to inflammation
- **Indications:** Severe, chronic inflammation (e.g., rheumatoid arthritis, inflammatory bowel disease, systemic lupus erythematosus); immunosuppression
- **Contraindications:** Current infections (active, untreated); recent live vaccine administration; intolerance to tartrazine, bisulfate, or alcohol
- **Use with caution in patients with:** Hypothyroidism, stress, signs of infection, cirrhosis
- **Major interactions:** Digoxin, NSAIDs, thiazide and loop diuretics, vaccines, insulin, oral antidiabetic drugs
- **Administration options:** <u>Oral</u>, IV, IM
- **Notes for patient education:**
  - **Adverse effects:** Can cause insomnia, low potassium levels, headache, dizziness, nausea, bloating, and change in body shape or location of body fat.
  - Prednisone can increase your risk of infection; wash hands frequently and avoid crowds.
  - Take with food to avoid GI upset.
  - Call your doctor if you are exposed to chickenpox or measles.
  - May slow growth in children.
  - Wear a medical-alert bracelet or tag or carry a medical-alert card while taking this medication.
  - Do not stop taking suddenly; may cause withdrawal.
  - Avoid live vaccines.

Anti-Inflammatory & Pain Drugs

Aspirin

- **Action:** Inhibits prostaglandins to reduce inflammation, fever, pain, and platelet aggregation
- **Indications:** Mild to moderate fever, inflammation, or pain; myocardial infarction; ischemic attacks; angina; arthritis
- **Contraindications:** Thrombocytopenia, bleeding disorders, viral infections in children and young adults, hypersensitivity
- **Use with caution in patients with:** Alcoholism, ulcer or GI bleeding disorders (past or present), severe hepatic or renal disease
- **Major interactions:** Warfarin, ibuprofen, corticosteroids
- **Administration options:** Oral
- **Notes for patient education:**
  - **Side effects:** Can cause nausea, heartburn, gastric pain, headache, dizziness, tinnitus, drowsiness, and increased bleeding time.
  - Take with a full glass of water.
  - GI perforation, ulceration, or bleeding may occur with long-term or high-dose use.
  - Do not give to children or teenagers without first consulting a doctor; use in children can lead to Reye syndrome.
  - Aspirin should not be used by patients with bleeding disorders.
  - Avoid alcohol, which may increase risk of GI bleeding.

Ibuprofen

- **Action:** Inhibits cyclooxygenase, an enzyme responsible for inflammation, fever, and pain
- **Indications:** Mild to moderate fever, inflammation, or pain; dysmenorrhea; myocardial infarction prevention; angina; arthritis
- **Contraindications:** Hypersensitivity to aspirin
- **Use with caution in patients with:** Severe renal, hepatic, or cardiovascular disease; bleeding disorder (past or present); GI bleeding (past or present)
- **Major interactions:** ACE inhibitors, beta-blockers, digoxin, anticoagulants, aminoglycosides, phenobarbital, rifampin, salicylates, fluconazole, ritonavir, lithium
- **Administration options:** Oral
- **Notes for patient education:**
  - **Side effects:** Can cause nausea, heartburn, gastric pain, headache, dizziness, tinnitus, drowsiness, and vertigo.
  - May increase risk of heart attack or stroke, especially with long-term use.
  - GI perforation, ulceration, or bleeding may occur with long-term or high-dose use.
  - Ibuprofen should not be used by patients with bleeding disorders.
  - Avoid alcohol, which may increase risk of GI bleeding.

Acetaminophen

- **Action:** Acts on the CNS to reduce synthesis of prostaglandin
- **Indications:** Mild to moderate fever or pain, arthritis
- **Contraindications:** Hypersensitivity
- **Use with caution in patients with:** Alcoholism or chronic alcohol use, hepatic or renal disease, malnutrition
- **Major interactions:** Warfarin
- **Administration options:** Oral
- **Notes for patient education:**
  - Acetaminophen should not be taken by people with liver disease.
  - Toxicity may cause liver disease.
  - Avoid alcohol.

Opioid Agonists

Prototype: Morphine

Other examples: Codeine, meperidine, fentanyl, methadone, oxycodone

- **Action:** Stimulates mu (μ) and kappa (κ) receptors in the brain to produce sedation and analgesic effects
- **Indications:** Moderate to severe pain
- **Contraindications:** Hypersensitivity
- **Use with caution in patients with:** Severe hepatic, pulmonary, or renal dysfunction; elevated intracranial pressure; head injury; hypothyroidism; adrenal insufficiency; undiagnosed abdominal pain; prostatic hyperplasia; use of a rapid-acting analgesic; substance abuse (past or present)
- **Major interactions:** CNS depressants, antihypertensives, anticholinergics, MAOIs
- **Administration options:** <u>Oral</u>, <u>IV</u>, subcut, IM, epidural, intrathecal
- **Notes for patient education:**
  - **Side effects:** Can cause sedation, depressed heart rate, hypotension, flushing, constricted pupils, constipation, decreased urine output, nausea, euphoria or dysphoria, cough suppression, elevated intracranial pressure, urinary retention, vomiting, sweating, headache, and abnormal dreams.
  - Overdose can lead to severe respiratory depression and death.
  - Avoid alcohol and other CNS depressants.

- Do not take morphine within 14 days of taking an MAOI.
- Stand slowly to reduce dizziness or lightheadedness.
- Can become habit-forming.
- Do not stop taking suddenly; may cause withdrawal.

Antibiotics

Note: Excessive use of antibiotics or stopping a regimen of antibiotics too early increases the risk of antibiotic resistance, which will decrease the effectiveness of antibiotics in the future.

Penicillins

Prototype: Penicillin V
Other examples: Amoxicillin, ampicillin, oxacillin, ticarcillin

- **Action:** Disrupts cell wall formation in bacterial cells
- **Indications:** Bacterial infections
- **Contraindications:** Hypersensitivity
- **Use with caution in patients with:** Renal impairment
- **Major interactions:** Aminoglycosides, probenecid
- **Administration options:** Oral, IV
- **Notes for patient education:**
  - **Side effects:** Can cause nausea, vomiting, epigastric disturbances, diarrhea, fever, and rash.
  - If diarrhea occurs, contact your doctor; do not treat with over-the-counter (OTC) drugs.
  - Take 1 hour before or 2 hours after meals.
  - Take with a full glass of water.
  - Take all the medication as prescribed, even if you feel well.
  - May make oral contraceptives less effective.

Aminoglycosides

Prototype: Gentamicin
Other examples: Tobramycin, amikacin, neomycin

- **Action:** Inhibits protein synthesis in bacterial cells
- **Indications:** Bacterial infections
- **Contraindications:** Intestinal obstruction (neomycin), hypersensitivity
- **Use with caution in patients with:** Hearing or renal impairment, neuromuscular disorders, obesity
- **Major interactions:** Penicillins, ototoxic drugs, nephrotoxic drugs, cephalosporins, vancomycin, skeletal muscle relaxants
- **Administration options:** IV, IM, oral, topical
- **Notes for patient education:**
  - **Side effects:** Can cause nausea, vomiting, and diarrhea.
  - Take all the medication as prescribed, even if you feel well.
  - Contact your doctor if you experience any of the following:
    - Nausea or vomiting
    - Fatigue
    - Pale skin
    - Hearing loss
    - Dizziness
    - Numbness or tingling
    - Muscle twitching
    - Seizures

Cephalosporins

Prototype: Cefadroxil
Other examples: Cephalexin, cefoxitin, cefotaxime, cefepime

- **Action:** Disrupts cell wall formation in bacterial cells
- **Indications:** Bacterial infections
    - **First generation:** Cephalexin; most effective against gram-positive bacteria
    - **Second generation:** Cefoxitin; most effective against gram-negative and an-aerobic bacteria
    - **Third generation:** Cefotaxime; broad-spectrum effectiveness
    - **Fourth generation:** Cefepime; broad-spectrum effectiveness
- **Contraindications:** Cross-sensitivity to penicillin, hypersensitivity
- **Use with caution in patients with:** GI bleeding or disease (past or present), renal impairment
- **Major interactions:** Probenecid, NSAIDs, thrombolytics, anticoagulants, antiplatelet drugs
- **Administration options:** <u>Oral</u>, IV, IM
- **Notes for patient education:**
    - **Side effects:** Can cause nausea, vomiting, diarrhea, and confusion.
    - If diarrhea occurs, contact your doctor; do not treat with OTC drugs.
    - Take with a full glass of water.
    - Take with food or milk to avoid GI symptoms.
    - Take all the medication as prescribed, even if you feel well.
    - May make oral contraceptives less effective.

Tetracyclines
Prototype: Tetracycline hydrochloride
Other examples: Oxytetracycline, demeclocycline, minocycline, doxycycline
- **Action:** Inhibits protein synthesis in bacterial cells
- **Indications:** Bacterial infections, including urinary tract infections, acne, gonorrhea, and chlamydia
- **Contraindications:** Hypersensitivity
- **Use with caution in patients with:** Renal or hepatic impairment, nephrogenic diabetes insipidus, debilitation
- **Major interactions:** Antacids, iron or calcium supplements, laxatives with magnesium
- **Administration options:** <u>Oral</u>, IV, IM
- **Notes for patient education:**
    - **Side effects:** Can cause nausea, vomiting, epigastric disturbances, diarrhea, cramping, photosensitivity, and dizziness.
    - Avoid excessive sunlight; wear sunscreen when outdoors.
    - Do not take antacids, vitamins, calcium tablets, iron supplements, or laxatives within 2 hours of taking tetracycline.
    - If diarrhea occurs, contact your doctor; do not treat with OTC drugs.
    - Take with a full glass of water.
    - Take at least 1 hour before or 2 hours after meals.
    - Take all the medication as prescribed, even if you feel well.

Macrolides
Prototype: Erythromycin
Other examples: Azithromycin, clarithromycin, dirithromycin
- **Action:** Inhibits protein synthesis in bacterial cells
- **Indications:** Bacterial infections, including bronchitis; diphtheria; Legionnaires' disease; pertussis; pneumonia; rheumatic fever; some types of venereal disease; ear, intestine, lung, urinary tract, and skin infections
- **Contraindications:** Alcohol or tartrazine sensitivity or intolerance, use of pimozide, hypersensitivity
- **Use with caution in patients with:** Hepatic or renal disease

- **Major interactions:** Warfarin, theophylline, carbamazepine, clindamycin, chloramphenicol, verapamil, diltiazem, azole antifungals, human immunodeficiency virus (HIV) protease inhibitors
- **Administration options:** <u>Oral</u>, IV
- **Notes for patient education:**
  - **Side effects:** Can cause nausea, vomiting, epigastric disturbances, diarrhea, fever, and rash.
  - Avoid fruit juice during treatment.

Estrogens & Progestins

Noncontraceptive
- **Action:** Mimics the actions of the natural hormones estrogen and progestin
- **Indications:** Postmenopausal hormone therapy (maintain reproductive organs, lower low-density lipoprotein cholesterol, increase bone mass), estrogen deficiency or imbalance
- **Contraindications:** Undiagnosed vaginal bleeding, breast cancer (past or present), thromboembolic disease, hepatic dysfunction
- **Use with caution in patients with:** Cardiovascular disease, hypertriglyceridemia
- **Major interactions:** Warfarin, insulin, oral antidiabetics
- **Administration options:** <u>Oral</u>, transdermal, vaginal, IV
- **Notes for patient education:**
  - **Side effects:** Can cause nausea, diarrhea, vomiting, anorexia, dizziness, headache, depression, breakthrough bleeding, acne, weight changes, and hypertension.
  - Postmenopausal women taking estrogens and progestins have an increased risk of heart attack, stroke, breast cancer, and blood clots.
  - Estrogens and estrogen with progestin should be used at the lowest dose for the shortest duration.
  - Women treated with combination estrogen plus progestin have a greater risk of developing dementia.

Oral Contraceptive
- **Action:** Exact mechanism unknown; acts to inhibit ovulation and thickens mucus in cervix
- **Indications:** Contraception, heavy menstrual bleeding, premenstrual dysphoric disorder, acne
- **Contraindications:** Pregnancy; thromboembolic or valvular heart disease (past or present); uncontrolled hypertension; estrogen-dependent breast or endometrial cancer; hepatic disease; diabetes with vascular involvement; abnormal vaginal bleeding; hypersensitivity
- **Use with caution in patients with:** Hypertension, obesity, hyperglycemia, history of or current cigarette smoking habit, diabetes, anticoagulant use, bleeding disorders, headaches
- **Major interactions:** Penicillins, tetracyclines, barbiturates, rifampin, antiepileptics, St. John's wort, warfarin, imipramine, theophylline
- **Administration options:** Oral
- **Notes for patient education:**
  - **Side effects:** Can cause nausea, bloating, weight gain, breast tenderness, fatigue, depression, increased appetite, migraine, and polyposis.
  - Take pill at the same time each day.
  - The use of oral contraceptives is associated with increased risk of heart attack, blood clots, stroke, liver tumors, and gallbladder disease; these risks are

Women who have a history of breast cancer, endometrial cancer, undiagnosed vaginal bleeding, liver disease, or risk of stroke should not take oral contraceptives.

higher in women with high blood pressure, high cholesterol, or diabetes and in those who smoke cigarettes.
- ○ Many antibiotics reduce contraceptive effectiveness.

Cancer Drugs

Cytotoxic Agents (Antineoplastics)

Prototype: Cyclophosphamide
Other examples: Busulfan, cisplatin, methotrexate, floxuridine, pentostatin, daunorubicin, vinblastine, etoposide, altretamine

- **Action:** Disrupts the replication of proliferating neoplastic cells (high growth fraction); may target proliferating nonneoplastic cells as well (e.g., hair follicles, bone marrow)
  - ○ **Cell cycle phase–specific (schedule-dependent) drugs:** Disrupt the replication of cells at a specific phase of the cell cycle (DNA synthesis, M phase, etc.)
  - ○ **Cell cycle phase–nonspecific drugs:** Disrupt the replication of cells at any phase of the cell cycle
- **Indications:** Cancer (lymphomas, leukemias, tumors)
  - ○ Combinations of different cytotoxic agents are used to treat specific cancers and malignancies based on type, location, progression, and so forth
- **Contraindications:** History of bone marrow suppression, hypersensitivity
- **Use with caution in patients with:** Debilitating illnesses, active infections, depleted bone marrow reserve, radiation therapy
- **Major interactions:** Drugs that suppress bone marrow, nephrotoxic agents (interactions vary widely among individual cytotoxic agents)
- **Administration options:** <u>Oral</u> (cyclophosphamide), <u>IV</u> (other cytotoxic agents), IM
- **Notes for patient education:**
  - ○ **Side effects:** Can cause severe nausea and vomiting, diarrhea, stomatitis, and hair loss.
  - ○ Drink plenty of fluids for the first 48 hours after treatment.
  - ○ May cause permanent sterility in men.
  - ○ Suppression of bone marrow increases risk of infections, uncontrolled bleeding, and anemia.
  - ○ May increase risk of developing secondary cancers.
  - ○ Cytotoxic agents often cause extreme nausea and vomiting; therefore, they are frequently prescribed with antiemetics.
  - ○ Avoid live vaccines.

Cytotoxic agents may be carcinogenic, teratogenic, or mutagenic; administer with extreme care.

MEDICATION ADMINISTRATION & LABORATORY VALUES

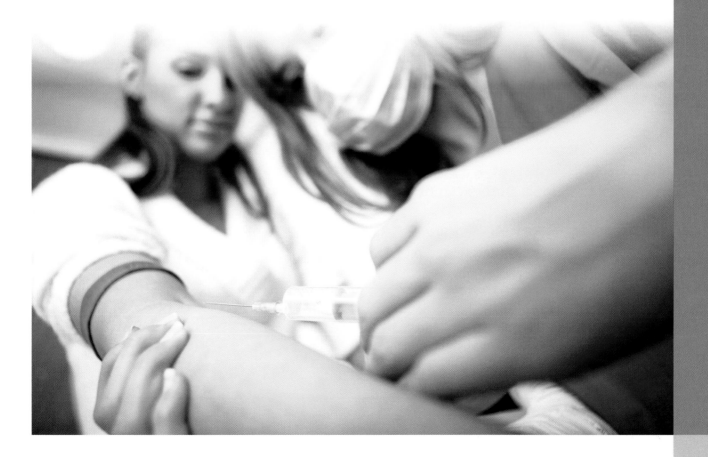

7

Introduction

Medications save lives. But if they are not administered correctly, they can also be deadly. That is why it is extremely important to have a good understanding of medication administration practices before you begin your career as a nurse. This chapter provides detailed information on how to properly administer medications. It includes dosage calculations, formulas, injection sites, intravenous (IV) flow rates, IV drip rates, and more. It also includes information about laboratory tests and common laboratory values.

Medication Administration

Routes of Administration

- **Oral:** Capsule, tablet, or liquid; absorbed in the gastrointestinal (GI) tract
- **Intravenous (IV):** Injection into the bloodstream via a vein
- **Intradermal:** Injection into the dermal layer of the skin
- **Intramuscular (IM):** Injection into muscle; can use large doses; fast systemic action
- **Intrathecal:** Injection into the spinal canal; affects spinal fluid
- **Subcutaneous (subcut):** Injection into the tissue below the dermis
- **Sublingual:** Absorbed under the tongue
- **Rectal or vaginal:** Suppositories or creams; usually for local distribution
- **Inhalation:** Absorbed in the lungs; gaseous form; rapid absorption

Five Rights of Medication Administration

1. Right patient
2. Right dose
3. Right route
4. Right time
5. Right medication

Formulas
Amount to Administer

$$\frac{\text{Dose Ordered}}{\text{Dose on Hand}} = \text{Amount to Administer}$$

Solution Concentration

$$\frac{\text{Dosage in Solution}}{\text{Volume of Solution}} = \text{Solution Concentration}$$

Body Size Calculations
Ideal Body Weight (IBW)

The Dr. Devine formula is used to calculate the dosage of certain medications:
- **For males:** 50 kg + 2.3 kg × [ht (inches) − 60] = IBW
- **For females:** 45.5 kg + 2.3 kg × [ht (inches) − 60] = IBW

Example
What is the IBW of a male who is 5'9" tall?
1. Convert height to inches: 5 ft × 12 in = 60 in + 9 in = 69 in
2. 50 kg + 2.3 kg × (69 − 60) = 50 kg + (2.3 kg × 9) = 50 kg + 20.7 kg = 70.7 kg
3. To convert to pounds (if needed): 1 kg = 2.2 lb, so 70.7 kg = 155.5 lb

---

Adjusted Body Weight (ABW)

IBW + 0.4(Actual Body Weight − IBW) = ABW

Example

What is the ABW of a female who is 5'3" and weighs 136 lb?

1. Convert height to inches: 5 ft × 12 in = 60 in + 3 in = 63 in
2. Convert weight to kilograms: 136 lb ÷ 2.2 lb/kg = 61.8 kg
3. Calculate IBW: 45.5 kg + 2.3 kg × (63 − 60) = 45.5 kg + (2.3 kg × 3) = 45.5 kg + 6.9 kg = 52.4 kg
4. Now calculate ABW: 52.4 + 0.4(61.8 − 52.4) = 52.4 + 0.4(9.4) = 52.4 + 3.8 = 56.2 kg
5. To convert to pounds (if needed): 1 kg = 2.2 lb, so 56.2 kg = 123.6 lb

Body Surface Area (BSA)

BSA is important to know when calculating dosages for many drugs; use one of the following equations to determine a patient's BSA:

$$\sqrt{\frac{\left[\text{ht (centimeters)} \times \text{wt (kilograms)}\right]}{3600}} = \text{BSA (m}^2\text{)}$$

$$\sqrt{\frac{\left[\text{ht (inches)} \times \text{wt (pounds)}\right]}{3131}} = \text{BSA (m}^2\text{)}$$

Body weight, not BSA, should be used in determining drug dosages for premature or full-term neonates.

Example

If a woman is 65" tall and weighs 145 lb, then what is her BSA in m²?

$$\sqrt{\frac{\left[\text{ht (inches)} \times \text{wt (pounds)}\right]}{3131}} = \sqrt{\frac{65 \text{ in} \times 145 \text{ lb}}{3131}} = \sqrt{\frac{9425}{3131}} = 1.74 \text{ m}^2$$

Body Mass Index (BMI)

$$\frac{\text{wt (kilograms)}}{\text{ht (meters)}^2} = \text{BMI}$$

BMI Values	
Value	**Condition**
<17.5	Anorexic
17.5–20	Underweight
20–25	Normal weight
25–30	Overweight
30–40	Obese
>40	Severe obesity

Example

What is the BMI of a male who is 6'1" and weighs 202 lb?

1. Convert height to meters: 6 ft × 12 in = 72 in + 1 in = 73 in ÷ 39.37 = 1.85 m
2. Convert weight to kilograms: 202 lb ÷ 2.2 lb/kg = 91.8 kg
3. Calculate BMI: kg/m^2 = 91.8 kg/[(1.85 m)^2] = 91.8 kg/3.42 m^2 = 26.8

Household & Metric Equivalents

Household		Metric
Volume		
—	=	1 mL*
1 tsp	=	5 mL
1 Tbsp	=	15 mL
1 cup	=	240 mL
1 pt	=	480 mL
1 qt	=	960 mL
Weight		
—	=	60–65 mg
—	=	1 g
—	=	4 g
2.2 pounds	=	1 kg
Length		
1 inch	=	2.54 cm
39.37 inches	=	1 m
*mL and cc are equivalent		

Conversion Factors

Weight		
1 gr	=	60–65 mg
1 mg	=	1000 mcg
1 g	=	1000 mg
1 kg	=	1000 g
Volume		
1 mL*	=	16 minims
5 mL	=	1 fl dr
15 mL	=	4 fl dr
30 mL	=	8 fl dr; 1 fl oz
Temperature		
°C		°F
37.0	=	98.6
37.8	=	100
38.4	=	101.1
39	=	102.2
39.6	=	103.3
°F	=	$([°C]×1.8)+32$
°C	=	$([°F]-32)÷1.8$
*mL and cc are equivalent		

Pediatric Dosage Calculations

Clark's Rule

(Weight of Child/150 lb) × Adult Dose = Child's Dose

Fried's Rule

(Age of Child in Months/150 lb) × Average Adult Dose = Child's Dose

Using BSA

BSA of Child m^2 × Average Dose per m^2 = Estimated Child's Dose

[BSA of Child m^2/Mean BSA of Adult (1.7)] × Average Adult Dose = Estimated Child's Dose

Oral Medication Dosage Calculations

Liquids

Use the following formula to find the dosage for liquids:

(Desired/Have) × Quantity = Liquid Dosage

Dosage Cup

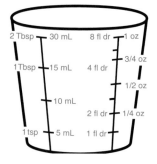

Example

Order: amoxicillin 500 mg orally (PO) daily; available: amoxicillin oral suspension
200 mg/5 mL
Use $(D/H) \times Q$:
$(500/200) \times 5$ = Liquid Dosage
$2.5 \times 5 = 12.5$ mL

Tablets & Capsules

There are two types of capsules:

- A capsule with a hard two-piece gelatin shell that may, in some cases, be opened to release powder or pellets (to be combined with soft food)
- A capsule with a soft gelatin shell

Use the following formula to find the dosage for tablets and capsules:
(Desired/Have) × Quantity = Tablet or Capsule Dosage

> Capsules should never be split, crushed, or altered; scored tablets may be split, but unscored tablets should never be split, crushed, or altered.

Example

Order: ibuprofen 1000 mg PO daily; available: ibuprofen 200 mg tablets
Use $(D/H) \times Q$:
$(1000/200) \times 1$ = Tablet Dosage
$5 \times 1 = 5$ tablets

Parenteral Medication Dosage Calculations

Parenteral medications are any medications not given through the GI tract, including IV, IM, and subcut. Use the following formula to find the dosage for liquids:
(Desired/Have) × Quantity = Liquid Dosage

Example

Order: oxacillin sodium (Bactocill) 300 mg IM every 8 hours; available: oxacillin sodium (Bactocill) 1 g/3 mL

1. First, make any necessary conversions: 1 g = 1000 mg
2. Then use $(D/H) \times Q$: $(300/1000) \times 3 = 0.3 \times 3 = 0.9$ mL
3. Because the answer is less than 1 mL, round to the nearest hundredth: 0.90 mL

> For amounts less than 1 mL, round to the nearest hundredth; for amounts greater than 1 mL, round to the nearest tenth.

Age- & Weight-Adjusted Dosage Calculations

Often, dosages are adjusted based on weight, especially for pediatric and geriatric patients.

Geriatric Example

An 82-year-old man weighs 174 pounds and is ordered amikacin sulfate. The ordered dose is 7.5 mg/kg IM twice daily (BID); the available dose is amikacin sulfate 250 mg/mL.

1. Convert weight to kilograms: 2.2 lb = 1 kg, so 174 lb = 79.0909… kg, or 79.1 kg
2. To find the dose, multiply 7.5 mg/kg by 79.1 kg: $7.5 \times 79.1 = 593.3$ mg
3. Then use $(D/H) \times Q$: $(593.3/250) \times 1 = 2.373 \times 1 = 2.4$ mL

> Other considerations must be taken into account for geriatric patients, especially any other medications that are being taken, frailty, or disease of other organs.

Pediatric Example

A 14-month-old child weighs 25 pounds and is ordered oxacillin sodium. The ordered dose is 50 mg/kg every 6 hours; the available dose is 250 mg/5 mL.

1. Convert weight to kilograms: 2.2 lb = 1 kg, so 25 lb = 11.3636… kg, or 11.4 kg
2. To find the dose, multiply 50 mg/kg by 11.4 kg: $50 \times 11.4 = 570$ mg
3. Then use $(D/H) \times Q$: $(570/250) \times 5 = 2.28 \times 5 = 11.4$ mL every 6 hours

Syringes

A syringe is an instrument used to inject or withdraw fluids. The open end of the syringe may be fitted with a hypodermic needle, a nozzle, or tubing to help direct the flow into and out of the barrel. Syringes are often used to administer injections. Types of syringes include the following:

- **Hypodermic syringe:** Used with a hypodermic needle for hypodermic injections and for aspiration because of its calibrated barrel, plunger, and tip. Syringe sizes may vary from 0.25 to 450 mL and can be made of glass or assorted plastics.
- **Insulin syringe:** Marked in insulin "units." Syringes for insulin users are designed for standard U-100 insulin. The dilution of insulin is such that 1 mL of insulin fluid has 100 standard units of insulin. Because insulin vials are typically 10 mL, each vial has 1000 units. Insulin syringes are made specifically for self-injections and have unique features: shorter needles, as insulin injections are subcut (under the skin) rather than IM; fine-gauge needles, for less pain; and markings in insulin units to simplify drawing a measured dose of insulin.
- **Oral syringe:** Handles oral medication delivery. It is available in 10 mL, 5 mL, 3 mL, and 1 mL sizes. The oral dispenser is designed to meet the demanding needs of safety, ease of use, and accuracy of dose.
- **Tuberculin (TB) syringe:** A 1 mL syringe with a fixed needle. Not to be used as an insulin syringe.

Choosing a Needle

Needles come in different lengths and gauges. The higher the gauge, the thinner the needle. The size you will need to use will depend on the type of injection you are giving and the size of the patient. Larger patients with a lot of tissue will require a larger needle.

Selecting a Needle Size & Gauge		
Type of Injection	**Length of Needle (in inches)**	**Gauge**
Intradermal	½	26–28
Subcut	½–⅝	25–30
IM	1–1½	20–22

Intradermal Injection Sites

Intradermal injections are normally done for allergy testing and for TB screening. The needle is inserted at a 10- to 15-degree angle into the dermal layer of the skin.

Inner Forearm

The inner forearm is the most common transdermal injection site. The injection is given on the flat portion of the inner surface of the forearm. The patient should be seated with the palm facing upward and the arm braced or supported.

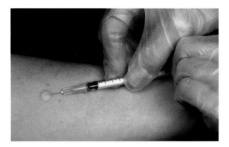

Subscapular Region

An injection in the subscapular region is given on the upper back below the shoulder blades.

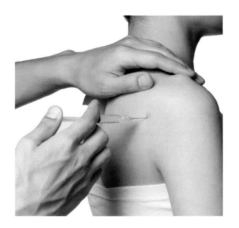

Subcutaneous Injection Sites

Subcutaneous injections are used to administer medications that need to be absorbed slowly. The needle is inserted at a 45- to 90-degree angle in the fatty tissue just under the skin.

Arm

An arm injection is given in the lateral aspect of the upper arm, at least one hand's width below the shoulder and one hand's width above the elbow.

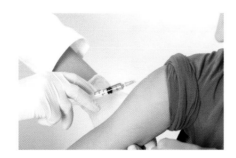

Thigh

A thigh injection is given anywhere between the middle of the anterior thigh and the middle of the lateral thigh, at least one hand's width below the hip and one hand's width above the knee.

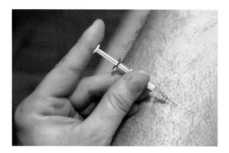

Abdomen

An abdomen injection is given between the waist and the hip, from where the abdomen begins to curve to approx. 2 inches from the center.

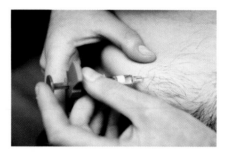

Insulin Types & Action Times				
Action	**Type of Subcut Insulin**	**Onset**	**Peak**	**Duration**
Rapid	Lispro (Humalog)	<15 min	30–90 min	3–5 hr
	NovoLog	<20 min	40–50 min	3–5 hr
Short	Regular	0.5–1 hr	2–4 hr	5–8 hr
	Semilente	1–1.5 hr	5–10 hr	12–16 hr
Intermediate	NPH	1–1.5 hr	4–12 hr	18–24 hr
	Lente	1–2.5 hr	7–15 hr	18–24 hr
Long	Lantus	1–1.5 hr	No true peak	20–24 hr
	Ultralente	30 min–3 hr	10–20 hr	20–36 hr
Premixed	Humulin/Novolin/ NovoLog	10–30 min	1–12 hr	14–24 hr

Intramuscular Injection Sites

Intramuscular injections are used to administer fast-acting medications. The needle is inserted at a 90-degree angle into the muscle.

Mid-Deltoid Area

The recommended boundaries of the injection area form a rectangle bounded by the lower edge of the acromion process on the top to a point on the lateral side of the arm opposite the axilla (armpit) on the bottom. Avoid the acromion and humerus, as well as the brachial veins and arteries. Limit the number of injections here, as the area is small and cannot tolerate repeated injections or quantities of medications greater than 1 mL.

Ventrogluteal Area

This is the site of choice for adults and infants older than 12 months, as it is removed from major nerves and vascular structures. Palpate to find the greater trochanter, the anterior superior iliac spine, and the iliac crest. When injecting into the left side of the patient, place the palm of the right hand on the greater trochanter and the index finger on the anterior superior iliac spine. Spread the middle finger posteriorly away from the index finger as far as possible along the iliac crest, as shown in the figure. A "V" space or triangle between the index and middle finger is formed. The injection is made in the center of the triangle, with the needle directed slightly upward, toward the crest of the ilium. When injecting into the right side of the patient, use your left hand for placement.

Vastus Lateralis Area

This is a relatively safe injection site, free from major nerves and blood vessels. This injection area is bounded by the mid-anterior thigh on the front of the leg, the mid-lateral thigh on the side, a hand's width below the greater trochanter of the femur at the proximal end, and another hand's width above the knee at the distal end.

Mid-Deltoid Injection

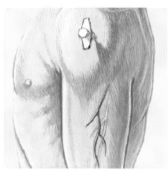

Ventrogluteal Injection

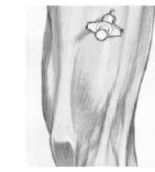

Vastus Lateralis Injection

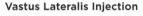

Z-Track Technique

A Z-track technique is used for administering any irritating fluid to "seal" medication in the muscle (see figure). Retract the tissue, insert the needle, administer the medication, remove the needle, and release the tissue. In the figure, note the tissue relationships after the angled Z-track left by the needle.

Z-Track Technique

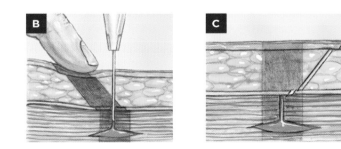

Common IV Solutions

- **Isotonic:** Dextrose 5% in water (D_5W); 0.9% sodium chloride (NaCl); lactated Ringer's (LR) solution
- **Hypertonic:** $D_{10}W$; 3% NaCl; 5% NaCl; D_5LR, $D_50.45\%$ NaCl; $D_50.9\%$ NaCl
- **Hypotonic:** $D_{2.5}W$; 0.45% NaCl; 0.33% NaCl

Catheters

A catheter is a small, flexible, tubular medical device for insertion into canals, vessels, passageways, or body cavities, usually to permit injection or withdrawal of fluids, to keep a passage open, or to obtain pressure readings. There are several types of catheters:

- **Arterial catheter, arterial line, or art-line:** A thin catheter inserted into an artery. It is most commonly used in intensive care medicine to monitor blood pressure (BP) in real time (rather than by intermittent measurement) and to obtain samples for arterial blood gas (ABG) measurements. It is not generally used to administer medication. An arterial line is usually inserted into the wrist (radial artery), but it can also be inserted into the elbow (brachial artery), groin (femoral artery), foot (pedal artery), or neck (carotid artery).
- **Butterfly catheter:** A metal needle with flexible plastic wings and a short length of tubing. The wings assist in placement in a vein and facilitate fixation with tape.
- **Central venous catheter, or central line:** A small, flexible plastic tube inserted into a large vein above the heart, usually the subclavian vein, to gain access to the bloodstream. This allows drugs and blood products to be given and blood samples to be painlessly withdrawn. Some of the catheters have more than one lumen (channel), either a double or triple, and can be used to administer more than one drug simultaneously. Such catheters can be left in place for many weeks to months.
- **Epidural catheter:** A thin plastic catheter placed between two bones in the back by an anesthesiologist. Where the catheter is placed in the back depends on the type of surgery or procedure planned and the medicine to be received.
- **Groshong catheter:** A tunneled IV catheter used for central venous access. Groshong lines may be left in place for extended periods and are used when long-term IV therapy is needed, such as for chemotherapy. The tip of the catheter is in the superior vena cava, and the catheter is tunneled under the skin to an incision on the chest wall. Where the distal end of the catheter exits the body, the Groshong line has a three-way valve that allows infusion, as well as blood aspiration, while reducing the risk of clotting, air embolism, and blood reflux.
- **Over-the-needle catheter:** A catheter that is introduced into the vein by a needle, which is subsequently removed; the catheter remains in place. An incision is made over the filled vein, and the needle cannula is inserted; the stylet is withdrawn first, then the needle, leaving the plastic cannula in situ.
- **Peripheral venous catheter (PVC), peripheral venous line, or peripheral venous access catheter:** A small, flexible catheter placed into a peripheral vein to administer medication or fluids. Once placed, the line can also be used to draw blood. The catheter is introduced into the vein by a needle (similar to blood drawing), which is subsequently removed while the small tube of the cannula remains in place. The catheter is then fixed by taping it to the patient's skin.
- **Peripherally inserted central catheter (PICC) line:** A form of IV access that can be used for a prolonged period of time (e.g., for chemotherapy regimens, extended antibiotic therapy, or total parenteral nutrition). It is an alternative to subclavian lines, internal jugular lines, or femoral lines, which have higher rates of infection. A PICC is inserted in a peripheral vein, such as the cephalic vein, basilic vein, or brachial vein, and then advanced through increasingly larger veins toward the heart until the tip rests in the distal superior vena cava or cavoatrial junction.

- **Port or Port-A-Cath:** A small medical appliance that is installed beneath the skin. A catheter connects the port to a vein. Under the skin, the port has a septum through which drugs can be injected and blood samples can be drawn many times, usually with less discomfort for the patient than a more typical needle stick.
- **Swan-Ganz catheter:** A soft, flow-directed catheter with a balloon at the tip for measuring pulmonary arterial pressures.
- **Umbilical catheter:** A catheter placed in the vessels of a neonate's umbilical cord.
  - **Umbilical artery catheter (UAC):** Allows blood to be taken from an infant at different times, without repeated needle sticks. It can also be used to continuously monitor a baby's BP. A UAC is most often used if a neonate needs mechanical ventilation or very strong medicines to treat BP problems.
  - **Umbilical venous catheter (UVC):** Allows fluids and medications to be given without having to frequently replace an IV line. This type of catheter may be used if a neonate is very premature, has bowel problems that prevent feeding, or needs very strong medicines to treat BP problems.

IV Flow Rate

IV flow rate can be measured in drops per minute (gtt/min) or milliliters per hour (mL/hr).

Measuring gtt/min

Calculation: Total Volume to Be Given (in mL)/Time (in Minutes) × Drop Factor = gtt/min

Example

Order: nicardipine 10 mg in 25 mL over 1 hour; drop factor = 15
1. First, convert hours to minutes: 1 hour = 60 minutes

2. Then calculate rate: $\dfrac{25 \text{ mL}}{60} \times 15 = 6.25$

3. Round to the nearest whole number: 6 gtt/min

Measuring mL/hr

Calculation: Total Volume to Be Given (in mL)/Infusion Time (in Hours) = mL/hr

Example

Order: IV saline 1000 mL over 4 hours

Calculation: $\dfrac{1000 \text{ mL}}{4 \text{ hr}} = 250 \text{ mL/hr}$

Solution Preparation Calculations

Directions for reconstitution of solutions give volumes of fluids to be added; once they are added, those volumes do not matter. Calculate dosages using the same formula method as for other parenteral or oral liquid medications:

(Desired/Have) × Quantity = Dosage

Example

Order: cefazolin 0.3 g IM; available: cefazolin 500 mg powder; add 2 mL of sterile water to obtain a concentration of 225 mg/mL

1. First, make any necessary conversions: 0.3 g = 300 mg
2. Then use $(D/H) \times Q$: $(300/225) \times 1 = 1.3333\ldots$ mL
3. Since the answer is greater than 1 mL, round to the nearest tenth: 1.3 mL

Laboratory Values

Laboratory Tests

- **Arterial blood gas (ABG):** Used to determine the concentrations of gases, such as carbon dioxide, oxygen, and bicarbonate, in blood, as well as its pH. It involves puncturing an artery with a thin needle and syringe, and then drawing a small volume of blood. The most common puncture site is the radial artery at the wrist, but sometimes the femoral artery in the groin or other sites are used.
- **Basic metabolic panel (BMP):** A set of eight blood chemical tests, including four electrolytes (sodium [Na^+], potassium [K^+], chloride [Cl^-], and bicarbonate [HCO_3^-]), blood urea nitrogen (BUN), creatinine, glucose, and calcium.
- **Bleeding time:** A test to assess platelet function.
- **Blood culture:** A test to check for bacteria or other microorganisms in a blood sample. Most cultures check for bacteria. A minimum of 10 mL of blood is taken through venipuncture and injected into two or more "blood bottles" with specific media for aerobic and anaerobic organisms.
- **Cerebrospinal fluid (CSF) culture:** A laboratory test to look for bacteria, fungi, and viruses in the clear fluid that moves in the space surrounding the spinal cord.
- **Coagulation screen:** A series of laboratory tests to determine how well the blood is clotting. A coagulation screen is used to determine the effectiveness of anticoagulant therapy, to diagnose clotting disorders, and to check blood clotting ability prior to surgery.
- **Complete blood count (CBC):** A test that gives information about the cells in a patient's blood. The cells that circulate in the bloodstream are generally divided into three types: white blood cells (WBCs; leukocytes), red blood cells (RBCs; erythrocytes), and platelets (thrombocytes). Abnormally high or low counts may indicate the presence of many forms of disease. Hence, blood counts are among the most commonly performed blood tests, as they can provide an overview of a patient's general health status.
- **Comprehensive metabolic panel:** A group of tests that provide an overall picture of the body's metabolism.
- **Erythrocyte sedimentation rate (ESR), or sedimentation rate:** The rate at which RBCs precipitate in a period of 1 hour. An ESR test indirectly measures the amount of inflammation in the body.
- **Fecal occult blood:** A term for checking for hidden (occult) blood in the stool (feces).
- **Glycated or glycosylated hemoglobin (hemoglobin A_{1c}, Hb_{1c}, Hb_{A1c}, A1C):** A form of hemoglobin used primarily to identify the average plasma glucose concentration over prolonged periods of time. It is formed in a nonenzymatic pathway by hemoglobin's normal exposure to high plasma levels of glucose.
- **Liver function tests (LFTs or LFs):** Groups of laboratory blood assays that include liver enzymes and are designed to give information about the state of a patient's liver. Most liver diseases cause only mild symptoms initially, so it is vital that these diseases be detected early. Hepatic involvement in some diseases can be of crucial

importance.

- **Platelet count:** A test to measure the number of platelets in the blood. If the number of platelets is too low, excessive bleeding can occur; however, if the number of platelets is too high, blood clots (thrombi) can form. These can block blood vessels and may cause a stroke or heart attack.
- **Serology:** The scientific study of blood serum. In practice, the term usually refers to the diagnostic identification of antibodies in the serum. Such antibodies are typically formed in response to infection, invasion of foreign proteins (e.g., in response to a mismatched blood transfusion), or autoimmune disease. Serologic tests may be performed for diagnostic purposes when an infection is suspected, in rheumatic illnesses, and in many other situations, such as checking an individual's blood type. Serology blood tests help to diagnose patients with certain immune deficiencies associated with the lack of antibodies.
- **Serum total protein, or total protein:** A biochemical test for measuring the total amount of protein in blood plasma or serum.

CBC & Differential		
CBC Component	**Adult**	
	Male	**Female**
RBCs	$4.7–6 \times 10^6$/mcL	$4.2–5.4 \times 10^6$/mcL
Hematocrit (Hct)	42%–52%	37%–47%
Hemoglobin (Hgb)	13.5–18 g/dL	12–16 g/dL
RBC indices		
Mean corpuscular volume (MCV)	78–100 fL	
Mean corpuscular Hgb (MCH)	27–31 pg	
Mean corpuscular Hgb conc. (MCHC)	33–37 g/dL	
WBCs	4K–10.5K/mcL	
Differential WBCs		
Neutrophils	1.5K–6.6K/mcL	
Bands	<1K/mcL	
Eosinophils	<0.7K/mcL	
Basophils	<0.1K/mcL	
Monocytes	<1K/mcL	
Lymphocytes	1.5K–3.5K/mcL	
T lymphocytes	60%–80% of lymphocytes	
B lymphocytes	4%–16% of lymphocytes	
Platelets	150K–300K/mcL	

Comprehensive Metabolic Panel

	Normal Adult Range*	Conditions with Abnormal Findings	
		Increased	Decreased
Blood urea nitrogen (BUN)	6–20 mg/dL	Congestive heart failure (CHF), excessive protein in the GI tract, GI bleeding, heart attack, hypovolemia, kidney disease, kidney failure, shock, urinary tract obstruction	Liver failure, low protein diet, malnutrition, overhydration
Sodium (Na)	135–145 mEq/L	CHF, dehydration, diabetes, diaphoresis, diarrhea, hypertension, ostomies, toxemia, vomiting	Ascites in cardiac failure, bowel obstruction, burns, diarrhea, cirrhosis, emphysema, GI malabsorption
Potassium (K)	3.7–5.2 mEq/L	Acidosis, adrenocortical insufficiency, anemia, anxiety, asthma, burns, dialysis, dysrhythmias, hypoventilation	Alcoholism, alkalosis, bradycardia, CHF, chronic cirrhosis, colon cancer, Crohn disease, diarrhea, diuretics, GI suction, intestinal fistulas, vomiting
Glucose	70–100 mg/dL (fasting)	Prediabetes, diabetes, hyperthyroidism, pancreatic cancer, pancreatitis	Hyperinsulinism, hypopituitarism, hypothyroidism, insulin overdose, malnutrition, transient hypoglycemia
Creatinine	0.6–1.3 mg/dL	ATN, CHF, dehydration, diabetic nephropathy, glomerulonephritis, kidney failure, muscular dystrophy, preeclampsia, pyelonephritis, rhabdomyolysis, shock, urinary tract obstruction	Muscular dystrophy (late stage), myasthenia gravis
Calcium (Ca)	8.5–10.2 mg/dL	ATN, bacteremia, chronic hepatic disease, respiratory acidosis	Alkalosis, burns, cachexia, celiac disease, chronic renal disease, diarrhea, GI malabsorption
Albumin	3.4–5.4 g/dL	Dehydration	Kidney disease, liver disease

Comprehensive Metabolic Panel (continued)

	Normal Adult Range*	Conditions with Abnormal Findings	
		Increased	Decreased
Total bilirubin	0.3–1.9 mg/dL	Biliary stricture, cirrhosis, gallstones, Gilbert disease, hepatitis, pancreatic or gallbladder cancer	N/A
Aspartate transaminase/serum glutamic-oxaloacetic transaminase (AST/SGOT)	10–34 U/L	Acute pancreatitis, cirrhosis, heart attack, hepatitis, kidney failure, liver cancer, mononucleosis	N/A
Alanine aminotransaminase/serum glutamic-pyruvic transaminase (ALT/SGPT)	7–56 U/L	Acute pancreatitis, cirrhosis, heart attack, hepatitis, liver cancer, mononucleosis	N/A
Alkaline phosphatase	44–147 U/L	Biliary obstruction, bone cancer, cirrhosis, hepatitis, hyperparathyroidism, Paget disease, leukemia, lymphoma	Malnutrition, protein deficiency, Wilson disease

* Ranges may vary by lab.

Lipid Profile	
Total cholesterol	<200 mg/dL
High-density lipoprotein	40–60 mg/dL
Low-density lipoprotein	<130 mg/dL
Triglycerides	<150 mg/dL

Drugs

Most Dangerous Drugs	
Drug Type	**Examples**
Anticoagulants	Heparin, warfarin
Antimicrobials	Cephalosporins, penicillins, sulfonamides
Bronchodilators	Theophylline, sympathomimetics
Cardiac drugs	Quinidine, digoxin, diuretics, antihypertensives
Central nervous system drugs	Sedative-hypnotics, neuroleptics, anticonvulsants, analgesics
Diagnostic agents	Radiographic contrast media
Hormones	Insulin, estrogens, corticosteroids

Drugs Causing Confusion in Older Adults

Antiarrhythmics, anticholinergics, antiemetics, antihistamines, antihypertensives, anti-parkinsonian agents, antipsychotics, diuretics, histamine blockers, opioid analgesics, sedative-hypnotics, and tranquilizers can all cause confusion in older adults.

Pharmacokinetics in Older Adults

The ways in which older adults absorb, distribute, metabolize, and eliminate drugs may affect the efficacy of their medications.

- **Absorption:** Change in quantity and quality of digestive enzymes, increased gastric pH, decreased number of absorbing cells, decreased GI motility, decreased intestinal blood flow, decreased GI emptying time
- **Distribution:** Decreased cardiac output and reserve; decreased blood flow to liver, kidneys, and target tissues; decreased distribution area and space; decreased lean body mass; increased stores of adipose; decreased plasma protein; decreased total body water
- **Metabolism:** Decreased microsomal metabolism of drug, decreased hepatic biotransformation
- **Elimination:** Decreased renal excretion of drug, decreased glomerular filtration, decreased renal tubular secretion

SPECIALTY NURSING

8

Introduction

Nurses can work in a variety of settings. Many work in hospital medical-surgical units; others choose to specialize. This chapter will discuss some of the more common nursing specialties. It includes information about pediatric nursing, obstetrics, and surgical nursing.

Pediatric Nursing

Pediatric nurses care for children and their families. Some pediatric nurses work in hospitals; others work in physicians' offices, ambulatory care centers, or home health care.

Classifications of Young Patients	
Age	**Classification**
<38 weeks' gestation	Premature or preterm infant
<1 month	Neonate or newborn infant
1 month to 1 year	Infant
1 year to 12 years	Child

Expected Growth Rates for Infants & Children	
Age	**Expected Growth Rate per Year**
1–6 months	18–22 cm
6–12 months	14–18 cm
Second year	11 cm
Third year	8 cm
Fourth year	7 cm
Fifth to tenth years	5–6 cm

Timeline of Childhood Milestones	
Age	**Milestone**
2 months	Smiles at the sound of a familiar voice
3 months	Raises head and chest when lying on stomach, grasps objects, smiles at other people
4 months	Babbles, laughs, tries to imitate sounds
6 months	Rolls from back to stomach

Human Growth & Development

The **cephalocaudal principle** describes the progression of a child's development. Remember *cephalo-* refers to the head and *caudal* refers to the tail or base of the spine.

- **Infancy:** Gains control of eye movements; smiles, coos, grasps objects, rolls over, sits; birth weight doubles.
- **Early childhood:** Walks, talks, identifies common objects, undergoes toilet training.
- **Preschool:** Develops gross motor skills (pedaling, hopping on one foot, kicking, catching a ball) and fine motor skills (drawing, using scissors, dressing self), follows commands.
- **School age:** Has strong motor skills; grammar and pronunciation become normal.
- **Adolescence:** Experiences rapid growth, understands abstract ideas, establishes relationships.
  - **Girls:** Breast development, hair growth (pubic, armpits, arms, legs), menarche.

- **Boys:** Genital growth, hair growth (pubic, armpits, arms, legs, chest, face); voice changes.
- **Young adulthood:** Experiences minimal physical growth, develops lasting relationships; physical performance, strength, and flexibility peak.
- **Middle adulthood:** Experiences hair loss and graying, develops fine lines and wrinkles; hearing and eyesight decline, menopause occurs (in women).
- **Late adulthood:** Slowing of all major organs and systems.

Erikson's Stages of Psychosocial Development
- **Trust versus mistrust (birth–18 months):** When needs are met, the child develops trust; if the caregiver is unreliable or inconsistent, mistrust develops.
- **Autonomy versus shame and doubt (18 months–3 years):** Successfully conquering new skills leads to a sense of autonomy; a lack of success in learning new skills can lead to shame and doubt.
- **Initiative versus guilt (3–5 years):** The child becomes more assertive in order to feel more in control over his or her environment; if the parents approve of the child's attempts to take the initiative, the child develops a sense of purpose. Disapproval can lead to feelings of guilt.
- **Industry versus inferiority (6–11 years):** The child goes to school and begins to acquire new social and learning skills; failure can lead to feelings of inferiority.
- **Identity versus role confusion (12–18 years):** The adolescent or teen begins to develop a sense of self or identity; failure can lead to confusion or identity crisis.
- **Intimacy versus isolation (19–40 years):** The adult forms intimate relationships with others; failure can lead to feelings of isolation.
- **Generativity versus stagnation (40–65 years):** Those in middle adulthood need to feel that they are doing something worthwhile that will outlast them; failure may lead to a societal disconnect and shallow relationships.
- **Ego integrity versus despair (65 years and older):** Older adults need to look back and feel that their lives were well-lived and had meaning; failure can lead to feelings of despair.

Common Childhood Diseases
- **Chickenpox:** A highly contagious virus that is characterized by itchy, fluid-filled blisters on the skin. A vaccine is available for the prevention of chickenpox.
- **Respiratory syncytial virus (RSV):** A respiratory virus that infects the lungs and airways. Symptoms may include runny nose, decreased appetite, coughing, sneezing, fever, and wheezing.
- **Whooping cough (pertussis):** A highly contagious respiratory disease that is characterized by uncontrollable, violent coughing fits followed by a "whooping" sound. A vaccine is available for the prevention of whooping cough.
- **Fifth disease (erythema infectiosum):** A virus that is characterized by a red facial rash that is known as a "slapped cheek" rash. Other symptoms may include runny nose, fever, and headache.
- **Hand, foot, and mouth disease:** A virus that is characterized by blister-like sores in the mouth and a skin rash (usually on the hands and/or feet). Other symptoms may include fever and malaise.
- **Croup:** An infection that is characterized by a "barking cough." Other symptoms may include cold-like symptoms and difficulty breathing.
- **Scarlet fever:** A strep infection that is characterized by a red rash that feels like sandpaper. Other symptoms may include sore throat, fever, chills, vomiting, and abdominal pain.
- **Impetigo:** A skin infection that is characterized by itchy, pus-filled blisters. Other symptoms may include a rash that spreads with scratching and swollen lymph nodes.

Childhood Immunizations

Recommended Immunizations for Birth–6 Years

Birth	1 mo	2 mo	4 mo	6 mo	12 mo	15 mo	18 mo	19–23 mo	2–3 yr	4–6 yr
HepB	HepB			HepB						
		RV	RV	RV						
		DTaP	DTaP	DTaP		DTaP				DTaP
		Hib	Hib	Hib	Hib					
		PCV	PCV	PCV	PCV					
		IPV	IPV	IPV						IPV
				Influenza (yearly)						
					MMR					MMR
					Varicella					Varicella
					HepA					

Key: Shaded boxes indicate the vaccine can be given during shown age range.

Recommended Immunizations for Ages 7–18 Years

7–10 yr	11–12 yr	13–18 yr
Tdap	Tdap	Tdap
	HPV (3 doses)	HPV
MCV4	MCV4 dose 1	MCV4 dose 1 / Booster at age 16 yr
Influenza (yearly)		
PCV		
HepA		
HepB		
IPV		
MMR		
Varicella		

Key:
Yellow: These shaded boxes indicate when the vaccine is recommended for all children unless a doctor says the child cannot safely receive the vaccine.
Green: These shaded boxes indicate the vaccine should be given if a child is catching up on missed vaccines.
Purple: These shaded boxes indicate the vaccine is recommended for children with certain health conditions that put them at high risk for serious diseases. Note that healthy children can get the HepA series.

Vaccine abbreviation key: DTaP = Diphtheria, pertussis, and tetanus; HepA = Hepatitis A; HepB = Hepatitis B; Hib = *Haemophilus influenzae* type b; HPV = Human papillomavirus; IPV = Polio; MCV4 = Meningococcal conjugate vaccine; MMR = Measles, mumps, rubella; PCV = Pneumococcal conjugate vaccine; RV = Rotavirus; Tdap = Tetanus, diphtheria, and pertussis.

Note: Tdap vaccine is a combination vaccine that is recommended at age 11 or 12 to protect against tetanus, diphtheria, and pertussis. If a child has not received any or all of the DTaP vaccine series or if the parent or guardian does not know if the child has received these shots, the child needs a single dose of Tdap when he or she is 7–10 years old. Check with the child's health care provider to find out if the child needs additional catch-up vaccines.

Source: Centers for Disease Control and Prevention, 2013.

Obstetrics

Obstetrical nurses care for patients who are pregnant, who are in the process of giving birth, or who have just given birth. Obstetrical nurses may work in a hospital (labor and delivery), a doctor's office, or an outpatient clinic.

Definitions

- **Perinatal**
  - **Perinatal period:** From before birth through day 28 after birth
  - **Prematurity:** Birth prior to completion of 37 weeks' gestation
  - **Low birth weight (LBW):** Baby born weighing less than 2500 grams (5 lb, 8 oz)
  - **Full term:** Gestation week 38–40 (266–280 days)
- **Prenatal periods**
  - **Embryonic period:** Gestation week 2–8
  - **Fetal period:** Gestation week 9 through delivery
- **Postpartum period:** First 6 weeks after childbirth
  - **Puerperium period:** From the end of labor until the uterus returns to normal size (typically 3–6 weeks)

Common Pregnancy Complications

Complication	Symptoms	Potential Causes
Bleeding	Vaginal bleeding	Vaginal bleeding during pregnancy (especially during the first trimester) is common and may not be a sign of a problem; potential problems include miscarriage, premature labor, ectopic pregnancy, placenta previa, cervical cancer
Gestational hypertension	High blood pressure during pregnancy; usually no symptoms, but may have headache, blurred vision	Unknown
Gestational diabetes	High blood sugar during pregnancy; usually no symptoms, but may have fatigue, increased thirst, increased urination, weight loss	Hormonal changes that lead to progressive impaired glucose intolerance
Eclampsia	Seizures that are not related to a preexisting brain condition; muscle pain; agitation; loss of consciousness	Blood vessel problems, neurological factors, genetics
Ectopic pregnancy	Pregnancy outside the uterus (usually in the fallopian tube); symptoms may include vaginal bleeding, abdominal or pelvic pain	Damage to the fallopian tube due to previous infection, endometriosis, or pelvic surgery
Preterm labor	Labor before 37 weeks' gestation; symptoms may include abdominal cramping, pressure in the abdomen or pelvis, contractions, vaginal bleeding, lower back pain	Smoking, drug abuse, multiple pregnancy (more than one fetus), infection, hypertension, diabetes
Placenta previa	Placenta covering the cervix; symptoms may include cramps, vaginal bleeding in the second or third trimester	Abnormal shape or size of uterus; multiple pregnancy (more than one fetus); uterine scarring from previous pregnancies, C-section, or surgery
Preeclampsia	Hypertension and proteinuria after the 20th week of pregnancy; symptoms may include edema, sudden weight gain, pain in the right upper quadrant, decreased urine output, nausea and vomiting, headaches, vision problems	Autoimmune disorders, poor nutrition, blood vessel damage

Nursing Care during Labor

- Monitor fetal heart rate via auscultation or external fetal monitor. (Optimal is 120–160 beats per minute [bpm].)
- Monitor mother's vital signs.
- Assess frequency, duration, and intensity of contractions by palpating uterine fundus.
- Perform vaginal examination; assess:
  - Dilation (use index and middle fingers to measure the size of the opening)
  - Effacement (thinning and shortening of the cervix)
  - Membrane status (ruptured or intact)
  - Station (the relationship between the baby's presenting part and the mother's ischial spines)
  - Fetal presentation and position (via vaginal examination and Leopold maneuvers)
  - Bloody show (amount and character)

Postpartum Care

Assess:
- **Uterus:** Fundal height, involution
- **Perineum:** Edema, infection, hematoma
- **Lochia:** Color, amount
- **Breasts:** Engorgement
- **Voiding:** Frequency, amount, bladder distention
- **Pain:** Location, intensity, duration

Newborn Assessment

- APGAR score
- Weight
- Measurement
- Vital signs
  - **Blood pressure (BP):** 65–85/45–55 mm Hg
  - **Pulse:** 120–160 bpm
  - **Respiratory rate (RR):** 30–50 breaths per minute
  - **Temperature:** 98.6°F–99.8°F (37°C–37.7°C)
- General appearance
- Skin
- Head and neck (appearance, shape, fontanels)
- Breath sounds
- Heart sounds
- Gastrointestinal (GI) and genitourinary (GU) systems
- Extremities

APGAR Score			
Signs	**0**	**1**	**2**
Activity	No muscle tone	Some muscle tone	Active motion
Pulse	No pulse	<100 bpm	>100 bpm
Grimace (reflex in response to stimulation)	No reaction	Grimace	Grimace and cough, sneeze, or cry
Appearance	Pale blue body and extremities	Pink body, blue extremities	Pink body and extremities
Respiration	No breathing	Slow or irregular breathing	Strong cry
Note: A normal APGAR score is 7–9.			

Surgical Nursing

Surgical nurses provide care and support to patients before, during, and after surgery. Surgical nurses may work in pre- or postoperative care units, as well as in operating rooms (ORs); they are a critical part of the surgical care team. Surgical nurses may be employed by freestanding surgery clinics, hospital trauma or emergency centers, or hospital surgical suites.

Categories of Surgical Procedures

- **Diagnostic:** Procedures performed to determine the origin and cause of a disorder or the cell type of a cancer. Examples include the following:
  - Breast biopsy
  - Exploratory laparotomy
- **Curative:** Procedures performed to resolve a health problem by repairing or removing the cause. Examples include the following:
  - Cholelithotomy
  - Mastectomy
  - Hysterectomy
- **Restorative:** Procedures performed to improve a patient's functional ability. Examples include the following:
  - Total knee replacement(s)
  - Finger reimplantation
- **Palliative:** Procedures performed to relieve symptoms of, but not cure, a disease process. Examples include the following:
  - Tumor debulking
  - Ileostomy
  - Nerve root resection
- **Cosmetic:** Procedures performed primarily to alter or enhance a person's appearance. Examples include the following:
  - Rhinoplasty
  - Liposuction
  - Blepharoplasty
  - Breast augmentation
- **Minimally invasive:** Procedures performed using a laparoscopic device or remote-controlled instrument manipulation with indirect observation of the surgical field through an endoscope or other device. Examples include the following:
  - Gastric banding
  - Tubal ligation

> Happiness is not a feeling; it is a choice. Choose to be a happy nurse. Happiness is contagious. Your coworkers, superiors, and patients will catch your happiness.

Urgency of Surgery

- **Elective:** Procedures that are planned in advance and intended to correct nonacute problems. Examples include the following:
  - Cataract removal
  - Hernia repair
  - Total joint replacement
- **Urgent:** Procedures for conditions that require prompt intervention and whose delay may be life threatening. Examples include the following:
  - Bowel obstruction
  - Wound dehiscence
  - Kidney stones
- **Emergency:** Procedures for conditions that require immediate intervention because of life-threatening consequences. Examples include the following:
  - Gunshot or stab wound
  - Severe bleeding

Classification of Surgery

- **Clean surgery:** No viscera opened (e.g., hernia repair)
  - **Infection rate:** Typically 1%–2%
- **Clean-contaminated:** Viscera opened but no spillage of gut contents (e.g., right hemicolectomy)
  - **Infection rate:** Usually <10%
- **Contaminated:** Viscera opened with inflammation or spillage of contents (e.g., colectomy for obstruction)
  - **Infection rate:** Typically 15%–20%
- **Dirty:** Intraperitoneal abscess formation or visceral perforation (e.g., ruptured appendix)
  - **Infection rate:** 40%

Common Drugs That Can Cause Surgical Complications

- **Aminoglycosides (amikacin, gentamicin, kanamycin, neomycin, streptomycin, tobramycin):** Greater risk of neuromuscular blockade, respiratory paralysis
- **Antianxiety drugs (diazepam [Valium]):** Excessive sedation; preoperative or postoperative nausea and vomiting; local tissue irritation (with intravenous [IV] administration)
- **Antiarrhythmics (all types):** Intensified cardiac depression and reduced cardiac output; laryngospasm
- **Antibiotics (all types):** Masked infection symptoms
- **Anticholinergics (atropine sulfate):** Increased intraocular pressure (IOP); dilated pupils; blurred vision; excessive mouth dryness, tachycardia, and flushing and decreased sweating; urine retention; agitation and delirium in elderly patients
- **Anticoagulants (heparin sodium, warfarin [Coumadin]):** Increased hemorrhage risk
- **Anticonvulsants (magnesium sulfate):** Increased neuromuscular blockade risk
- **Antidiabetics (insulin):** Increased requirement for insulin during stress and healing; decreased requirement for insulin during fasting
- **Antihypertensives (all types):** Hypotension
- **Central nervous system (CNS) depressants (alcohol, sedative hypnotics):** Increased risk of respiratory depression, hypotension, or apnea if given with general anesthetics
- **Corticosteroids (betamethasone, cortisone, dexamethasone, hydrocortisone, methylprednisolone, prednisolone, prednisone, triamcinolone):** Acute adrenal insufficiency risk, delayed wound healing, masked infection symptoms, increased risk of infection, increased risk of hemorrhage
- **Diuretics (furosemide [Lasix], potassium-wasting diuretics):** Increased risk of complications associated with hypokalemia; increased risk of hypotension if given with certain anesthetics
- **Erythromycin (Erythrocin, E-Mycin):** Prolonged action of opiates
- **Glycopyrrolate (Robinul):** Increased IOP; urine retention; excessive mouth dryness, tachycardia, flushing, and decreased sweating
- **Histamine 2 (H$_2$) receptor antagonists (cimetidine [Tagamet], ranitidine [Zantac]):** Decreased clearance of all drugs, especially propranolol, diazepam, and lidocaine
- **Hydroxyzine hydrochloride (Vistaril):** Dry mouth and drowsiness
- **Midazolam hydrochloride:** Respiratory depression (with high doses)
- **Miotics (demecarium, echothiophate, isoflurophate):** Increased risk of neuromuscular blockade, cardiovascular collapse, apnea, or prolonged respiratory depression if given with succinylcholine
- **Nonsteroidal anti-inflammatory drugs (celecoxib, ibuprofen, meloxicam, naproxen, rofecoxib):** Increased risk of bleeding or hemorrhage

Be cautious, but do not be afraid. Challenge yourself, and present yourself with confidence.

- **Opiates (all types):** Increased risk of respiratory depression, hypotension, or apnea if given with certain IV anesthetics, such as midazolam, propofol, droperidol, and thiopental
- **Opioids (meperidine hydrochloride [Demerol], morphine):** Sweating, dizziness, and tachycardia; depressed respiration, gastric motility, and circulation; pre- or postoperative nausea and vomiting; excitement, hypotension, and restlessness
- **Procainamide:** Hypotension; enhanced or prolonged effects of neuromuscular blockers
- **Propranolol (Inderal):** Depressed myocardial function, enhanced or prolonged effects of neuromuscular blockers, hypotension, laryngospasm
- **Scopolamine bromide:** Increased IOP; blurred vision; dilated pupils; excessive mouth dryness, tachycardia, and flushing; excessive drowsiness and urine retention; agitation and delirium in elderly patients
- **Sedative-hypnotics (pentobarbital sodium [Nembutal]):** Excitement or confusion, particularly in elderly patients or patients with severe pain
- **Thyroid hormones (all types):** Increased risk of hypertension and tachycardia if given with ketamine
- **Tranquilizers (promethazine hydrochloride [Phenergan]):** Postoperative hypotension

Preoperative Surgical Period
The preoperative surgical period begins with the decision to have surgery and ends when the patient is transferred to the OR table or bed.

Preoperative Assessment
A preoperative nursing history should include the following:
- Past medical history:
  - Bleeding disorders
  - Cardiac disease
  - Renal disease
  - Chronic respiratory disease
  - Diabetes mellitus
  - Liver disease
  - Uncontrolled hypertension
  - Upper respiratory infection
- Past surgical history, which includes previous surgical procedures and their outcomes (e.g., success and complications)
- Allergies
- Lifestyle, including smoking and alcohol habits
- Current medications, with particular attention to those that may interact with anesthetic agents or increase risk during surgery
- Use of natural or herbal agents:
  - Several herbs and natural remedies have anticlotting properties and can lead to excessive bleeding (e.g., feverfew, garlic, ginger, ginkgo, vitamin E).
  - Some herbs and natural remedies increase postoperative inflammation (e.g., echinacea, goldenseal, licorice), which can delay healing, increase scarring, and increase the risk of postoperative infection.
  - Some herbs and natural remedies can elevate BP (e.g., ephedra, ginseng, licorice).
  - A few herbs and natural remedies (e.g., kava kava, St. John's wort, valerian) have sedative effects, which have been shown to prolong the effects of certain types of anesthesia.
- Patient's and significant others' emotional well-being:
  - Understanding of the surgery
  - Feelings about the surgery

- ○ Coping mechanisms
- ○ Description of changes to self-concept and body image
- Comprehensive physical assessment

Surgical Risk Factors
- Age
- Nutritional status
- Obesity
- Fluid and electrolyte imbalance
- Cardiac or respiratory problems

Presurgical Diagnostic Screenings
- Laboratory screenings:
  - ○ **Complete blood count (CBC):** To identify anemia, conditions that would alter clotting, infection-fighting abilities, or oxygen transport
  - ○ **Serum electrolyte studies:** To identify altered levels and potential for acid-base alterations
  - ○ **Urinalysis:** To identify bacterial colonization or presence of urinary tract alteration
  - ○ **Type and crossmatch:** To be prepared in case a transfusion is needed
- Radiologic screenings:
  - ○ **Chest X-ray:** To assess respiratory and cardiac structures
  - ○ **Magnetic resonance imaging (MRI) and computed tomography (CT) scan:** May or may not be done, depending on the type of surgery planned
- **Electrocardiogram (ECG):** To assess cardiac function

In the preoperative setting, the surgical nurse monitors the patient and confirms that the patient is ready, both physically and psychologically, for the procedure.

Ensuring Informed Consent
Informed consent is the process by which a patient makes an informed decision about whether to undergo a medical treatment or procedure. There are four components to the informed consent process:
- **Decision-making capacity:** The person signing the consent form must have the ability to make an informed decision.
- **Disclosure:** During the process of obtaining an informed consent, the nurse should give the patient information about his or her diagnosis, the reason for the treatment or procedure, the potential benefits of the procedure, any potential risks or complications associated with the procedure, any potential risks of not undergoing the procedure, and the risks and benefits of alternative treatments.
- **Comprehension:** The person signing the consent form must have the ability to comprehend the information given during the disclosure.
- **Voluntary participation:** The person signing the consent form must consent voluntarily, without coercion.

Preoperative Teaching
Preoperative teaching should be done with the patient and significant others, as appropriate.
- **Preoperative routines:** Preparations before the surgery
  - ○ Change in diet
  - ○ Change in medication or treatment schedule
  - ○ Specific preparations for the surgery
- **Postoperative routines:** Preparations for after the surgery
  - ○ Pain relief
  - ○ Postoperative exercises:
    - – Breathing exercises
    - – Incentive spirometry
    - – Splinting the incision when the patient coughs
    - – Leg exercises

Using the SOLER System for Good Communication

S	Sit to make the patient feel more comfortable.
O	Open your posture; do not sit with arms crossed.
L	Lean forward.
E	Make eye contact.
R	Relax your posture and attitude.

– Early ambulation range of motion (ROM) exercises
- ○ Postoperative equipment and procedures
- ○ Access devices:
  – IV equipment (peripheral, central venous pressure, pulmonary arterial)
  – Catheters and nasogastric tubes
  – Drains (Penrose, T-tube, Jackson-Pratt, Hemovac)
- ○ Oxygenation equipment (nasal cannula, face mask)
- ○ Lower extremity pressure devices (sequential compression devices [SCDs] or thromboembolic deterrent [TED] stockings)

Discharge Planning
- Evaluation of the home environment
- Description of the patient's self-care capabilities
- Presence or absence of significant others and support systems

Day of Surgery: Completing the Preoperative Assessment Sheet
- Assess vital signs.
- Promote relaxation.
- Provide personal hygiene:
  - ○ Prepare hair and remove cosmetics.
  - ○ Remove dentures.
- Remove prostheses.
- Have the patient void (if catheter is not inserted).
- Safeguard the patient's valuables.
- Administer preoperative medications as needed to:
  - ○ Reduce oral secretions.
  - ○ Reduce anxiety.
  - ○ Promote relaxation.
  - ○ Prevent laryngospasm.
  - ○ Inhibit gastric secretions.
  - ○ Minimize amount of anesthetic required for induction and maintenance of anesthesia.

Categories of Preoperative Medications
- **Sedatives (pentobarbital, secobarbital, chloral hydrate):** Drugs that calm down the patient, easing agitation and permitting sleep
- **Tranquilizers (chlorpromazine, hydroxyzine, diazepam):** Drugs used to reduce tension or anxiety, increasing drowsiness as potency increases
- **Opioid analgesics (meperidine, morphine, hydromorphone):** Drugs that decrease perception of pain and reaction to pain, as well as increase pain tolerance
- **Anticholinergics (atropine, scopolamine):** Medications that inhibit the transmission of parasympathetic nerve impulses and thereby reduce spasms of smooth muscle (e.g., muscle in the bladder)
- **H_2-receptor antagonists (cimetidine, ranitidine, famotidine):** Drugs used to block the action of histamine on parietal cells in the stomach, decreasing the production of acid by these cells
- **Antiemetics (metoclopramide, droperidol, promethazine):** Drugs that are effective against vomiting and nausea

Identification of Person & Surgical Site
- All patients should have at least two corroborating patient identifiers to confirm identity; acceptable patient identifiers include the following:
  - ○ Name, as stated by the patient (name should always be used as one patient identifier)

- Assigned identification or medical records number
- Date of birth
- Address
- Social security number
- Photograph
- Surgical procedure

- All patients must be properly identified by the surgical team members at multiple points prior to transporting the patient to the OR; verify the patient's identity at each of these key points:
  - When the surgery is scheduled
  - When the patient is admitted to the health care facility
  - Any time the patient's care is transferred to another caregiver
  - Prior to sedation
  - Prior to the patient's entry into the OR
- All patients should be asked to state their name.
- If the patient is mentally incapacitated:
  - Verify the patient's identity by asking a family member or designee to state the patient's full name and date of birth.
  - Verify that the information on the patient's wristband is the same as the information in the patient's chart.
- Take a time-out just before entering the OR; ask the patient to state his or her name, date of birth, and site of surgical procedure; then match personal identifying information as stated by the patient to that on the wristband and match the surgical procedure as stated by the patient with the data on the OR schedule and in the chart.
- All patients undergoing a surgical procedure should wear an identifying marker to prevent wrong-patient and wrong-site surgery; verification of the correct operative site is the responsibility of the surgical team.
  - Mark the surgical site to identify the intended site of skin incision.
  - No marks of any type should be made on nonoperative sites.
  - Each facility should have a policy for indicating the types of mark and methods of marking to promote continuity among the various departments of the facility.
  - The individual performing the surgical procedure should be responsible for marking the surgical site.
  - Site marking takes place when the patient is conscious, alert, oriented, and able to indicate the surgical site.
  - Use permanent markers, which will remain visible after the skin prep is performed.
  - The mark must be visible after the sterile surgical drapes have been placed.

> Take a time-out immediately before surgery is started, in the OR, so that the entire team can confirm the following: correct patient, correct surgical procedure, correct surgical site, correct patient position, and correct equipment.

Preparation of Skin for Surgery

The goals of skin preparation are to remove soil and transient microbes from the skin, reduce the residual microbial count to subpathogenic amounts in a short period of time and with the least amount of skin-tissue irritation, and inhibit rapid rebound growth of microbes. Skin preparation should be done as ordered by the surgeon but may include the following:

- Cleaning the skin over the surgical site with an antimicrobial solution, such as povidone-iodine
- Removing hair over the surgical site if necessary
  - Clipping of hair is becoming more popular than shaving the hair; clipping causes less damage to the underlying skin barrier.
- Applying, or "painting," an antimicrobial solution to the skin over the surgical site

Intraoperative Surgical Period

The intraoperative surgical period begins when the patient is transferred to the OR bed and ends when the patient is admitted to the postanesthesia care unit (PACU).

Nursing Roles during Surgery

Circulating Nurse

The circulating nurse is responsible for patient safety during the surgical procedure. The circulating nurse coordinates care of the patient with the surgeon, scrub nurse or tech, and anesthesia provider. The circulating nurse also provides assistance to the surgical team throughout the surgical procedure. Duties include the following:

- Setting up the OR
  - Ensuring that needed supplies and equipment are available, safe, and functional
  - Preparing the OR bed with gel, heating pads, and grounding pad, as appropriate to the situation
- Greeting the patient
- Verifying the patient's identity, the surgical procedure, and the surgical site
- Assisting the OR team in transferring the patient onto the OR bed
- Positioning the patient for the surgical procedure
- Performing the surgical skin preparation
- Draping the surgical site
- Opening and dispensing sterile supplies during the surgery
- Managing catheters, tubes, drains, and specimens during the procedure
- Adding medication and solutions to the sterile field as needed
- Assessing the amount of urine and blood loss and reporting the findings to the surgeon and anesthesiologist
- Reviewing results of diagnostic tests or laboratory test results and reporting the findings to the surgeon and anesthesiologist
- Maintaining a safe, aseptic environment:
  - Limiting traffic in the OR
  - Ensuring that the surgical team maintains sterile technique and a sterile field
- Maintaining a timeline of the surgery:
  - Time on table
  - Time of first incision
  - Time of skin closure
  - Time off table
- Performing "sharps," sponge, and instrument counts
- Documenting all care events, findings, and patient responses during the surgery

> The circulating nurse is in charge of maintaining sterility and monitoring the use of surgical instruments, sponges, and other materials so that nothing is left inside the patient.

Scrub Nurse

The scrub nurse supports the surgeon during the operation. Duties include the following:

- Handing instruments to the surgeon
- Helping set up the sterile field
- Helping drape the patient

Registered Nurse First Assistant (RNFA)

The RNFA is a perioperative registered nurse who functions in an expanded role by working in collaboration with the surgeon and health care team members to achieve optimal patient outcomes. The RNFA performs:

- Preoperative patient management in collaboration with other health care providers, including but not limited to:
  - Performing a preoperative evaluation or focused nursing assessment
  - Communicating and collaborating with other health care providers regarding the patient plan of care
  - Writing preoperative orders according to established protocols
- Intraoperative surgical first assisting, including but not limited to:
  - Using instruments and medical devices
  - Providing exposure
  - Handling and cutting tissue

- Providing hemostasis
- Suturing
- Postoperative patient management in collaboration with other health care providers in the immediate postoperative period and beyond, including but not limited to:
    - Writing postoperative orders or operative notes according to established protocols
    - Participating in postoperative rounds
    - Assisting with discharge planning and identifying appropriate community resources as needed

Certified Registered Nurse Anesthetist (CRNA)
- Administers anesthetic drugs to induce and maintain anesthesia
- Administers other medications as indicated to support the patient's physiologic status during surgery

Types of Anesthesia
General Anesthesia
General anesthesia produces total loss of consciousness by blocking awareness centers in the brain, thereby inducing amnesia, hypnosis, and relaxation.
- Stages of general anesthesia:
    - Analgesia, sedation, and relaxation
    - Excitement
    - Light to deep anesthesia
    - Overdose
- Administration of general anesthesia:
    - Inhalation of gases or volatile agents through an endotracheal tube or face mask
    - IV infusion of barbiturates or nonbarbiturates
- Adjuncts to general anesthetic agents:
    - Hypnotics
    - Opioid analgesics
    - Neuromuscular blocking agents
- Complications of general anesthesia:
    - Malignant hyperthermia, a life-threatening reaction to general anesthetic agents
    - Overdosage
    - Complications related to a reaction to a specific anesthetic agent
    - Complications of the endotracheal intubation process

Local or Regional Anesthesia
Local or regional anesthesia reduces the sensation of pain in a region of the body without inducing unconsciousness.
- Administration of local anesthesia:
    - **Topical local anesthesia:** Application of an anesthetic agent directly to the surface of the tissue to be anesthetized; produces anesthesia by inhibiting sensory system conduction of pain from the local nerves supplying the tissue to be anesthetized
    - **Infiltration local anesthesia:** Injection of an anesthetic agent intracutaneously and subcutaneously directly into the tissue to be anesthetized; produces anesthesia by inhibiting sensory system conduction of pain from the local nerves supplying the tissue to be anesthetized
- Administration of regional anesthesia:
    - **Nerve block:** Injection of an anesthetic agent into or around a specific nerve or nerve trunk or several groups of nerve trunks supplying the tissue to be anesthetized; produces anesthesia by inhibiting sensory system conduction of pain from the local nerves in the tissue to be anesthetized
    - **Spinal anesthesia:** Injection of an anesthetic agent into the cerebrospinal fluid in the subarachnoid space around the nerve roots supplying the tissue to be

anesthetized; produces anesthesia by inhibiting sensory system conduction of pain from nerve roots supplying the tissue to be anesthetized by acting on them as they exit the spinal cord, before they leave the spinal canal through the intervertebral foramina

- ○ **Epidural anesthesia:** Injection of an anesthetic agent into the epidural space surrounding the dura mater around the nerve roots supplying the tissue to be anesthetized; produces anesthesia by inhibiting sensory system conduction of pain from nerve roots supplying the tissue to be anesthetized by acting on them as they leave the spinal canal through the intervertebral foramina
- Adjuncts to local or regional anesthetic agents:
  - ○ Opioid analgesics
  - ○ Hypnotics
- Complications of local or regional anesthesia:
  - ○ Overdosage
  - ○ Incorrect administration technique
  - ○ Systemic absorption
  - ○ Patient sensitization to the anesthetic agent
- Complications of spinal anesthesia:
  - ○ Hypotension
    - – **Cause:** Paralysis of vasomotor nerves
    - – **Interventions:** Administer oxygen as ordered; administer vasoactive drugs as ordered; Trendelenburg position if level of anesthesia is fixed
  - ○ Nausea and vomiting
    - – **Cause:** Hypotension; traction placed on various structures within the abdomen
    - – **Interventions:** Position to decrease pressure and hypotension; administer antinausea medications as ordered
  - ○ Respiratory paralysis
    - – **Cause:** Spread of drug to the upper thoracic and cervical area; excessive concentrations of anesthesia administered
    - – **Interventions:** Provide artificial respiration; teach slow breathing and relaxation exercises
  - ○ Neurologic complications (e.g., paraplegia, severe muscle weakness in legs), very low incidence
    - – **Cause:** Edema and pressure on the spinal nerves; direct injury
    - – **Interventions:** Listen for patient sensations experienced during the procedure; monitor for changes in neurologic or motor function

Teamwork in the OR
The Preoperative Briefing
The preoperative briefing brings all the participants together (the surgeon, anesthesia provider, surgical technician, nurses, residents, students, and any others who may be involved in the surgery). Before the patient is wheeled into the OR, the team sets the stage for the surgery. The goal is for everyone to be aware of who is on the team for that case, to discuss any potential safety issues or medical conditions that might affect surgery, and to review the planned procedure.

- Team members can verify that safety checks have been completed and that the right equipment, instruments, medications, and any special requirements for the case are ready.
- The preoperative briefing provides an opportunity to ask questions or clarify misunderstandings in an atmosphere devoid of the tension that may exist during the procedure itself.

The Debriefing
The debriefing should take place as soon as possible after the operation is complete. All team members should be present. During the debriefing, team members give each other

feedback and review what could have been done better. Debriefing is an excellent time to discuss any near misses ("good catches") and error-prone points that were encountered during the procedure. During the debriefing, the following questions should be explored:

- Are sponge, needle, and instrument counts correct?
- Are specimens labeled correctly?
- What went well?
- What could have been done better or differently?
- Is there anything that someone wanted to bring up but did not or brought up but was ignored?
- Is there a system change that could make this operation safer for the next patient?

The Whiteboard

The whiteboard in the OR is a simple yet effective innovation that increases situational awareness among the OR team members. It provides:

- A means of knowing what is going on around team members, which is critical in a complex environment like the OR
- A display of vital information about the patient, the procedure, and the team

> Adverse events occur more often with surgical patients than with those of any other clinical specialty, and disproportionately greater harm results from surgical errors.

Postoperative Surgical Period

The postoperative surgical period begins with the admission of the patient to the PACU, and ends with the discharge of the patient from the hospital or the facility providing care.

Immediate Postoperative Nursing Care in the PACU

Respiratory Status

- Assessment:
  - Respiratory pattern, including rate, rhythm, and depth
  - Patency of airway
  - Presence of oral or artificial airway
  - Presence and character of breath sounds
  - Use of accessory muscles
  - Skin color
  - Ability to cough
  - Arterial blood gases
  - Pulse oximetry for oxygen saturation
- Interventions:
  - Ask the patient to expel the artificial airway.
  - Position the patient on his or her side to prevent aspiration.
  - Suction the artificial airway and oral cavity as necessary.
  - Ask the patient to perform respiratory exercises.
  - Administer oxygen as needed.
  - Turn the patient every 1–2 hours to mobilize respiratory secretions.

Circulatory Status

- Assessment:
  - Heart rate
  - BP
  - Skin color
  - Heart sounds
  - Peripheral pulses
  - Capillary refill
  - Edema
  - Skin temperature
  - Urine output
  - Homans sign
  - Change in vital signs indicating shock
  - Type, amount, color, odor, and character of drainage from tubes, drains, catheters, or incisions

- Interventions:
  - Check for pooling of blood under the patient and in dependent areas.
  - Check dressings, tubes, drains, and catheters for blood.
  - Monitor for changes in heart rate and BP.
  - Position the patient in bed to promote circulation to extremities.
  - Encourage leg exercises.
  - Apply SCDs.
  - Maintain an adequate state of hydration.
  - Administer anticoagulants as ordered.

Thermoregulatory Status
- Assessment:
  - Temperature
  - Shivering
- Intervention:
  - Apply warming blankets.

CNS Status
- Assessment:
  - Level of consciousness
  - Mental status
  - Movement and sensation in extremities
  - Presence of gag and corneal reflexes
- Interventions:
  - Orient patient to PACU environment.
  - Protect eyes if corneal reflex is absent.
  - Protect airway if gag reflex is absent.

Wound Status
- Assessment:
  - Warmth, swelling, tenderness, or pain at incision site
  - Type, amount, color, odor, and character of drainage on surgical dressing
  - Amount, consistency, and color of drainage in wound drains or tubes
- Interventions:
  - Reinforce dressing as needed.
  - Contact surgeon if there is excessive drainage on surgical dressing.

Urinary Status
- Assessment:
  - Presence of bladder distention
  - Amount, color, odor, and character of urine from Foley catheter if present or from spontaneous voiding
- Interventions:
  - Catheterize as needed.
  - Notify surgeon if urinary output is less than 30 mL/hr.
  - Assist the patient into an upright position during voiding.

GI Status
- Assessment:
  - Abdominal distention
  - Presence of nausea or vomiting
  - Presence of bowel sounds
  - Passage of flatus
  - Type, amount, color, odor, and character of drainage from nasogastric tube
- Interventions:
  - Promote adequate fluid intake via IV or orally (PO), as appropriate to general condition.
  - Progress diet as ordered and tolerated.

- o Encourage ambulation.
- o Administer fiber supplements, stool softeners, enemas, and rectal suppositories as ordered.

Fluid & Electrolyte Status
- Assessment:
  - o Intake and output
  - o Color and appearance of mucous membranes
  - o Skin turgor, tenting, and texture
  - o Status of IVs and type of fluid being infused
  - o Type, amount, color, odor, and character of drainage from tubes, drains, catheters, and incisions
- Interventions:
  - o Record and monitor details of fluids administered.
  - o Progress to oral fluids when patient is hemodynamically stable and has adequate bowel sounds.
  - o Administer isotonic, hypotonic, or hypertonic IV fluids based on type of surgical procedure and individual patient needs.
  - o Monitor loss of electrolytes in body secretions or drainage, and replace as needed.

Comfort
- Assessment:
  - o Patient's statement of pain or request for medication
  - o Facial grimacing
  - o Guarding or protecting of the operative site
  - o Change in vital signs or behavior
- Interventions:
  - o Administer pain medications as ordered.
  - o Use music, touch, or distraction to help the patient relax.

Preventing Postoperative Complications
Wound Infection
- Causes:
  - o Break in aseptic technique
  - o Dirty wound
  - o Predisposing factors, such as diabetes, anemia, obesity, malnutrition, and corticosteroid therapy
- Clinical manifestations:
  - o Fever
  - o Foul-smelling, greenish-white drainage from wound
  - o Persistent edema
  - o Redness
- Interventions:
  - o Perform culture and sensitivity reports of wound drainage.
  - o Administer antibiotics as ordered.
- Prevention:
  - o Keep a strict aseptic technique in the OR.
  - o Keep the wound clean and dry during the postoperative period.

Wound Dehiscence & Evisceration
- Causes:
  - o Inadequate surgical closure
  - o Increased intraabdominal pressure from coughing, vomiting, or straining with defecation
  - o Poor wound healing conditions caused by malnutrition, poor circulation, old age, or obesity

- Clinical manifestations:
  - Discharge of serosanguineous drainage from the wound
  - Patient's sensation that "something gave" or "something let go"
- Interventions:
  - Have the patient lie flat in bed.
  - Cover the wound with sterile, saline-soaked gauze.
  - Prepare the patient for immediate return to the OR for repair.
  - Monitor for signs of shock.
- Prevention:
  - Splint incision line when the patient coughs or vomits.
  - Medicate to decrease nausea and vomiting.
  - Teach the patient and patient's family the signs, symptoms, and emergent nature of this situation, as the highest risk is during days 5–8 of the postoperative period.

Elevated Temperature

- Causes:
  - Infection
  - Dehydration
  - Response to stress and trauma
  - Prolonged hypotension
  - Transfusion reaction
  - Respiratory congestion
  - Thrombophlebitis
- Clinical manifestations:
  - Temperature ≥99.5°F (37.5°C)
  - Elevated pulse and RR
  - Diaphoresis
  - Lethargy
- Interventions:
  - Increase fluids.
  - Give tepid sponge baths.
  - Administer antipyretics as ordered.
  - Implement preventive measures for causative factors.

Urinary Retention

- Causes:
  - Lack of urge to void because of anesthetic, narcotic, or anticholinergic drugs
  - Surgery in the abdominal, pelvic, or perineal area, resulting in edema in the area of the bladder
  - Contamination of the urinary tract
- Clinical manifestations:
  - Mild fever
  - Dysuria
  - Hematuria
  - Malaise
- Interventions:
  - Maintain adequate hydration.
  - Promote good bladder drainage.
  - Administer antibiotics (as ordered based on cultures and sensitivity reports).
- Prevention:
  - Encourage fluid intake.
  - Encourage early ambulation and spontaneous voiding.
  - Avoid catheterization.

Adhesions
- Causes:
  - Overhealing of tissue; may be more extensive if inflammatory process is present
  - Other unknown factors
- Clinical manifestations:
  - Bowel obstruction
  - Pain
- Intervention and prevention:
  - Prepare for surgery for lysis of adhesions.
  - Minimize inflammation with use of aseptic technique in the OR and during incisional care.

Pneumonia
- Causes:
  - Aspiration
  - Infection
  - Decreased cough reflex
  - Increased secretions from anesthesia
  - Dehydration
  - Immobilization
  - Atelectasis
- Clinical manifestations:
  - Increased temperature
  - Productive cough with purulent sputum
  - Crackles
  - Wheezes
  - Dyspnea
  - Chest pain
  - Tachypnea
  - Increased secretions
- Interventions:
  - Promote full aeration of lungs by positioning the patient in semi-Fowler or Fowler position.
  - Administer oxygen as ordered.
  - Maintain fluid status.
  - Administer antibiotics, expectorants, and analgesics as ordered.
  - Perform chest physical therapy to mobilize secretions.
- Prevention:
  - Assist with turning, coughing, and deep breathing.
  - Perform frequent position changes.
  - Promote early ambulation.
  - Encourage breathing exercises.

Atelectasis
- Causes:
  - Secretions obstructing airway
  - Collapse of the bronchioles as a result of shallow breathing or failure to periodically hyperventilate
- Clinical manifestations:
  - Decreased breath sounds in affected area
  - Dyspnea
  - Cyanosis
  - Crackles
  - Restlessness

- Apprehension
- Fever
- Tachypnea
- Interventions:
    - Encourage lung expansion by positioning the patient in semi-Fowler or Fowler position.
    - Administer oxygen as ordered.
    - Maintain hydration.
    - Administer analgesics as ordered.
    - Perform chest physical therapy.
    - Perform suctioning as needed.
    - Administer bronchial dilators and mucolytics via nebulizer as ordered.
- Prevention:
    - Promote early ambulation.
    - Assist with turning, coughing, and deep breathing.
    - Encourage the patient to perform incentive spirometry.

Paralytic Ileus

- Causes:
    - Anesthetic agents
    - Manipulation of bowel
    - Wound infection
    - Electrolyte imbalance
- Clinical manifestations:
    - Absent bowel sounds
    - No passage of flatus or feces
    - Abdominal distention
- Interventions:
    - Perform nasogastric suction.
    - Administer and maintain IV fluids for hydration and electrolyte correction.
    - Insert rectal tube.
    - Promote ambulation.
- Prevention:
    - Promote early ambulation.
    - Assist with abdominal-tightening exercises.
    - Keep NPO (i.e., nothing by mouth) if bowel sounds are absent.

Bowel Obstruction

- Causes:
    - Intestinal adhesions
    - Manipulation of bowel during surgery
- Clinical manifestations:
    - Absent bowel sounds
    - No passage of flatus or feces
    - Abdominal distention
- Interventions:
    - Initiate bowel decompression as ordered.
    - Prepare for surgical correction.
- Prevention:
    - Promote early ambulation.
    - Assist with abdominal-tightening exercises.
    - Keep NPO if bowel sounds are absent.

Pulmonary Embolism

- Causes:
  - Venous thrombus, usually originating in the legs, pelvis, or right side of the heart; thrombus travels to the pulmonary circulation
- Clinical manifestations:
  - Dyspnea
  - Sudden severe chest pain or tightness
  - Cough
  - Pallor or cyanosis
  - Increased respirations
  - Anxiety
  - Hypotension
  - Restlessness
- Interventions:
  - Contact physician STAT.
  - Maintain bed rest in semi-Fowler position.
  - Maintain fluid balance.
  - Administer oxygen as ordered.
  - Administer anticoagulants and analgesics as ordered.
- Prevention:
  - Assist with passive and active ROM leg exercises.
  - Provide antiembolic stockings.
  - Administer low-dose heparin if predisposing factors are present.
  - Promote early ambulation.

Hematoma

- Causes:
  - Imperfect hemostasis
  - Use of anticoagulants
  - Coagulation disorders
- Clinical manifestations:
  - Excessive bleeding
- Interventions:
  - Elevate the wound.
  - Prepare for surgical evacuation for large hematomas exerting pressure on other structures.
- Prevention:
  - Maintain pressure dressing over operative site as ordered.
  - Maintain patency of the wound drainage system if applicable.

Hypovolemic Shock

- Causes:
  - Excessive bleeding
- Clinical manifestations:
  - Decreased BP
  - Cold, clammy skin
  - Weak, rapid, thready pulse
  - Deep, rapid respirations
  - Decreased urinary output
  - Thirst
  - Apprehension
  - Restlessness
- Interventions:
  - Elevate legs 45 degrees.

As members of the health care team, surgical nurses play a critical role in ensuring a safe journey for all patients who are undergoing surgery.

- Administer fluid resuscitation, including whole blood or its components as ordered.
  - Administer oxygen.
  - Maintain warmth.
  - Anticipate return to the OR to find source of excessive blood loss.
- Prevention:
  - Administer IV fluids as ordered.

Thrombophlebitis

- Causes:
  - Venous stasis caused by prolonged immobilization or pressure from leg straps on the operating table
- Clinical manifestations:
  - Pain and cramping in the calf of the involved extremity
  - Redness or swelling in the affected area of the involved extremity
  - Increased temperature of the involved extremity
  - Increased local temperature
  - Increased diameter of the involved extremity
- Interventions:
  - Administer analgesics as ordered.
  - Measure bilateral calf or thigh circumference.
  - Administer anticoagulants as ordered.
  - Maintain bed rest.
  - Apply moist heat on affected extremity as ordered.
- Prevention:
  - Provide antiembolic stockings or sequential compression stockings.
  - Assist with postoperative leg exercises.
  - Promote early ambulation.

MEDICAL TERMINOLOGY, ABBREVIATIONS & ACRONYMS

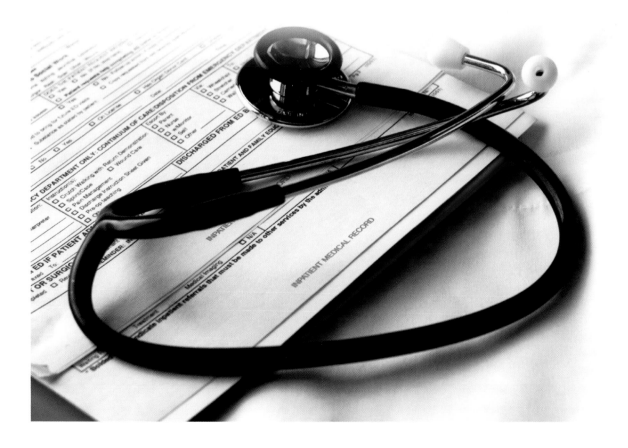

Introduction

To interpret physician orders and patient charts, you will need to be able to speak the language. This chapter will give you an overview of how medical words are structured. It also includes an A–Z list of medical terms, as well as an extensive list of medical abbreviations and acronyms.

Medical Terms

Structure of Medical Words
Most medical words are composed of two or more terms; to define a medical word:
- Divide the word into its terms: Term + Term = Medical Word
- Analyze the terms.
- Define the word.

Examples
Pericarditis
- *peri* = around; *card* = heart; *itis* = inflammation
- **Definition:** Inflammation around the heart

Oncology
- *onco* = tumor, mass; *logy* = study of
- **Definition:** Study of tumors

There are four categories of terms:
- **Prefix:** The beginning of a word (e.g., *pre-*, *post-*), designated by a hyphen before the root word
- **Suffix:** The ending of a word (e.g., *-stomy*, *-itis*), designated by a hyphen after the root word
- **Root:** The foundation, or base, of a word (e.g., *hepat*, *gastr*)
- **Combining form:** A vowel (usually *o*) added to a root (e.g., *gastro*); use a combining form when joining:
  - A root to another root (e.g., *gastrohepatitis*)
  - A root to a suffix beginning with a consonant (e.g., *cardiomegaly*)

Examples
Hyperleukocytosis
- *hyper* (prefix) = excessive
- *leuko* (combining form) = white
- *cyt* (root) = cell
- *osis* (suffix) = condition of
- **Definition:** Condition of excessive white [blood] cells (leukocytes)

Hematotoxic
- *hemato* (combining form) = blood
- *tox* (root) = poison
- *ic* (suffix) = pertaining to
- **Definition:** Pertaining to blood poisoning

Some terms have more than one definition; to determine the correct definition in a particular medical word, analyze the other terms in the word.

Examples
Poliomyelitis
- *polio* (prefix) = gray matter
- *myel* (root) = spinal cord *or* bone marrow
- *itis* (suffix) = inflammation
- **Definition:** Inflammation of the gray matter of the spinal cord; the bone marrow does not have gray matter.

Some terms may function as a root or combining form in one word and as a suffix in another word; classification depends on the specific medical word.

Examples
Cytology
- *cyto* (combining form) = cell
- *logy* (suffix) = study of
- **Definition:** Study of cells

Erythrocyte
- *erythro* (combining form) = red
- *cyte* (suffix) = cell
- **Definition:** Red blood cell

Terminology Sets

Directional Terms

ab-: away from
ad-: toward, near
ambi-: around, on both sides, about
amphi-: around, on both sides
ana-: up, backward, against
ante-: before, forward
anter/o: front
anti-: against
apo-: away, separated
cata-: down, under
circum-: around
contra-: against, opposite
dextr/o: right
dia-: through, throughout
dis-: apart, to separate
dist/o: distant
ec-, ecto-: outside, out
en-, endo-: inside, within
epi-: above, over, upon
eso-: within

ex-: out, away from
exo-: outside, outward
extra-: outside
fore-: before, in front
hyper-: above, excessive, beyond
hypo-: under, deficient, below
infra-: below, beneath
inter-: between
intra-: within
juxta-: near
later/o: side
levo-: left
medi/o: middle
meso-: middle
para-: alongside, near, beyond, abnormal
per-: through, throughout
peri-: around, surrounding
post-: after, behind
poster/o: behind, toward the back
pre-: before, in front of
pro-: before
pros/o: forward, anterior

proxim/o: near
re-: back, again
retro-: behind, backward
sinistr/o: left
sub-: under, beneath
super-: above, beyond
supra-: above, beyond
tel/e: distant, end
trans-: across
ultra-: beyond, excess

Numerical Values

half: demi-, hemi-, semi-
one: mono-, uni-
one and a half: sesqui-
two: bi-, di-
three: tri-
four: tetra-, quadri-
five: quinque-, penta-
six: hex-, hexa-, sex-
seven: hepta-, sept-, septi-
eight: octa-, octi-
nine: noni-
ten (10^1): deca-
hundred (10^2): hecto-
thousand (10^3): kilo-
million (10^6): mega-
billion(10^9): giga-
trillion (10^{12}): tera-
quadrillion (10^{15}): peta-
quintillion (10^{18}): exa-
one-tenth (10^{-1}): deci-
one-hundredth (10^{-2}): centi-
one-thousandth (10^{-3}): milli-
one-millionth (10^{-6}): micro-
one-billionth (10^{-9}): nano-
one-trillionth (10^{-12}): pico-
one-quadrillionth (10^{-15}): femto-
one-quintillionth (10^{-18}): atto-

Colors

alb/o, albin/o: white
chlor/o: green
cirrh/o: orange-yellow
cyan/o: blue
eosin/o: red, rosy, dawn-colored
erythr/o: red
flav/o: yellow
fusc/o: dark brown
glauc/o: gray, bluish green
jaund/o: yellow
leuk/o: white
lute/o: yellow
melan/o: black
poli/o: gray

purpur/i: purple
rhod/o: red, rosy
rose/o: rosy
rubr/o, rubr/i: red
tephr/o: gray, ashen
xanth/o: yellow

Pathogens

acar/o: mites
arachn/o: spider
bacteri/o: bacteria
-coccus: berry-shaped bacterium
fung/i: fungus, mushroom
helminth/o: worm
hirud/i, hirudin/i: leech
ixod/i: ticks
myc/o: fungus
parasit/o: parasite
pedicul/o: louse
scolec/o: worm
verm/i: worm
vir/o: virus

Diagnostic Procedures

aspir/o, aspirat/o: removal
-assay: to examine, to analyze
auscult/o, auscultat/o: to listen
echo-: reverberating sound
electr/o: electricity
-gram: written record
-graph: instrument for recording
-graphy: process of recording
-meter: instrument for measuring
-metry: process of measuring
-opsy: to view
palp/o, palpat/o: to touch gently
percuss/o: to tap
radi/o: X-ray, radiation
-scope: instrument for visual
    examination
-scopy: visual examination
-tome: instrument for cutting

Surgical Procedures

-centesis: surgical puncture of a cavity
-desis: surgical fixation, fusion
-ectomy: surgical removal
-pexy: fixation
-plasty: surgical correction or repair
-rrhaphy: suture
-sect: to cut
-stomy: surgical opening
-tomy: surgical incision
-tripsy: crushing, breaking

Five Rrh's

-rrhagia, -rrhage: excessive flow, profuse fluid discharge
-rrhaphy: suture
-rrhea: flow, discharge
-rrhexis: rupture
rrhythm/o: rhythm

Five Senses

hearing: acous/o, acoust/o, audi/o, audit/o, -cusis
smell: olfact/o, -osmia, osm/o, -osphresia, osphresi/o
taste: -geusia, gustat/o, gust/o
touch: haph/e, pselaphes/o, tact/o, thigm/o
vision: -opia, -opsia, opt/o

Synonyms

abdomen: abdomin/o, celi/o, lapar/o
air: aer/o, phys/o, pneum/o, pneumon/o
all: pan-, pant/o
bile: bil/i, chol/e
bladder: cyst/o, vesic/o
blood: hem/o, hemat/o, sangu/i, sanguin/o
body: corpor/o, somat/o, -some
breast: mamm/o, mast/o
breath: -pnea, respir/o, respirat/o, spir/o
cecum: cec/o, typhl/o
chest: pector/o, steth/o, thorac/o
childbirth: -para, -parous, -partum, -tocia, toc/o
cornea of the eye: corne/o, kerat/o
death: mort/o, necr/o, thanat/o
different: allo-, hetero-
disease: nos/o, path/o
dry: kraur/o, xer/o
ear: aur/o, auricul/o, ot/o
eardrum: myring/o, tympan/o
eye: ocul/o, ophthalm/o, opt/o
eyelid: blephar/o, palpebr/o
face: faci/o, op/o, prosop/o
fat: adip/o, lip/o, pimel/o, steat/o
feces: copr/o, scat/o, sterc/o
fever: febr/i, pyr/o, pyret/o
first: arch/e, arch/i, -arche, primi-, prot/o
foot: ped/o, pod/o
hair: pil/o, trich/o
half: demi-, hemi-, semi-
hearing: acous/o, acoust/o, audi/o, audit/o, -cusis
heart: cardi/o, coron/o

heat: calor/i, therm/o
huge: gigant/o, mega-, megalo-
itching: prurit/o, psor/o
kidney: nephr/o, ren/o
lens of the eye: phac/o, phak/o
life: bio-, vit/o, viv/i
ligament: desm/o, ligament/o, syndesm/o
lip: cheil/o, chil/o, labi/o
little, small: -ole, -ule
lung: pneum/o, pneumon/o, pulmon/o
milk: galact/o, lact/o
mind: ment/o, -noia, phren/o, psych/o
mouth: or/o, stomat/o
mucus: blenn/o, muc/o, myx/o
muscle: muscul/o, my/o, myos/o
nail: onych/o, ungu/o
night: noct/i, nyct/o
nose: nas/o, rhin/o
nucleus: kary/o, nucle/o
oil: ele/o, ole/o
ovary: oophor/o, ovari/o
pain: -algia, dolor/o, -dynia
palate: palat/o, uran/o
pregnancy: -cyesis, gravid/o
pupil: cor/o, pupill/o
rectum: proct/o, rect/o
saliva: ptyal/o, sial/o
same: homeo-, homo-, ipsi-, tauto-
skin: cutane/o, derm/o, dermat/o
sound: son/o, phon/o
specialist: -ician, -ist, -logist
stone: lith/o, petr/o
straight: ithy, orth/o
strength: dynam/o, -sthenia, sthen/o
sugar: gluc/o, glyc/o, sacchar/o
sweat: hidr/o, sud/o
swelling: -edema, -tumescence, tumesc/o
tear: dacry/o, lacrim/o
thick: pachy-, pycn/o, pykn/o
time: chron/o, temp/o, tempor/o
tongue: gloss/o, lingu/o
tooth: dent/i, odont/o
tumor/mass: -oma, onc/o
uterus: hyster/o, metr/o, uter/o
vagina: colp/o, vagin/o
vein: phleb/o, ven/o
vertebral/spinal column: rachi/o, spin/o, spondyl/o
vessel: angi/o, vas/o
vulva: episi/o, vulv/o
water: aque/o, hydr/o

Term Glossary

A

a-, an-: without, not
ab-: away from
abdomin/o: abdomen
ablat/o: to remove, to take away
abrad/o, abras/o: to scrape off
acanth/o: thorny, spiny
acar/o: mites
acid/o: acid, sour, bitter
acous/o: hearing
acoust/o: hearing, sound
acr/o: extremities
actin/o: ray, radiation
acu-: needle
acu/o, acut/o: sharp, severe
ad-: toward, near
aden/o: gland
adenoid/o: adenoids
adip/o: fat
adren/o: adrenal glands
aer/o: air, gas
agglutin/o: clumping
agit/o: rapidity, restlessness
-agogue: producer, leader
-agra: severe pain
alb/o, albin/o: white
albumin/o: albumin
-algesia, alges/o: pain sensitivity
-algia: pain
allo-: other, different
alveol/o: alveolus
ambi-: around, on both sides, about
ambly/o: dim, dull
ambul/o: to walk
ammon/o: ammonium
amni/o: amnion
amphi-: around, on both sides
amyl/o: starch
an/o: anus
ana-: up, backward, against
andr/o: male
aneurysm/o: aneurysm
angi/o: vessel
anis/o: unequal
ankyl/o: stiff, crooked, bent
anomal/o: irregular
ante-: before, forward
anter/o: front
anthrac/o: coal, carbon, carbuncle
anthrop/o: man, human being
anti-: against

antr/o: antrum
aort/o: aorta
-apheresis: separation, removal
aphth/o: ulcer
apic/o: apex
apo-: away, separation
aque/o: water
arachn/o: spider
arch/i, arch/e, -arche: first
arsenic/o: arsenic
arteri/o: artery
arteriol/o: arteriole
arthr/o: joint
articul/o: joint
aspir/o, aspirat/o: inhaling, removal
-assay: to examine, to analyze
-asthenia, asthen/o: weakness
astr/o: star, star-shaped
atel/o: incomplete, imperfect
ather/o: fatty substance, plaque
atmo-: steam, vapor
-atresia: closure, occlusion
atreto-: closed, lacking an opening
atri/o: atrium
atto-: one-quintillionth (10^{-18})
audi/o, audit/o: hearing
aur/o, auricul/o: ear
auscult/o, auscultat/o: to listen
auto-: self
aux/o: growth, acceleration
axi/o: axis
axill/o: armpit
azot/o: nitrogen, urea

B

bacteri/o: bacteria
balan/o: glans penis
balne/o: bath
bar/o: weight, pressure
bary-: heavy, dull, hard
bas/o, basi/o: base, foundation
-basia: walking
bathy-, batho-: deep, depth
bi-: two
bibli/o: books
bil/i: bile
bio-, bi/o: life, living
blast/o, -blast: early embryonic stage, immature
blenn/o: mucus
blephar/o: eyelid
brachi/o: arm
brachy-: short

brady-: slow
brom/o: bromine-containing compound, odor
bronch/o: bronchus
bronchiol/o: bronchiole
bucc/o: cheek
-bulia, -boulia: will
burs/o: sac

C

cac/o: bad, ill
calcane/o: heel
calci/o: calcium
calcul/o: stone
cali/o: calyx
calor/i: heat
campt/o: bent
-capnia, capn/o: carbon dioxide
capsul/o, caps/o: capsule, container
carb/o: carbon
carcin/o: cancer
cardi/o: heart
cari/o: caries
carp/o: wrist
cata-: down, under
-cataphasia: affirmation
cathar/o, cathart/o: cleansing, purging
-cathisia, -kathisia: sitting
caud/o: tail
caus/o, cauter/o: burn, burning
cavit/o, cav/o: hollow, cavity
cec/o: cecum
-cele: hernia, swelling
celi/o: abdomen
-centesis: surgical puncture of a cavity
centi-: one-hundredth (10^{-2})
centr/o: center
cephal/o: head
-ceptor: receiver
cerebell/o: cerebellum
cerebr/o: cerebrum, brain
cervic/o: neck, cervix
-chalasia: relaxation
cheil/o, chil/o: lip
chem/o: chemical, chemistry
-chezia, -chesia: defecation
chir/o, cheir/o: hand
chlor/o: green
chol/e: gall, bile
choledoch/o: common bile duct
chondr/o: cartilage
chori/o: chorion
-chroia: skin coloration

chrom/o: color
chron/o: time, timing
chrys/o: gold
chyl/o: chyle
-cide: killing, agent that kills
cine-: movement
circum-: around
cirrh/o: orange-yellow
-clasis, -clasia: break
cleid/o: clavicle
clin/o: to slope, to bend
-clysis: irrigation, washing
coagul/o: coagulation, clotting
-coccus: berry-shaped bacterium
coccyg/o: coccyx
cochle/o: cochlea
-coimesis: sleeping
col/o: colon
colp/o: vagina
com-: with, together
coma: deep sleep
con-: with, together
coni/o: dust
conjunctiv/o: conjunctiva
consci/o: awareness, aware
constrict/o: narrowing, binding
contra-: against, opposite
contus/o: to bruise
cor/o: pupil
corne/o: cornea
coron/o: heart
corpor/o: body
cortic/o: cortex
cost/o: rib
cox/o: hip
crani/o: skull
-crasia: mixture (good or bad), temperament
cric/o: ring
crin/o: secrete, separate
-crit: separate
critic/o: crisis, dangerous
cry/o: cold
crypt/o: hidden, concealed
crystall/o: crystal, transparent
cubit/o: elbow, forearm
culd/o: cul-de-sac
cune/o: wedge, wedge shaped
cupr/o: copper
-cusis: hearing
cutane/o: skin
cyan/o: blue
cycl/o: ciliary body, circular
-cyesis: pregnancy

cyst/o: bladder, cyst
cyt/o, -cyte: cell

D

dacry/o: tears
dactyl/o: digit (finger or toe)
deca-: ten (10^1)
deci-: one-tenth (10^{-1})
demi-: half
dem/o: people
dent/i: tooth
derm/o, dermat/o: skin
desicc/o: to dry
-desis: surgical fixation, fusion
desm/o: ligament
deuter/o: second, secondary
dextr/o: right
di-: two
dia-: through, throughout
didym/o: a twin, testis
-didymus: conjoined twin
dilat/o: to enlarge, to expand
dipl/o: double
dips/o: thirst
dis-: apart, to separate
dist/o: distant
dolich/o: long
dolor/o: pain
dors/o: back
drom/o, -drome: running
duct/o: to lead
duoden/o: duodenum
dynam/o: power, strength
-dynia: pain
dys-: bad, difficult, painful

E

ec-, ecto-: outside, out
echin/o: spiny, prickly
echo-: reverberating sound
eco-: environment
-ectasis, -ectasia: dilation, expansion
-ectomy: surgical removal
ectr/o: congenital absence
-edema: swelling
ele/o: oil
electr/o: electricity
embol/o: embolus
embry/o: embryo
-emesis: vomiting
-emia: blood condition
emmetr/o: the correct measure, proportioned
-emphraxis: stoppage, obstruction
en-, endo-: inside, within

enanti/o: opposite, opposed
encephal/o: brain
enter/o: intestines (small intestines)
eosin/o: red, rosy, dawn-colored
epi-: above, over, upon
epididym/o: epididymis
epiglott/o: epiglottis
episi/o: vulva
equi-: equality, equal
erethism/o: irritation
erg/o: work
erythem/o: flushed, redness
erythr/o: red
eschar/o: scab
eso-: within
esophag/o: esophagus
esthesi/o, -esthesia: sensation, feeling
eti/o: cause
eu-: good, normal, well
eury-: wide, broad
ex-: out, away from
exa-: quintillion (10^{18})
excit/o: to arouse
exo-: outside, outward
extra-: outside

F

faci/o: face
-facient: to cause, to make happen
fasci/o: fascia
febr/i: fever
femor/o: femur
femto-: one-quadrillionth (10^{-15})
ferr/i, ferr/o: iron
fet/o: fetus
fibr/o: fiber, fibrous
fibul/o: fibula
fil/o, fil/i, filament/o: thread, threadlike
flav/o: yellow
flex/o, flect/o: bend
flu/o, flux/o: flow
fluor/o: fluorine
follicul/o: small sac, follicle
fore-: before, in front
-form: specified shape, form
frig/o, frigid/o: cold
funct/o: performance
fung/i: fungus, mushroom
fusc/o: dark brown

G

galact/o: milk
galvano-: direct electric current
gamet/o: gamete
gam/o: marriage, sexual union

gangli/o, ganglion/o: ganglion
gastr/o: stomach
ge/o: earth, soil
gel/o: to freeze, to congeal
gemell/o: twins
-gen, gen/o: producing, generating
-genesis: production, formation
-genic: produced by, forming
geni/o: chin
genit/o: reproduction
ger/o, geront/o: aged, old age
gest/o, gestat/o: to bear
-geusia: taste
giga-: billion (10^9)
gigant/o: huge
gingiv/o: gums
glauc/o: gray, bluish green
gli/o: glue, neuroglia
-globin: protein
glomerul/o: glomerulus
gloss/o: tongue
gluc/o: glucose, sugar
glyc/o: glucose, sugar
gnath/o: jaw
gnos/o: knowledge
gon/o: genitals, semen
gonad/o: gonads
goni/o: angle
-grade: step
-gram: written record
granul/o: granules
-graph: instrument for recording
graph/o: writing
-graphy: process of recording
gravid/o: pregnancy
-gravida: pregnant woman
gustat/o, gust/o: taste
gynec/o: woman, female
gyr/o: circle, spiral

H

haph/e: touch
hapl/o: simple, single
hect/o: hundred (10^2)
helc/o: ulcer
heli/o: sun
helminth/o, -helminth: worm
hemi-: half
hem/o, hemat/o: blood
hepat/o: liver
hepta-: seven
heredo-: heredity
hetero-: different, other
hex-, hexa-: six

-hexia: condition
hidr/o: sweat
hirsut/o: hairy
hirud/i, hirudin/i: leech
hist/o: tissue
holo-: entire, complete
homeo-: likeness, constant, sameness
homo-: same, similar
hormon/o: hormone
humer/o: humerus
hyal/o: resembling glass, glassy
hydr/o: water, hydrogen
hygr/o: moisture
hymen/o: hymen
hyper-: above, excessive, beyond
hypn/o: sleep
hypo-: under, deficient, below
hypothalam/o: hypothalamus
hypsi-: high
hyster/o: uterus

I

iatr/o: treatment, physician
ichthy/o: fish
-ician: specialist
icter/o: jaundice
ide/o: idea, mental images
idi/o: individual, distinct, unknown
ile/o: ileum
ili/o: ilium
immun/o: protection, immunity
infra-: below, beneath
inguin/o: groin
inter-: between
intra-: within
iod/o: iodine
ion/o: ion
ipsi-: same
ir/o, irid/o: iris
isch/o: suppress, restrain
ischi/o: ischium
is/o: equal
-ist: specialist
ithy-: erect, straight
-itis: inflammation
ixod/i: ticks

J

jaund/o: yellow
jejun/o: jejunum
juxta-: near

K

kal/i: potassium
kary/o: nucleus

kel/o: tumor, fibrous growth
ken/o: empty
kerat/o: horny tissue, cornea
keraun/o: lightning
keton/o: ketones
kilo-: thousand (10^3)
kinesi/o, -kinesia, -kinetic: movement
klept/o: theft, stealing
koil/o: hollow, concave, depressed
kraur/o: dry
kym/o: waves
kyph/o: humpback

L

-labile: unstable, perishable
lacrim/o: tear, lacrimal duct
lact/o: milk
lal/o, -lalia: speech, babble
lamin/o: lamina
lampr/o: clear
lapar/o: abdomen, abdominal wall
laryng/o: larynx
later/o: side
laxat/o: to slacken, to relax, to loosen
lecith/o: yolk, ovum
-legia: reading
lei/o: smooth
-lemma: confining membrane
lepid/o: flakes, scales
lepr/o: leprosy
-lepsy: seizure
lept/o: slender, thin, delicate
letharg/o: drowsiness
leuk/o: white
levo-: left
-lexia: speech, word
lien/o: spleen
ligament/o: ligament
ligat/o: binding, tying
lim/o: hunger
lingu/o: tongue
lip/o: fat
-lipsis: to omit, to fail
-listhesis: slipping
lith/o: stone, calculus
lob/o: lobe
logad/o: whites of the eyes
log/o, -log, -logue: word, speech, thought
-logist: specialist
-logy: study of
loph/o: ridge
lord/o: curvature, bending
lox/o: oblique, slanting

-lucent: light-admitting
luc/i: light
lucid/o: clear
lumb/o: loin
lumin/o: light
lute/o: yellow
luxat/o: dislocate
ly/o: to dissolve, to loosen
lymph/o: lymph
-lysis: dissolution, breakdown

M

-malacia: softening
mamm/o: breast
-mania: madness, obsessive preoccupation
-masesis: mastication, chewing
mast/o: breast
maxill/o: maxilla
medi/o: middle
mediastin/o: mediastinum
medic/o: to heal, healing
medull/o: medulla, marrow
mega-: million (10^6)
mega-, megalo-: large
-megaly: enlargement
mel/o: limb
melan/o: black
meli-, melit/o: honey, sugar
men/o: menses, menstruation
mening/o: meninges, membranes
ment/o: mind
mer/o: part
meso-: middle
meta-: after, beyond, change
metall/o: metal
-meter: instrument for measuring
method/o: procedure, technique
metr/o: uterus
-metry: process of measuring
mi/o: less, smaller
micro-: one-millionth (10^{-6}), small
milli-: one-thousandth (10^{-3})
-mimesis: imitation, simulation
mis/o: hatred of, aversion to
-mnesia: memory
mogi-: difficult
mono-: one
morph/o: shape, form
mort/o: death
-motor: movement, motion
muc/o: mucus
multi-: many, much
muscul/o: muscle
mutilat/o: to maim, to disfigure

my/o, myos/o: muscle
myc/o: fungus
myel/o: bone marrow, spinal cord
myring/o: eardrum
myx/o: mucus

N

nano-: one-billionth (10^{-9})
narc/o: numbness, stupor
nas/o: nose
nat/o: birth
natr/o: sodium
necr/o: death
neo-: new
nephr/o: kidney
neur/o: nerve
neutr/o: neutral
nev/o: mole, birthmark
noci-: to cause harm, injury or pain
noct/i: night
nod/o: knot
-noia: mind, will
nom/o: custom, law
nomen-: name
noni-: nine
norm/o: normal, usual
nos/o: disease
not/o: the back
nucle/o: nucleus
nulli-: none
nutri/o, nutrit/o: nourish
nyct/o: night

O

obstetr/o: midwife
oct-, octa-, octi-: eight
ocul/o: eye
odont/o: tooth
-oid: resembling
-ole: little, small
ole/o: oil
olfact/o: smell
olig/o: scanty, few, little
-oma: tumor, mass
om/o: shoulder
omphal/o: navel
onc/o: tumor, mass
onych/o: nail
o/o: egg, ovum
oophor/o: ovary
ophry/o: eyebrow
ophthalm/o: eye
-opia, -opsia: vision
opisth/o: backward, behind
op/o: juice, face

-opsy: to view
opt/o: eye, vision
or/o: mouth
orch/o, orchi/o, orchid/o: testis
-orexia: appetite
organ/o: organ
ornith/o: bird
orth/o: straight, normal, correct
osche/o: scrotum
oscill/o: to swing
-osis: condition, status, abnormal increase
osm/o, -osmia: sense of smell, odor, impulse
osphresi/o, -osphresia: sense of smell, odor
oste/o: bone
ot/o: ear
ov/o, ov/i: egg, ovum
ovari/o: ovary
ox/o, -oxia: oxygen
oxy-: sharp, quick, sour

P

pachy-: thick
-pagus: conjoined twins
palat/o: palate
pale/o: old
palin-, pali-: recurrence, repetition
palliat/o: to soothe, to relieve
palp/o, palpat/o: to touch gently
palpebr/o: eyelid
palpit/o, palpitat/o: flutter, throbbing
pan-: all
pancreat/o: pancreas
pant/o: all, whole
papill/o: nipple-like, papilla
papul/o: papule, pimple
para-: alongside, near, beyond, abnormal
-para, -parous: to bear, to bring forth
parasit/o: parasite
parathyroid/o: parathyroid
-paresis: partial paralysis
-partum: childbirth, labor
patell/o: patella
path/o: disease
-pause: cessation
pector/o: chest
ped/o: foot, child
pedicul/o: louse
pel/o: mud
pelv/i: pelvis
-penia: deficiency

pent-, penta-: five
-pepsia: digestion
per-: through, throughout
percuss/o: to tap
peri-: around, surrounding
perine/o: perineum
peritone/o: peritoneum
per/o: deformed, maimed
perone/o: fibula
perspir/o: to breathe through, sweat
pest/i: plague, pests
peta-: quadrillion (10^{15})
-petal: moving toward, seeking
petr/o: stone, petrous region of temporal bone
-pexy: fixation
phac/o: lens
phag/o, -phagia: eating, ingestion
phak/o: lens
phalang/o: phalanges
phall/o: penis
phaner/o: visible, apparent
pharmac/o: drugs
phas/o, -phasia: speech
phe/o: dusky
phen/o: appearance
-pheresis: removal
-phil, -philia: affinity for, tendency toward
phim/o: muzzle
phleb/o: vein
-phobia, phob/o: fear, aversion
phon/o, -phonia: voice, sound
-phore, phor/o: bearer, processor
-phoresis: bearing, transmission
phosphat/o: phosphate
phot/o: light
phren/o: mind, diaphragm
phyc/o: seaweed, algae
phyl/o: race, species, type
-phylaxis: protection
phyll/o: leaf, leaf-like
-phyma: tumor, growth
physic/o: physical, natural
physi/o: nature
phys/o: air, gas
-physis: growth, growing
phyt/o, -phyte: plant
pico-: one-trillionth (10^{-12})
picr/o: bitter
piez/o, pies/i, -piesis: pressure
pil/o: hair
pimel/o: fat, fatty
pin/o: to drink
pineal/o: pineal gland

pituitar/o: pituitary gland
plagi/o: slanting, oblique
plan/o: flat, level, wandering
plant/o: sole of the foot
-plasm: formation, growth
plasm/o: plasma, formative substance
-plasty: surgical correction, repair
platy-: broad, flat
ple/o: more
-plegia: paralysis
plesi/o: nearness, similarity
pless/i: striking
pleur/o: pleura
plex/o: network of nerves or vessels, plexus
plic/o, plicat/o: to fold, to pleat
-ploid, -ploidy: number of chromosome sets
pluri-: more, several
-pnea: to breathe
pneum/o: lung, air
pneumon/o: lung, air
pod/o: foot
-poiesis: formation
poikil/o: variation, irregular
poli/o: gray matter
poly-: many, much
pon/o: fatigue, overwork, pain
-pore, por/o: opening, passageway
-porosis: porosity, decrease in density
-posia: drinking
posit/o: arrangement, place
post-: after, behind
poster/o: behind, toward the back
potenti/o: power, strength
-prandial: meal
-praxia: action, activity
pre-: before, in front of
presby-: aging, elderly
primi-: first
-privia: loss, deprivation
pro-: before
proct/o: rectum, anus
pros/o: forward, anterior
prosop/o: face
prostat/o: prostate gland
prote/o: protein
prot/o: first
proxim/o: near
prurit/o: itching
psamm/o: sand, sand-like
pselaphes/o: to touch
pseudo-: false
psor/o: itching
psych/o: mind

psychr/o: cold
pteryg/o: wing shaped
-pterygium: abnormality of the conjunctiva
-ptosis: prolapse, drooping
ptyal/o: saliva
-ptysis: spitting
pub/o: pubis
pulmon/o: lung
puls/o, pulsat/o: to beat, beating
-puncture: to pierce a surface
pupill/o: pupil
purgat/o: cleansing
purpur/i: purple
purul/o: pus formation
py/o: pus
pyel/o: renal pelvis
pyg/o: buttocks
pykn/o, pycn/o: thick, dense
pyl/e: portal vein
pylor/o: pylorus
pyret/o: fever
pyrex/o: feverishness, fever
pyr/o: heat, fire, fever

Q

quadri-: four
quinque-: five
quint/i: fifth

R

rachi/o: spine
radi/o: X-ray, radiation
radicul/o: nerve root
ram/i: branch
re-: back, again
-receptor: receiver
rect/o: rectum
reflex/o, reflect/o: to bend back
registrat/o: recording
relaps/o: to slide back
ren/o: kidney
respir/o, respirat/o: to breathe, breathing
resuscit/o: to revive
reticul/o: netlike
retin/o: retina
retract/o: drawing back
retro-: behind, backward
rhabd/o: rod
rhabdomy/o: striated or skeletal muscle
rhe/o: flow, current, stream
rhin/o: nose
rhiz/o: root
rhod/o: red, rosy

rhytid/o: wrinkle
rose/o: rosy
rot/o, rotat/o: to turn, to revolve
-rrhagia, -rrhage: excessive flow, profuse fluid discharge
-rrhaphy: suture
-rrhea: flow, discharge
-rrhexis: rupture
rrhythm/o: rhythm
-rubr/o, rubr/i: red

S

sacchar/o: sugar
sacr/o: sacrum
salping/o: fallopian tube
sangu/i, sanguin/o: blood
sanit/a: health
sap/o: soap
sapr/o: rotten, decaying
sarc/o: flesh
saur/o: lizard
scaph/o: scapha, boat shaped
scapul/o: scapula
scat/o: feces
scel/o, -scelia: leg
schist/o, -schisis: split, cleft
schiz/o: split, division
scint/i: spark
scirrh/o: hard
scler/o: sclera
-sclerosis: hardening
scolec/o: worm
scoli/o: crooked, twisted
-scope: instrument for visual examination
-scopy: visual examination
scot/o: darkness
scrib/o, script/o: to write
seb/o: sebum
-sect: to cut
secund/i: second
sedat/o: to calm
semi-: half
semin/i: semen
senil/o: old, old age
sens/o, sensat/o: feeling, perception
sensor/i: sensory
-sepsis, septic/o: putrefaction, putrefying
sept-, septi-: seven
sept/o: partition
ser/o: serum, serous
sesqui-: one and a half
sex-: six
sial/o: saliva

sicc/o: to dry
sider/o: iron
sigmoid/o: sigmoid colon
silic/o: silica, quartz
sinistr/o: left
sinus/o, sin/o: cavity, sinus
sit/o: food
skelet/o: skeleton
soci/o: social, society
sodi/o: sodium-containing compound
solut/o: dissolved
somat/o: body
-some: body
somn/i, -somnia: sleep
son/o: sound
span/o: scanty, scarce
-spasm, spasm/o: involuntary contraction
spectr/o: image, spectrum
sperm/o, spermat/o: spermatozoa
sphen/o: wedge, sphenoid bone
spher/o: round, sphere
sphygm/o: pulse
-sphyxia: pulse
spin/o: spinal cord, spine
spir/o: to breathe
splanchn/o: viscera
splen/o: spleen
spondyl/o: vertebrae, spinal column
spongi/o: spongelike, spongy
spor/o: spore, seed
squam/o: squamous, scales
-stabile: stable, fixed
-stalsis: contraction
staped/o: stapes
staphyl/o: uvula, grape-like clusters
-stasis: standing still, standing
-stat: device or instrument for keeping something stationary
steat/o: fat
-stenosis, sten/o: narrowed, constricted
stere/o: solid, three-dimensional
steril/o: barren
stern/o: sternum
steth/o: chest
sthen/o, -sthenia: strength
stich/o, -stichia: rows
stigmat/o: mark, point
stomat/o: mouth
-stomy: surgical opening
strat/i: layer
strept/o: twisted, curved
strict/o: to tighten, to bind
-stroma: supporting tissue of an organ
stroph/o: twisted

sub-: under, beneath
succ/o: juice
suct/o: to suck
sud/o: sweat
sulc/o: furrow, groove
super-: above, beyond
supra-: above, beyond
suspend/o, suspens/o: to hang up, to suspend
sym-, syn-: with, together
symptom/o: occurrence
synaps/o, synapt/o: point of contact, to join
syndesm/o: ligament, connective tissue
synov/o: synovia, synovial membrane
syphil/o: syphilis
syring/o: tube, fistula
system/o: system
systol/o: contraction
syzygi/o: bound together, conjunction

T

tachy-: fast
tact/o: to touch
tal/o: talus
taph/o: grave
tapin/o: low
tars/o: tarsus, edge of eyelid
tauto-: identical, same
-taxia, tax/o: arrangement, coordination
techn/o: skill, art
tect/o: rooflike
tegment/o: covering
tel/e: end, distant
tel/o: end
tele/o: perfect, complete
temp/o, tempor/o: period of time, the temples
ten/o: tendon
tenont/o: tendon
-tension, tens/o: stretched, strained
tephr/o: gray (ashen)
tera-: trillion (10^{12})
terat/o: monster
termin/o: boundary, limit
terti-: third
test/o, testicul/o: testis
tetan/o: tetanus
tetra-: four
thalam/o: thalamus
thanat/o: death
thec/o: sheath
thel/o: nipple
theor/o: speculation

-therapy, therapeut/o: treatment
theri/o: animals
therm/o: heat
thigm/o: to touch
thio-: presence of sulfur
thorac/o: chest
thromb/o: clot, thrombus
-thymia: mind, emotions
thym/o: thymus gland
thyr/o: thyroid gland
tibi/o: tibia
toc/o, -tocia: childbirth, labor
-tome: instrument for cutting
tom/o: a cutting (section or layer)
-tomy: surgical incision
ton/o: tone, tension
tonsill/o: tonsils
top/o: particular place or area
torpid/o: sluggish, inactive
tors/o: twisting, twisted
tox/o, toxic/o: poison
trachel/o: neck
trache/o: trachea
trachy-: rough
trans-: across
traumat/o: trauma, injury, wound
trem/o, tremul/o: shaking, trembling
-tresia: opening, perforation
tri-: three
tri/o: to sort out, sorting
trich/o: hair
-tripsy: crushing, breaking
-trophy, troph/o: nourishment, growth
-tropia: to turn
tubercul/o: tubercle, tuberculosis
tub/o: tube
-tumescence, tumesc/o: swelling
turbid/i: cloudy, confused
turg/o, turgid/o: to swell, swollen
tympan/o: eardrum (tympanic
   membrane)
-type, typ/o: class, representative form
typhl/o: cecum, blindness
typh/o: typhus, typhoid
tyr/o: cheese, caseous

U

-ule: little, small
ul/o: scar, scarring
ultra-: beyond, excess
un-: not, reversal
ungu/o: nail
uni-: one
uran/o: palate
-uresis: urination
ureter/o: ureter

urethr/o: urethra
-uria: urine condition
uric/o: uric acid
urin/o: urine
ur/o: urine
uter/o: uterus
uve/o: uvea
uvul/o: uvula

V

vaccin/o: vaccine
vag/o: vagus nerve
vagin/o: vagina
valv/o, valvul/o: valve
varic/o: varix, varicose vein
vari/o, variat/o: to change, to vary
vas/o: vessel, vas deferens
vascul/o: blood vessel
ven/o: vein
venere/o: sexual intercourse
ventil/o: to aerate, to oxygenate
ventr/o: belly, front of the body
ventricul/o: ventricle of the heart or
   brain
venul/o: venule
verm/i: worm
verruc/i: wart
vers/o, -verse: turn, turning
vertebr/o: vertebra
vesic/o: urinary bladder
vesicul/o: seminal vesicle, a vesicle
vestibul/o: vestibule
vibr/o, vibrat/o: to quiver, to shake
viril/o: masculine, manly
vir/o: virus
viscer/o: internal organs
viscid/o, viscos/o: sticky, glutinous
vitell/o: yolk
vit/o, vital/o: life
vitre/o: glassy, vitreous body
viv/i: life, alive
-volemia: blood volume
volv/o, volut/o: to roll
vulv/o: vulva

X

xanth/o: yellow
xen/o: strange, foreign matter
xer/o: dry
xiph/o: sword shaped, xiphoid

Z

zon/i, zon/o: zone, encircling region
zo/o: animal
zyg/o: union, junction
zym/o: enzyme, ferment

Medical Abbreviations

An abbreviation is a shortened form of a word or phrase (e.g., cm = centimeter). An acronym is formed from the initial letters in a term and is pronounced as a single word (e.g., WHO = World Health Organization). Because there are thousands of medical abbreviations and acronyms, the purpose of this section is to present those most commonly used. Care must be exercised when using this shorthand communication format because many abbreviations and acronyms have multiple meanings. The correct definition is determined by the context of the material.

> Some abbreviations and acronyms may appear in either lower- or upper-case lettering and either with or without periods.

Dangerous Abbreviations

The most dangerous abbreviations, acronyms, and symbols (in handwriting or preprinted), according to The Joint Commission's Official "Do Not Use" List of abbreviations, are the following:

Official "Do Not Use" List[1]

Do Not Use	Potential Problem	Use Instead
U (unit)	Mistaken for "0" (zero), the number "4" (four) or "cc"	Write "unit"
IU (International Unit)	Mistaken for IV (intravenous) or the number 10 (ten)	Write "International Unit"
Q.D., QD, q.d., qd (daily)	Mistaken for each other	Write "daily"
Q.O.D., QOD, q.o.d, qod (every other day)	Period after the Q mistaken for "I" and the "O" mistaken for "I"	Write "every other day"
Trailing zero (X.0 mg)* Lack of leading zero (.X mg)	Decimal point is missed	Write X mg Write 0.X mg
MS	Can mean morphine sulfate or magnesium sulfate	Write "morphine sulfate" Write "magnesium sulfate"
MSO_4 and $MgSO_4$	Confused for one another	

[1] Applies to all orders and all medication-related documentation that is handwritten (including free-text computer entry) or on pre-printed forms.

*Exception: A "trailing zero" may be used only where required to demonstrate the level of precision of the value being reported, such as for laboratory results, imaging studies that report size of lesions, or catheter/tube sizes. It may not be used in medication orders or other medication-related documentation.

© The Joint Commission, 2013. Reprinted with permission.

Weights & Measurements

C: Celsius, centigrade
cc: cubic centimeter
Ci, c: Curie
cm: centimeter
dB: decibel
dl, dL: deciliter
dr: dram
F: Fahrenheit
fl dr: fluid dram
Fl, fld: fluid
fl oz: fluid ounce
g, gm: gram
Hz: hertz
IU: International Unit
kg: kilogram
km: kilometer
L, l: liter

L/min: liters per minute
lb: pound
M: mega-, million, molar
m: meter
mcg, μg: microgram
mCi, mc: millicurie
mEq: milliequivalent
mEq/L: milliequivalent per liter
mg, mgm: milligram
ml, mL: milliliter
mm: millimeter
mm Hg: millimeters of mercury
mol wt, MW, MWt: molecular weight
μ, mu: micron
mμ: millimicron
oz: ounce
ppm: parts per million
pt: pint

rad: radiation-absorbed dose
rev/min, rpm: revolutions per minute
SI: International System of Units
U: unit
V: volt
vol %: volume percent
v/v: volume per volume
W: watt
w/v: weight per volume

Pharmacology

Drugs

ACD: anticonvulsant drug
ADR: adverse drug reaction
ASA: acetylsalicylic acid (aspirin)
CD: curative dose
D, dos: dose, dosage
DAW: dispense as written
DAWN: Drug Abuse Warning Network
DIG: digitalis
DSB: drug-seeking behavior
IND: investigational new drug
INH: isoniazid (TB drug)
LD: lethal dose
MAOI: monoamine oxidase inhibitor
MAR: medication administration record
Meds: medications, medicines
NSAID: nonsteroidal anti-inflammatory drug
OD: (drug) overdose
OTC: over the counter
PCA: patient-controlled analgesia
PCN, PNC: penicillin
Rx: prescription, drug, medication
sig: label
TDM: therapeutic drug monitoring

Formulations

aer: aerosol
aq: water, aqueous
bol, pil: pill
cap: capsule
comp: compound
dil, dilut: dilute
elix, el: elixir
ext: extract
fld, FL: fluid
garg: a gargle
gtt, gt: drops, drop
linim: liniment
liq: liquid
lot: lotion
M: mixture, mix
pulv: powder

sol, soln.: solution
solv: dissolve
spt: spirit
supp: suppository
susp: suspension
syr: syrup
tab: tablet
tinct: tincture
ung: ointment

Medication Administration: Directions

ā: before
āā: of each
ac: before meals
ad lib.: freely, as desired
admov.: apply
AM: before noon
atc: around the clock
bib: drink
b.i.d.: twice a day
c̄: with
d: day
dc, D/C: discontinue
h: hour
h.s.: at bedtime
n.p.o., NPO: nothing by mouth
od: every day, daily
p, p.: after
pc: after meals
PM: afternoon, evening
prn, PRN: as required, as needed
q: every
qd: every day
qh: every hour
qid: four times a day
ql: as much as desired
qm: every morning
qn: every night
qod: every other day
qoh: every other hour
qon: every other night
qp: as much as desired
qpm, qn: every night, every evening
qs: quantity sufficient
s̄: without
semih: half an hour
sos: if necessary
s̄s̄, ss, s̄s̄: half
t.i.d.: three times a day
tin: three times a night
ut: as directed

Medication Administration: Routes

hypo: hypodermic
IC, ICAV: intracavitary
ID: intradermal

IM: intramuscular
inhal: inhalation
inj, inject: injection
IT, i-thec: intrathecal
IV: intravenous
IVP: intravenous push
IVPB: intravenous piggyback
MDI: metered-dose inhaler
parent, P: parenteral
po, PO: orally
pr: through rectum, per rectum
SL, subl: sublingual
SQ, SC, subq, subcu, subcut: subcutaneous
TDD: transdermal drug delivery
top: topically

References
NDC: National Drug Code
NF: National Formulary
PDR: *Physicians' Desk Reference*

Standards & Regulations
CDC: Centers for Disease Control and Prevention
DEA: Drug Enforcement Agency
FDA: Food and Drug Administration
USP: United States Pharmacopeia

Diagnostic Testing
ac phos, ACP: acid phosphatase
AFP: alpha fetoprotein
A/G: albumin-to-globulin ratio
alk phos, ALP: alkaline phosphatase
ALT: alanine aminotransferase (serum glutamic pyruvic transaminase [SGPT])
ANA: antinuclear antibody
APTT, aPTT: activated partial thromboplastin time
ASO, ASL-O: antistreptolysin-O
AST: aspartate aminotransferase (serum glutamic oxaloacetic transaminase [SGOT])
BT: bleeding time
BUN: blood urea nitrogen
Ca: calcium
CAT: computed axial tomography
CBC: complete blood count
CEA: carcinoembryonic antigen
CHOL: cholesterol
Cl: chloride
CPK: creatine phosphokinase
creat: creatinine
CRP: C-reactive protein
CT: computed tomography

CXR: chest X-ray
DEXA: dual energy X-ray absorptiometry
diff: differential (blood count)
DR: diagnostic radiography
DSA: digital subtraction angiography
ECG, EKG: electrocardiogram
ECHO: echocardiography
EEG: electroencephalogram
ESR, sed rate: erythrocyte sedimentation rate
FBS: fasting blood sugar
GTT: glucose tolerance test
HCT, crit: hematocrit
HDI: high-definition imaging
HDL: high-density lipoprotein
Hgb: hemoglobin
K: potassium
LDH: lactate dehydrogenase
LDL: low-density lipoprotein
lytes: electrolytes
MCH: mean corpuscular hemoglobin
MCHC: mean corpuscular hemoglobin concentration
MCV: mean corpuscular volume
MRI: magnetic resonance imaging
MUGA: multiple-gated acquisition scanning
Na: sodium
PCV: packed-cell volume
PET: positron emission tomography
PFT: pulmonary function test
pH: hydrogen ion concentration
plats, PLTs: platelets
PT, pro time: prothrombin time
PTT: partial thromboplastin time
RAIU, RIU: radioactive iodine uptake
RAST: radioallergosorbent test
RBC: red blood cell, red blood count
RDW: red blood cell distribution width
RIA: radioimmunoassay
SMA: sequential multiple analysis (clinical chemistry)
SPECT: single-photon-emission computed tomography
sp. gr., SG, SpG: specific gravity
T&C: type and crossmatch
TFT: thyroid function test
trig: triglycerides
TT: thrombin time
UA, U/A: urinalysis
U/S, US: ultrasound
VLDL: very-low-density lipoprotein
WBC: white blood cell, white blood count
XR: X-ray

Health Assessment

abn, abnorm: abnormal
amb: ambulatory
A&O x 4: alert and oriented to person, place, time, and date
A/O, A&O: alert and oriented
A&P: auscultation and palpation, auscultation and percussion
Asx, ASX: asymptomatic
ausc, auscul: auscultation
A&W: alive and well
BP: blood pressure
CA: chronological age
C&A: conscious and alert
CC, c/o: chief complaint, complains of
DOB, D/B: date of birth
DU: diagnosis undetermined
Dx, diag: diagnosis
Ex, exam: examination
F: female
FH, FHx: family history
FOD: free of disease
F/U, FU: follow-up
FUO: fever of unknown origin
h/o: history of
H&P: history and physical
Ht, h: height
Hx, H: history
IBW: ideal body weight
IPPA: inspection, palpation, percussion, and auscultation
IQ: intelligence quotient
L&W: living and well
LWD: living with disease
M: male
MA: mental age
MHx, MH: medical history
NAD: no appreciable disease, no apparent distress or disease, nothing abnormal detected
N/C, NC: no complaints
ND: not diagnosed
NDF: no disease found
NED: no evidence of disease
NKA: no known allergies
NKDA: no known drug allergies
norm: normal
NVS: neurologic vital signs
NYD: not yet diagnosed
P: pulse
P&A, P/A: percussion and auscultation
palp: palpation
PE, PEx, PX: physical examination
PH: poor health

PH, Px, PHx: past history
PI: present illness
PMH, PMHx: past medical history
PMI: past medical illness
PPHx: previous psychiatric history
prog, progn, Px: prognosis
Pt: patient
R: respiration
R/O, RO: rule out
ROS: review of systems
RVC: responds to verbal commands
SOAP: problem-oriented record that includes subjective data, objective data, assessment or analysis, and plan
SOI: severity of illness
SONP: soft organs not palpable
S/S: signs and symptoms
Sx: symptoms, signs
T: temperature
TPR: temperature, pulse, and respiration
Tx, treat, tr: treatment
UCHD, UCD: usual childhood diseases
U/O, UO: under observation
VS, v/s: vital signs
WDWN: well-developed, well-nourished
WNL: within normal limits
wt: weight
X&D: examination and diagnosis
y, yr: year
y/o: years old
YOB: year of birth

Locations & Directions

AAL: anterior axillary line
A&D: ascending and descending
AE: above the elbow
AK: above the knee
ant.: anterior
AP, A-P: anteroposterior
A&P: anterior and posterior
BE: below the elbow
bilat: bilateral
BK: below the knee
ext: exterior, external
ICS, IS: intercostal space
inf: inferior
int: interior, internal
L: left
LAD: left anterior descending
LAO: left anterior oblique
Lat, L: lateral

LE: lower extremity
LLE: left lower extremity
LLL: left lower lobe (lung)
LLQ: left lower quadrant
LPO: left posterior oblique
L&R: left and right
L-R: left to right
LRT: lower respiratory tract
L&U: lower and upper
LUE: left upper extremity
LUL: left upper lobe (lung)
LUQ: left upper quadrant
MCL: midclavicular line
ML: midline
MSL: midsternal line
PA, P-A: posteroanterior
post.: posterior
prox.: proximal
R: right
RAD: right anterior descending
RAO: right anterior oblique
R/L, R-L: right to left
RLE: right lower extremity
RLL: right lower lobe (lung)
RLQ: right lower quadrant
RML: right middle lobe (lung), right mediolateral
RPO: right posterior oblique
RUE: right upper extremity
RUL: right upper lobe (lung)
RUQ: right upper quadrant
sup: superior
U/L, U&L: upper and lower
UE: upper extremity
URT: upper respiratory tract

Professional Designations

ARNP: Advanced Registered Nurse Practitioner
ATR-BC: Registered Art Therapist, Board Certified
CCT: Certified Cardiographic Technician
CDA: Certified Dental Assistant
CDT: Certified Dental Technician
CMA: Certified Medical Assistant
CNMT: Certified Nuclear Medicine Technologist
CO: Certified Orthotist
COMT: Certified Ophthalmic Medical Technologist
COT: Certified Ophthalmic Technician
COTA: Certified Occupational
Therapy Assistant
CP: Certified Prosthetist
CPhT: Certified Pharmacy Technician
CPO: Certified Prosthetist and Orthotist
CRC: Certified Rehabilitation Counselor
CRT: Certified Respiratory Therapist
CST: Certified Surgical Technologist
CT (ASCP): Cytotechnologist (American Society for Clinical Pathology)
CTRS: Certified Therapeutic Recreation Specialist
DC: Doctor of Chiropractic
DDS: Doctor of Dental Surgery
DMD: Doctor of Dental Medicine
DO: Doctor of Osteopathy
DPM: Doctor of Podiatric Medicine
DTR: Dietetic Technician, Registered
EMT: Emergency Medical Technician
EMT-P: Emergency Medical Technician–Paramedic
HT (ASCP): Histologic Technician (American Society for Clinical Pathology)
HTL (ASCP): Histotechnologist (American Society for Clinical Pathology)
LCSW: Licensed Clinical Social Worker
LMHC: Licensed Mental Health Counselor
LPN: Licensed Practical Nurse
LVN: Licensed Vocational Nurse
MD: Doctor of Medicine
MLT (ASCP): Medical Laboratory Technician (American Society for Clinical Pathology)
MT (ASCP): Medical Technologist (American Society for Clinical Pathology)
MT-BC: Music Therapist, Board Certified
NA: Nursing Assistant
OD: Doctor of Optometry
OTR: Occupational Therapist, Registered
PA-C: Physician's Assistant, Certified
PT: Physical Therapist
PTA: Physical Therapist Assistant
RCIS: Registered Cardiovascular Invasive Specialist
RCS: Registered Cardiac Sonographer

RD: Registered Dietitian

RDH: Registered Dental Hygienist

RDMS: Registered Diagnostic Medical Sonographer

RHIA: Registered Health Information Administrator

RN: Registered Nurse

RPh: Registered Pharmacist

RRT: Registered Respiratory Therapist

RT(N): Radiologic Technologist (Nuclear Medicine)

RT(R): Radiologic Technologist (Radiographer)

RT(T): Radiologic Technologist (Radiation Therapist)

RVS: Registered Vascular Specialist

SCT (ASCP): Specialist in Cytotechnology (American Society for Clinical Pathology)

Specialized Areas & Facilities

ACC: ambulatory care center

ALF: assisted living facility

BB, BLBK: blood bank

BU: burn unit

CCRC: continuous care retirement community

CCU: coronary care unit, critical care unit

DR: delivery room

ECF: extended care facility

ED: emergency department

ER: emergency room

ETU: emergency trauma unit, emergency treatment unit

HDU: hemodialysis unit

ICF: intermediate care facility

ICU: intensive care unit, intermediate care unit

Lab: laboratory

LR: labor room

MHC: mental health center

MICU: medical intensive care unit

MRD: medical records department

NICU: neonatal intensive care unit

OPC: outpatient clinic

OPD: outpatient department

OPS: outpatient surgery, outpatient service

OR: operating room

OT: occupational therapy

PCC: poison control center

PCU: progressive care unit

Peds: pediatrics

Pharm: pharmacy

PICU: pediatric intensive care unit

PT: physical therapy

RPCH: rural primary care hospital

RR: recovery room

SICU: surgical intensive care unit

SNF: skilled nursing facility

TC: therapeutic community, trauma center

Agencies & Organizations

AHA: American Hospital Association

AMA: American Medical Association

CAAHEP: Commission on Accreditation of Allied Health Education Programs

CDC: Centers for Disease Control and Prevention

FDA: Food and Drug Administration

HCFA: Health Care Financing Administration

HHA: Home Health Agency

IOM: Institute of Medicine

NCI: National Cancer Institute

NHC: National Health Council

NIH: National Institutes of Health

NLN: National League for Nursing

NORD: National Organization for Rare Disorders

UNOS: United Network for Organ Sharing

USDHHS: U.S. Department of Health and Human Services

USPHS: U.S. Public Health Service

VNA: Visiting Nurse Association

WHO: World Health Organization

Managed Care

ASO: administrative services only, application services organization

cap: capitation (reimbursement)

CM: case management, case manager

COB: coordination of benefits

COBRA: Consolidated Omnibus Budget Reconciliation Act (1985)

COC: certificate of coverage

co-pay: copayment

DUR: drug utilization review

EOB: explanation of benefits

EPO: exclusive provider organization

ERISA: Employee Retirement Income Security Act (1974)

FFS: fee for service (reimbursement)

HEDIS: Health Employer Data and Information Set

HI: health insurance

HIPAA: Health Insurance Portability and Accountability Act (1996)
HMO: health maintenance organization
IPA: independent practice association
MCO: managed care organization
MCP: managed care plan
MIP: managed indemnity plan
MSP: Medicare secondary payor
NCQA: National Committee for Quality Assurance
PBM: pharmacy benefit management, pharmacy benefit manager

PCP: primary care provider, primary care physician
PHO: Physician-Hospital Organization
PMPM: per member per month (capitation)
POS: point of service
PPO: preferred provider organization
PPS: prospective payment system
SSO: second surgical opinion
TPA: third-party administrator
UCR: usual, customary, and reasonable (fees)
UR: utilization review

Terms & Abbreviations for Body Systems

Development of the Human Body

- **Cells:** Major components
  - Cell membrane
  - Cytoplasm
  - Nucleus
- **Tissues:** Primary types
  - Connective
  - Epithelial
  - Muscle
  - Nervous
- **Organs**
  - Composed of two or more different tissues
  - Have specific functions
    - **Systems:** Related organs with common functions
    - **Organism:** A living person

Cavities
Cavities are spaces containing organs.
- **Dorsal**
  - Cranial
  - Vertebral (spinal)
- **Ventral**
  - Abdominal
  - Pelvic
  - Thoracic

Planes
A plane is an imaginary flat surface.
- **Frontal:** Anterior/posterior
- **Sagittal:** Right/left
- **Transverse:** Upper/lower

Positions
A position is a reference point for location or direction.
- **Anterior/ventral:** Front of the body

- **Posterior/dorsal:** Back of the body
- **Deep:** Away from the surface
- **Superficial:** On the surface
- **Inferior:** Situated below
- **Superior:** Situated above
- **Lateral:** Pertaining to the side
- **Medial:** Pertaining to the middle
- **Prone:** Lying face down
- **Supine:** Lying face up
- **Distal:** Farther from the midline or center of the body
- **Proximal:** Closer to the midline or center of the body

Skeletal System
- **Bones**
  - Formation: Ossification
  - Types: Long, short, flat, irregular
  - Tissues: Compact, spongy (cancellous)
  - Markings: Depressions, openings, projections
  - Axial skeleton
    - Skull
    - Vertebral column
    - Thoracic cage
  - Appendicular skeleton
    - Upper extremities
    - Lower extremities
    - Pectoral girdle
    - Pelvic girdle
- **Joints/articulations**
  - Structural classification
    - Fibrous
    - Cartilaginous
    - Synovial

- ○ Functional classification
  - – Synarthroses
  - – Amphiarthroses
  - – Diarthroses

Terms

ankyl/o: stiff, crooked, bent; *ankylosis*
arthr/o: joint; *arthrodysplasia*
articul/o: joint; *articulation*
brachi/o: arm; *brachiocephalic*
burs/o: bursa; *bursolith*
calcane/o: heel; *calcaneodynia*
carp/o: wrist; *carpoptosis*
centr/o: center; *centrosclerosis*
cephal/o: head; *cephaledema*
cervic/o: neck, cervix; *cervicofacial*
chir/o, cheir/o: hand; *chiropodalgia*
chondr/o: cartilage; *chondrodystrophy*
cleid/o: clavicle; *cleidorrhexis*
coccyg/o: coccyx; *coccygodynia*
cost/o: rib; *costosternal*
cox/o: hip; *coxarthrosis*
crani/o: skull; *cranioclast*
cubit/o: elbow, forearm; *genucubital*
dactyl/o: digit (finger or toe);
  dactylospasm
eury-: wide, broad; *eurycephalic*
faci/o: face; *facioplasty*
femor/o: femur; *ischiofemoral*
fibul/o: fibula; *fibulocalcaneal*
geni/o: chin; *genioplasty*
gnath/o: jaw; *gnathoschisis*
gnos/o: knowledge; *acrognosis*
goni/o: angle; *goniometer*
gyr/o: circle, spiral; *gyrospasm*
holo-: entire, complete; *holarthritis*
humer/o: humerus; *humeroradial*
hypsi-: high; *hypsicephaly*
ili/o: ilium; *iliolumbar*
ischi/o: ischium; *ischiodynia*
kyph/o: humpback; *kyphoscoliosis*
lamin/o: lamina; *laminectomy*
lip/o: fat; *lipochondroma*
-listhesis: slipping; *spondylolisthesis*
lord/o: curvature, bending;
  lordoscoliosis
lox/o: oblique, slanting; *loxarthron*
lumb/o: loin; *lumbodynia*
maxill/o: maxilla; *maxillotomy*
mega-, megalo-: large; *megalopodia*
-megaly: enlargement; *dactylomegaly*
mel/o: limb, limbs; *melalgia*
om/o: shoulder; *omodynia*
opisth/o: backward, behind;
  opisthognathism

oste/o: bone; *osteochondroma*
pan-: all; *panarthritis*
patell/o: patella; *patellofemoral*
ped/o: foot, child; *pedal*
pelv/i: pelvis; *pelvimeter*
perone/o: fibula; *peroneotibial*
petr/o: stone, petrous region of
  temporal bone; *petromastoid*
phalang/o: phalanges; *phalangitis*
-physis: growth, growing; *diaphysis*
pod/o: foot; *podiatrist*
-porosis: porous, decrease in density;
  osteoporosis
pub/o: pubis; *pubovesical*
rachi/o: spine; *rachioplegia*
sacr/o: sacrum; *sacrocoxalgia*
scapul/o: scapula; *scapulopexy*
scoli/o: crooked, twisted; *scoliorachitic*
skelet/o: skeleton; *skeletogenous*
spin/o: spinal cord, spine;
  spinocerebellar
spondyl/o: vertebrae; *spondylopyosis*
stern/o: sternum; *sternocostal*
synov/o: synovia, synovial membrane;
  synovectomy
tal/o: talus; *talofibular*
tars/o: tarsus, edge of eyelid;
  tarsoclasis
tibi/o: tibia; *tibiotarsal*
vertebr/o: vertebra; *vertebrosternal*
xiph/o: sword-shaped, xiphoid;
  xiphocostal

Abbreviations

AEA: above-elbow amputation
AFO: ankle-foot orthosis
AKA: above-knee amputation
AROM: active range of motion
BEA: below-elbow amputation
BKA: below-knee amputation
BSF: basal skull fracture
C1–C7: cervical vertebrae
CDH: congenital dislocation of hip
CPM: continuous passive motion
DJD: degenerative joint disease
FRJM: full range of joint movement
FROM: full range of motion
Fx: fracture
HD: herniated disk
IVD: intervertebral disk
JRA: juvenile rheumatoid arthritis
jt, jnt: joint
KB: knee brace
KJ: knee jerk
L1–L5: lumbar vertebrae

LBP: low back pain
LOM: limitation or loss of motion or movement
LS: lumbosacral
OA: osteoarthritis
OAWO: opening abductory wedge osteotomy
OM: osteomalacia, osteomyelitis
ORIF: open reduction internal fixation
Ortho: orthopedics
PEMF: pulsing electromagnetic field
PKR: partial knee replacement
PROM: passive range of motion
RA: rheumatoid arthritis
RF: rheumatoid factor
ROM: range of motion
S1–S5: sacral vertebrae
sh, shld: shoulder
skel, sk: skeletal
T1–T12: thoracic vertebrae
THR: total hip replacement
TKA: total knee arthroplasty
TKR: total knee replacement
TMJ: temporomandibular joint
TX, Tx: traction

Nervous System

- Cells
    - Neuron: Dendrites, cell body, axon
    - Neuroglia (glial)
- Central nervous system (CNS)
    - Brain: Cerebrum, cerebellum, brain stem, diencephalon
    - Spinal cord: Ascending and descending tracts
    - Membranes (meninges): Dura mater, arachnoid, pia mater
    - Cerebrospinal fluid (CSF)
- Peripheral nervous system (PNS)
    - Cranial nerves (12 pairs)
    - Spinal nerves (31 pairs)
    - Afferent (sensory) division: Sensory receptors
    - Efferent (motor) division
        - Somatic nervous system (voluntary)
        - Autonomic nervous system (involuntary): Sympathetic nervous system and para-sympathetic nervous system

Terms

-algesia, alges/o: pain sensitivity; *analgesia*
astr/o: star, star-shaped; *astrocytoma*

atel/o: incomplete, imperfect; *atelomyelia*
-bulia, -boulia: will; *abulia*
cerebell/o: cerebellum; *cerebellospinal*
cerebr/o: cerebrum, brain; *cerebroid*
-crasia: mixture (good or bad), temperament; *eucrasia*
drom/o, -drome: running; *dromotropic*
encephal/o: brain; *encephalomalacia*
esthesi/o, -esthesia: sensation, feeling; *esthesioneurosis*
gangli/o, ganglion/o: ganglion; *gangliocytoma*
gli/o: glue, neuroglia; *gliocyte*
heli/o: sun; *heliophobia*
hydr/o: water, hydrogen; *hydrocephalocele*
hypn/o: sleep; *hypnogenic*
hypothalam/o: hypothalamus; *hypothalamohypophysial*
keraun/o: lightning; *keraunoneurosis*
klept/o: theft, stealing; *kleptomania*
-lemma: confining membrane; *epilemma*
-lepsy: seizure; *epilepsy*
-lexia: speech, word; *bradylexia*
log/o, -log, -logue: word, speech, thought; *logorrhea*
-mania: madness, obsessive preoccupation; *hypomania*
medull/o: medulla, marrow; *medulloblast*
mening/o: meninges, membranes; *meningocele*
ment/o: mind; *dementia*
-mnesia: memory; *ecmnesia*
myel/o: bone marrow, spinal cord; *myelocele*
narc/o: numbness, stupor; *narcoanesthesia*
neur/o: nerve; *neurotripsy*
noci-: to cause harm, injury or pain; *nociceptor*
-noia: mind, will; *paranoia*
-paresis: partial paralysis; *hemiparesis*
phaner/o: visible, apparent; *phaneromania*
-phobia, phob/o: fear, aversion; *phobophobia*
phren/o: mind, diaphragm; *tachyphrenia*
picr/o: bitter; *picrotoxin*
piez/o, pies/i, -piesis: pressure; *piesesthesia*
-plegia: paralysis; *quadriplegia*

poli/o: gray matter; *poliomyelitis*
-pore: opening, passageway; *neuropore*
-praxia: action, activity; *parapraxia*
psych/o: mind; *psychokinesis*
psychr/o: cold; *psychrophobia*
radicul/o: nerve root; *radiculitis*
rhiz/o: root; *rhizotomy*
schiz/o: split, division; *schizophasia*
somn/i, -somnia: sleep; *insomnia*
syring/o: tube, fistula; *syringomyelocele*
tauto-: identical, same; *tautomeral*
-taxia, tax/o: arrangement, coordination; *dystaxia*
tel/o: end; *telodendron*
tephr/o: gray, ashen; *tephromyelitis*
thanat/o: death; *thanatomania*
thec/o: sheath; *neurothecitis*
vag/o: vagus nerve; *vagolysis*

Abbreviations

ACh: acetylcholine
AD: Alzheimer disease
ADD: attention deficit disorder
ADHD: attention deficit hyperactivity disorder
ALD: adrenoleukodystrophy
ALS: amyotrophic lateral sclerosis (Lou Gehrig disease)
anesth, anes: anesthesia
ANS: autonomic nervous system
BAER: brainstem auditory evoked response
BBB: blood-brain barrier
BD: brain dead
BEAM: brain electrical activity mapping
CBF: cerebral blood flow
CJD: Creutzfeldt-Jakob disease (subacute spongiform encephalopathy; a.k.a. Mad Cow disease)
CNE: chronic nervous exhaustion
CNS: central nervous system
CP: cerebral palsy
CSF: cerebrospinal fluid
CVA: cerebrovascular accident
CVD: cerebrovascular disease
DAI: diffuse axonal injury
DT: delirium tremens
ECT: electroconvulsive therapy
EEG: electroencephalogram
EST: electroshock therapy
GAD: generalized anxiety disorder
GAS: general adaptation syndrome

HD: Huntington disease
ICH: intracerebral hemorrhage
ICP: intracranial pressure
IQ: intelligence quotient
LMN: lower motor neuron
LOC: level of consciousness; loss of consciousness
LP: lumbar puncture
MA: mental age
MBD: minimal brain dysfunction
MND: motor neuron disease
MS: multiple sclerosis
NCS: nerve conduction study
NF: neurofibromatosis
NGF: nerve growth factor
NTD: neural tube defect
OBS: organic brain syndrome
OCD: obsessive-compulsive disorder
OMD: organic mental disorder
PD: Parkinson disease, psychotic depression, psychotic dementia
PNI: peripheral nerve injury
PNS: peripheral nervous system
PTSD: posttraumatic stress disorder
RIND: reversible ischemic neurologic deficit
SAD: seasonal affective disorder
Sz: seizure
TBI: traumatic brain injury
TENS: transcutaneous electrical nerve stimulation
TGA: transient global amnesia
TIA: transient ischemic attack
UMN: upper motor neuron

Male Reproductive System

- **Scrotum:** Sac containing the testes
  - Testes
  - Seminiferous tubules: Spermatozoa
  - Interstitial cells: Testosterone
- **Ducts**
  - Epididymis
  - Vas deferens, ductus deferens
  - Ejaculatory duct
  - Urethra
- **Penis:** Erectile tissue
- **Glands**
  - Seminal vesicles
  - Prostate gland
  - Bulbourethral (Cowper) gland
- **Secretions**
  - Semen
  - Sperm
  - Glandular secretions

andr/o: male; *androgen*
balan/o: glans penis; *balanoblennorrhea*
-cele: hernia, swelling; *hydrocele*
-cide: killing, agent that kills; *spermicide*
crypt/o: hidden, concealed; *cryptorchism*
epididym/o: epididymis; *epididymectomy*
genit/o: reproduction; *genitourinary*
gon/o: genitals; *gonocyte*
gonad/o: gonads; *gonadogenesis*
olig/o: scanty, few, little; *oligospermia*
orch/o, orchi/o, orchid/o: testis; *orchidopexy*
osche/o: scrotum; *oscheoplasty*
phall/o: penis; *phallodynia*
phim/o: prepuce, muzzle; *paraphimosis*
prostat/o: prostate gland; *prostatocystotomy*
semin/i: semen; *seminiferous*
sperm/o, spermat/o: spermatozoa; *spermatogenesis*
test/o, testicul/o: testis; *testectomy*
vas/o: vas deferens, vessel; *vasovasostomy*
venere/o: sexual intercourse; *venereologist*
vesicul/o: seminal vesicle; *vasovesiculitis*
zo/o: animal; *azoospermia*

Abbreviations

AIH: artificial insemination by husband
BPH: benign prostatic hypertrophy
ED: erectile dysfunction
HSV: herpes simplex virus
NGU: nongonococcal urethritis
NPT: nocturnal penile tumescence
PSA: prostate-specific antigen
RPR: rapid plasma reagin (test)
SPP: suprapubic prostatectomy
STD: sexually transmitted disease
TDF: testes determining factor
TFS: testicular feminization syndrome
TSE: testicular self-examination
TUR, TURP: transurethral resection of the prostate
VD: venereal disease
VDG: venereal disease, gonorrhea
VDS: venereal disease, syphilis

Urinary System

- **Organs**
  - Kidneys: Cortex, medulla, nephron, collecting duct, renal pelvis
  - Ureters: Tubes
  - Bladder: Trigone
  - Urethra: Tube
- **Urine**
  - Formation: Filtration, reabsorption, secretion
  - Composition: Water, nitrogenous waste, salts, other substances

Terms

a-, an-: without, not; *anuria*
albumin/o: albumin; *albuminimeter*
ammoni/o: ammonium; *ammoniuria*
-atresia: closure, occlusion; *urethratresia*
atreto-: closed, lacking an opening; *atretocystia*
azot/o: nitrogen, urea; *azoturia*
calci/o: calcium; *hypocalciuria*
cali/o: calyx; *pyelocaliectasis*
cupr/o: copper; *cupruresis*
cyan/o: blue; *urocyanosis*
cyst/o: bladder, cyst; *cystogram*
-ectasis, -ectasia: dilation, expansion; *nephrectasia*
fusc/o: dark brown; *urofuscohematin*
glomerul/o: glomerulus; *glomerulopathy*
keton/o: ketones; *ketonuria*
lith/o: stone, calculus; *pyelolithotomy*
nephr/o: kidney; *nephrotoxic*
noct/i: night; *noctalbuminuria*
py/o: pus; *pyocalix*
pyel/o: renal pelvis; *pyelophlebitis*
ren/o: kidney; *renogastric*
ur/o: urine; *uroerythrin*
-uresis: urination; *diuresis*
ureter/o: ureter; *ureterocolostomy*
urethr/o: urethra; *urethrorrhagia*
-uria: urine condition; *pyuria*
uric/o: uric acid; *uricosuria*
urin/o: urine; *urinalysis*
vesic/o: urinary bladder; *vesicoclysis*

Abbreviations

AGN: acute glomerulonephritis
AHC: acute hemorrhagic cystitis
APD: adult polycystic disease
APORF: acute postoperative renal failure

ARF: acute renal failure
ATN: acute tubular necrosis
BUN: blood urea nitrogen
CAPD: continuous ambulatory
  peritoneal dialysis
cath.: catheter, catheterization
CRF: chronic renal failure
ESRD: end-stage renal disease
ESWL: extracorporeal shockwave
  lithotripsy
GFR: glomerular filtration rate
GU: genitourinary
HD: hemodialysis
IC: interstitial cystitis
I&O: intake and output
IVC: intravenous cholangiography
IVP: intravenous pyelography
IVU: intravenous urography
KUB: kidney, ureter, and bladder
NPN: nonprotein nitrogen
NSU: nonspecific urethritis
PD: peritoneal dialysis
PKD: polycystic kidney disease
PKU: phenylketonuria
RPF: renal plasma flow
RPG: retrograde pyelogram
RTA: renal tubular acidosis
RUG: retrograde urethrogram
TRBF: total renal blood flow
UA, U/A: urinalysis
UO, UOP: urinary output
urol: urology
UTI: urinary tract infection
VCUG: voiding cystourethrogram

Female Reproductive System

- **Ovaries**
  - Oocyte development
  - Ovulation
- **Fallopian tubes, uterine tubes:**
  Fertilization
- **Uterus**
  - Wall
    - Perimetrium
    - Myometrium
    - Endometrium
  - Parts
    - Fundus
    - Body
    - Cervix
- **Vagina:** Hymen
  - External genitalia/vulva
  - Labia majora and minora
  - Clitoris
  - Bartholin glands

- **Breasts**
  - Mammary glands
  - Nipple
  - Areola
  - Lactation
- **Menstrual cycle**
  - Phases
  - Hormonal interaction
  - Cessation

Terms

amni/o: amnion; *amnioscopy*
cervic/o: neck, cervix; *cervicovaginitis*
chori/o: chorion; *chorioadenoma*
-clasis, -clast, -clasia: break, breaking;
  cranioclasis
colp/o: vagina; *colporrhaphy*
culd/o: cul-de-sac; *culdoscopy*
-cyesis: pregnancy; *ovariocyesis*
embry/o: embryo; *embryopathy*
episi/o: vulva; *episiostenosis*
fet/o: fetus; *fetography*
galact/o: milk; *galactacrasia*
gravid/o: pregnancy; *gravidocardiac*
-gravida: pregnant woman; *unigravida*
gyn/e, gynec/o: woman, female;
  gynecography
helc/o: ulcer; *helcomenia*
hymen/o: hymen; *hymenitis*
hyster/o: uterus; *panhysterectomy*
lact/o: milk; *lactorrhea*
lecith/o: yolk, ovum; *centrolecithal*
-lipsis: omit, fail; *menolipsis*
mamm/o: breast; *mammography*
mast/o: breast; *mastalgia*
men/o: menses, menstruation;
  menorrhagia
metr/o: uterus; *myometritis*
nat/o: birth; *neonatology*
neo-: new; *neonatal*
nulli-: none; *nulliparity*
o/o: egg, ovum; *oogenesis*
obstetr/o: midwife; *obstetrician*
omphal/o: navel; *omphalocele*
oophor/o: ovary; *oophorohysterectomy*
ov/o, ov/i: egg, ovum; *ovicide*
ovari/o: ovary; *ovariocentesis*
-para, -parous: to bear, to bring forth;
  septipara
-partum: childbirth, labor; *postpartum*
perine/o: perineum; *colpoperineoplasty*
per/o: deformed, maimed; *peromelia*
phys/o: air, gas; *physometra*
sacchar/o: sugar;
  saccharogalactorrhea

salping/o: fallopian tube; *salpingocyesis*
terat/o: monster; *teratogenesis*
thel/o: nipple; *thelorrhagia*
toc/o, -tocia: childbirth, labor; *dystocia*
tub/o: tube; *tuboplasty*
uter/o: uterus; *uterolith*
vagin/o: vagina; *vaginography*
viv/i: life, alive; *viviparous*
vulv/o: vulva; *vulvopathy*

Abbreviations

Ab, AB: abortion
AFP: alpha fetoprotein
ARM, AROM: artificial rupture of membranes
ART: assisted reproductive technology
BSE: breast self-examination
BSO: bilateral salpingo-oophorectomy
BWS: battered woman syndrome
C section, CS: cesarean section
CVS: chorionic villus sampling
CX: cervix
D&C: dilation and curettage
D&E: dilation and evacuation
DUB: dysfunctional uterine bleeding
ECC: endocervical curettage
EDC: estimated date of confinement
EDD: estimated date of delivery
EFM: electronic fetal monitor
ERT: estrogen replacement therapy
FHR: fetal heart rate
FHT: fetal heart tone
FTND: full-term normal delivery
GDM: gestational diabetes mellitus
GIFT: gamete intrafallopian transfer
grav: pregnancy
GYN: gynecology
HCG: human chorionic gonadotropin
HDN: hemolytic disease of the newborn
HRT: hormone replacement therapy
HSG: hysterosalpingography
IDM: infant of a diabetic mother
IUD: intrauterine device
IUFD: intrauterine fetal distress
IUP: intrauterine pregnancy
IVF: in vitro fertilization
L&D: labor and delivery
LDRP: labor, delivery, recovery, and postpartum
LMP: last menstrual period
NB: newborn
ND: normal delivery
OB: obstetrics

OB/GYN: obstetrics and gynecology
OCP: oral contraceptive pills
Pap smear: Papanicolaou smear
para: number of viable births
PID: pelvic inflammatory disease
PIH: pregnancy-induced hypertension
PMS: premenstrual syndrome
POU: placenta, ovary, uterus
SAB: spontaneous abortion
SVD: spontaneous vaginal delivery
TAb, TAB: therapeutic abortion
TAH: total abdominal hysterectomy
TOP: termination of pregnancy
TSS: toxic shock syndrome
UC: uterine contraction
VH: vaginal hysterectomy
ZIFT: zygote intrafallopian transfer

Cardiovascular System

- **Heart**
  - Four chambers
    - Two upper (atria)
    - Two lower (ventricles)
  - Wall
    - Endocardium
    - Myocardium
    - Pericardium
  - Two partitions
    - Interatrial septum
    - Interventricular septum
  - Four valves
    - Atrioventricular: Tricuspid and bicuspid (mitral)
    - Semilunar: Pulmonary and aortic
- **Blood vessels**
  - Arteries, arterioles
  - Veins, venules
  - Capillaries
- **Circulation**
  - Pulmonary
  - Systemic
- **Blood pressure**
  - Systole (contraction)
  - Diastole (relaxation)
- **Pulse:** Rhythmical expansion and contraction of an artery as a result of heart contraction.
- **Electrical conduction system**
  - Components: sinoatrial (SA) node, atrioventricular (AV) node, bundle of His, bundle branches, Purkinje fibers
  - Measurement: ECG

Terms

aneurysm/o: aneurysm; *aneurysmectomy*

angi/o: vessel; *angioblast*

aort/o: aorta; *aortomalacia*

arteri/o: artery; *arteriolith*

arteriol/o: arteriole; *arteriolosclerosis*

ather/o: fatty substance, plaque; *atheroma*

atri/o: atrium; *atrioseptopexy*

brady-: slow; *bradycardia*

cardi/o: heart; *cardioptosis*

cine-: movement; *cineangiograph*

-clysis: irrigation, washing; *venoclysis*

coron/o: heart; *coronary*

embol/o: embolus; *embolectomy*

isch/o: to suppress, to restrain; *ischemia*

-megaly: enlargement; *atriomegaly*

mi/o: less, smaller; *miocardia*

-motor: movement, motion; *venomotor*

palpit/o, palpitat/o: flutter, throbbing; *palpitation*

phleb/o: vein; *phleborrhexis*

presby-: aging, elderly; *presbycardia*

rhe/o: flow, current, stream; *rheocardiography*

-spasm: involuntary contraction; *vasospasm*

sphygm/o: pulse; *sphygmoscope*

-sphyxia: pulse; *asphyxia*

-stenosis: narrowed, constricted; *aortostenosis*

tachy-: fast; *tachycardia*

tel/e: end, distant; *telecardiography*

-tension: stretched, strained; *hypertension*

valv/o, valvul/o: valve; *valvulotome*

varic/o: varicose veins; *varicophlebitis*

vas/o: vessel; *vasohypotonic*

vascul/o: vessel; *vasculitis*

ven/o: vein; *venography*

ventricul/o: ventricle; *ventriculogram*

venul/o: venule; *venular*

Abbreviations

ABP: arterial blood pressure

ACLS: advanced cardiac life support

AED: automated external defibrillator

AF, Afib, at fib: atrial fibrillation

AIVR: accelerated idioventricular rhythm

AMI: acute myocardial infarction

ang: angiogram

Ao: aorta

AR: aortic regurgitation

AS: aortic stenosis, arteriosclerosis

ASCVD: arteriosclerotic cardiovascular disease

ASD: atrial septal defect

ASHD: arteriosclerotic heart disease

AV, A-V: atrioventricular, arteriovenous

AVB: atrioventricular block

AVD: aortic valve disease

AVR: aortic valve replacement

AVS: arteriovenous shunt

BBB: bundle branch block

BCLS: basic cardiac life support

BP: blood pressure

BPd, DBP: blood pressure, diastolic

bpm: beats per minute

BPs, SBP: blood pressure, systolic

CA: cardiac arrest, cancer, cardiac arrhythmia

CABG: coronary artery bypass graft

CABS: coronary artery bypass surgery

CAD: coronary artery disease

CEA: carotid endarterectomy

CHB: complete heart block

CHD: congenital heart disease, coronary heart disease

CHF: congestive heart failure

CO: cardiac output

CoA: coarctation of the aorta

CP: chest pain, cardiopulmonary

CPA: cardiopulmonary arrest, carotid phonoangiography

CPR: cardiopulmonary resuscitation

CV: cardiovascular

CVP: central venous pressure

CVS: cardiovascular system

DNR: do not resuscitate

DVT: deep vein thrombosis

ECC: emergency cardiac care, extracorporeal circulation

ECG, EKG: electrocardiogram

ECHO: echocardiography

EF: ejection fraction

EPS: electrophysiologic study

ETT: exercise tolerance test, exercise treadmill test

HBP: high blood pressure

HCM: hypertrophic cardiomyopathy

HCVD: hypertensive cardiovascular disease

HF: heart failure

HR: heart rate

HTN: hypertension

IABP: intraaortic balloon pump
ICD: implantable cardiac defibrillator
ISH: isolated systolic hypertension
IV: intravenous, intraventricular
IVF: intravenous fluid, intravascular fluid
JVP: jugular venous pulse
LBBB: left bundle branch block
LBP: low blood pressure
LQTS: long QT syndromes
LVAD: left ventricular assist device
LVET: left ventricular ejection time
LVH: left ventricular hypertrophy
MI: myocardial infarction
MR: mitral regurgitation
MS: mitral stenosis
MVP: mitral valve prolapse
NSR: normal sinus rhythm
P: pulse
PAC: premature atrial contraction
PAD: peripheral arterial disease
PALS: pediatric advanced life support
PDA: patent ductus arteriosus
PEA: pulseless electrical activity
PPM: permanent pacemaker
PSVT: paroxysmal supraventricular tachycardia
PTCA: percutaneous transluminal coronary angioplasty
PVC: premature ventricular contraction
PVD: peripheral vascular disease
RBBB: right bundle branch block
RHD: rheumatic heart disease
S1, S2: heart sound (first, second)
SBE: subacute bacterial endocarditis
SSS: sick sinus syndrome
SVT: supraventricular tachycardia
TET: treadmill exercise test
tPA, TPA: tissue plasminogen activator
TR: tricuspid regurgitation
TT: thrombolytic therapy
VF, Vfib, vent fib: ventricular fibrillation
VHD: valvular heart disease, ventricular heart disease
VPC: ventricular premature contraction
VSP: ventricular septal defect
VT, Vtach: ventricular tachycardia
WPW: Wolff-Parkinson-White [syndrome]

Gastrointestinal System
- **Oral cavity**
  - Tongue, teeth, hard/soft palate, gums, salivary glands
- **Pharynx**
- **Esophagus**
- **Stomach:** Sphincter, fundus, body, pylorus
- **Small intestine:** Duodenum, jejunum, ileum
- **Liver:** Right and left lobes
- **Pancreas:** Endocrine and exocrine tissue
- **Large intestine:** Cecum, colon, rectum, anus

Terms

abdomin/o: abdomen; *abdominocentesis*
-agogue: producer, leader; *cholagogue*
-agra: severe pain; *dentagra*
amyl/o: starch; *amylolysis*
an/o: anus; *anorectocolonic*
arsenic/o: arsenic; *arsenicophagy*
atel/o: incomplete, imperfect; *ateloglossia*
bil/i: bile; *biligenesis*
bucc/o: cheek; *buccal*
cec/o: cecum; *cecoileostomy*
celi/o: abdomen; *celiomyositis*
cheil/o, chil/o: lip; *cheiloschisis*
-chezia, -chesia: defecation; *dyschezia*
chol/e: gall, bile; *cholangiostomy*
choledoch/o: common bile duct; *choledocholithiasis*
chyl/o: chyle; *chylopoiesis*
col/o: colon; *proctocolectomy*
dent/i: tooth; *dentalgia*
dips/o: thirst; *adipsia*
duoden/o: duodenum; *duodenohepatic*
-emesis: vomiting; *hyperemesis*
enter/o: intestine; *enteroclysis*
esophag/o: esophagus; *esophagocele*
gastr/o: stomach; *dextrogastria*
ge/o: earth, soil; *geophagia*
gingiv/o: gums; *gingivoplasty*
gloss/o: tongue; *glossolalia*
gluc/o: glucose, sugar; *glucokinetic*
glyc/o: glucose, sugar; *glycosialorrhea*
hepat/o: liver; *hepatosplenomegaly*
idi/o: individual, distinct, unknown; *idioglossia*
ile/o: ileum; *ileoileostomy*
jejun/o: jejunum; *jejunorrhaphy*
lapar/o: abdomen, abdominal wall; *laparoscope*
lingu/o: tongue; *retrolingual*
loph/o: ridge; *lophodont*
odont/o: tooth; *anodontia*

or/o: mouth; *intraoral*
-orexia: appetite; *hyperorexia*
orth/o: straight, normal, correct; *orthodontist*
palat/o: palate; *palatoplegia*
-pepsia: digestion; *dyspepsia*
peritone/o: peritoneum; *peritoneoclysis*
phag/o, phagia: eating, ingestion; *phagodynamometer*
-posia: drinking; *polyposia*
-prandial: meal; *postprandial*
proct/o: rectum, anus; *proctopexy*
ptyal/o: saliva; *ptyalogenic*
pyl/e: portal vein; *pylemphraxis*
pylor/o: pylorus; *pyloroplasty*
pyr/o: heat, fire, fever; *pyrosis*
rect/o: rectum; *rectocele*
sial/o: saliva; *sialolith*
sigmoid/o: sigmoid colon; *sigmoidoscope*
sit/o: food; *sitophobia*
splanchn/o: viscera; *splanchnoptosis*
-stalis: contraction; *peristalsis*
staphyl/o: uvula, grapelike clusters; *staphylorrhaphy*
stomat/o: mouth; *stomatomalacia*
-tresia: opening, perforation; *proctotresia*
typhl/o: cecum, blindness; *typhlectasis*
uran/o: palate; *uranoschisis*
zym/o: enzyme, ferment; *zymolysis*

Abbreviations

abd: abdomen, abdominal
BE: barium enema
BM: bowel movement
BS: bowel sounds
CAH: chronic active hepatitis
CBD: common bile duct
CUC: chronic ulcerative colitis
D&V: diarrhea and vomiting
DU: duodenal ulcer
EGD: esophagogastroduodenoscopy
ERCP: endoscopic retrograde cholangiopancreatography
ESO, esoph: esophagus
GB: gallbladder
GBS: gallbladder series
GERD, GRD: gastroesophageal reflux disease
GI: gastrointestinal
HAV: hepatitis A virus
HBV: hepatitis B virus
HCl: hydrochloric acid
HCV: hepatitis C virus

HDV: hepatitis D virus
HI: hepatic insufficiency
IBD: inflammatory bowel disease
IBS: irritable bowel syndrome
IH: infectious hepatitis
IVC: intravenous cholangiography
LES: lower esophageal sphincter
LFT: liver function tests
LGI: lower gastrointestinal
LSK: liver, spleen, and kidneys
NG, N-G: nasogastric (tube)
N/V: nausea and vomiting
OCG: oral cholecystogram
PEG: percutaneous endoscopic gastrostomy
PEM: protein-energy malnutrition
procto: proctoscopy
PU: peptic ulcer
PUD: peptic ulcer disease
RDA: recommended daily allowance, recommended dietary allowance
SBFT: small bowel follow-through
SBO: small bowel obstruction
SBS: small bowel series
TPN: total parenteral nutrition
UGI: upper gastrointestinal
VH: viral hepatitis

Blood System

- **Composition**
  - 55% plasma, a pale, yellow fluid
  - 45% formed elements (cells)
    - Erythrocytes (red blood cells)
    - Leukocytes (white blood cells): Granulocytes (eosinophils, basophils, neutrophils) and agranulocytes (monocytes, lymphocytes)
  - Thrombocytes (platelets)
- **Blood groups**
  - ABO group
    - Types: A, B, AB, O
    - Determined by antigen(s) on erythrocyte
  - Rh group
    - + or – Rh; presence or absence of Rh antigen on erythrocyte
- **Blood clotting (coagulation)**
  - Chemical reactions
  - Clot prevention
  - Clot retraction

agglutin/o: clumping; *agglutinophilic*
anis/o: unequal; *anisonormocytosis*
bas/o, basi/o: base, foundation; *basophil*
coagul/o: coagulation, clotting; *coagulopathy*
-crit: to separate; *thrombocytocrit*
-emia: blood condition; *erythremia*
eosin/o: red, rosy, dawn-colored; *eosinopenia*
erythr/o: red; *erythrocytoschisis*
ferr/i, ferr/o: iron; *ferrous sulfate*
gigant/o: huge; *gigantocyte*
-globin: protein; *hemoglobin*
granul/o: granules; *agranulocytosis*
hem/o, hemat/o: blood; *hemocytozoon*
kal/i: potassium; *hyperkalemia*
leuk/o: white; *leukocytotoxin*
myel/o: bone marrow, spinal cord; *myelocytosis*
natr/o: sodium; *hypernatremia*
neutr/o: neutral; *neutropenia*
norm/o: normal, usual; *normocytic*
-pheresis: removal; *plateletpheresis*
-phil, -philia: affinity for, tendency toward; *hemophilia*
-phore: bearer, processor; *siderophore*
-phoresis: bearing, transmission; *electrophoresis*
phosphat/o: phosphate; *phosphatemia*
poikil/o: variation, irregular; *poikiloblast*
pykn/o, pycn/o: thick, dense; *pyknocyte*
rhod/o: red, rosy; *rhodococcus*
sangu/i, sanguin/o: blood; *sanguiferous*
sapr/o: rotten, decay; *sapremia*
schist/o, -schisis: split, cleft; *schistocyte*
ser/o: serum, serous; *serosanguineous*
sider/o: iron; *sideropenia*
spher/o: round, sphere; *spherocytosis*
strept/o: twisted, curved; *streptococcemia*
thromb/o: clot, thrombus; *thromboelastogram*
-volemia: blood volume; *normovolemia*

ABMT: autologous bone marrow transplant
ABO: blood groups
AC: anticoagulant
ACT: anticoagulant therapy
agg, aggl: agglutination
AHF: antihemophilic factor
AIHA: autoimmune hemolytic anemia
ALL: acute lymphocytic leukemia
AML: acute myelogenous leukemia
APA: antipernicious anemia (factor)
AUL: acute undifferentiated leukemia
B, bl, bld: blood
baso: basophil
bl: bleeding
BMB: bone marrow biopsy
BMT: bone marrow transplant
CBC: complete blood count
CLL: chronic lymphocytic leukemia
CML: chronic myelogenous leukemia
coag: coagulation
DIC: disseminated intravascular coagulation
eos, eosins: eosinophil
EPO: erythropoietin
IF: intrinsic factor
ITP: idiopathic thrombocytopenia purpura
LIF: leukemia-inhibitory factor
lymphs: lymphocytes
mono: monocyte
PAF: platelet-activating factor
plat, PLT: platelet
PMN, polys, segs: polymorphonuclear neutrophils
PNH: paroxysmal nocturnal hemoglobinuria
PV: polycythemia vera
RBC: red blood cell, red blood cell count
retic: reticulocyte
Rh: Rhesus blood factor
SCT: sickle cell trait
T&C: type and crossmatch
TTP: thrombotic thrombocytopenia purpura
WBC: white blood cell, white blood cell count

Endocrine System

- **Characteristics**
  - Glands secrete hormones directly into the bloodstream.
  - Hormones affect growth and development, reproduction, and metabolism.

- **Endocrine glands**
  - Pituitary
    - Anterior
    - Posterior
  - Thyroid
  - Parathyroid
  - Adrenal
    - Medulla
    - Cortex
  - Pancreas
  - Testes
  - Ovaries
  - Pineal
  - Thymus

Terms

acr/o: extremities; *acrogeria*
aden/o: gland; *adenectopia*
adren/o: adrenal glands; *adrenomegaly*
cortic/o: cortex; *corticoadrenal*
crin/o: to secrete, to separate; *crinogenic*
hirsut/o: hairy; *hirsutism*
hormon/o: hormone; *hormonopoiesis*
medull/o: medulla, marrow; *medulloadrenal*
myx/o: mucus; *myxedema*
pancreat/o: pancreas; *pancreatolithotomy*
parathyroid/o: parathyroid; *parathyroidoma*
phe/o: dusky; *pheochromocytoma*
pineal/o: pineal gland; *pinealopathy*
pituitar/i: pituitary gland; *pituitarism*
thym/o: thymus gland; *thymotoxin*
thyr/o: thyroid gland; *thyrocele*
tox/o, toxic/o: poison; *thyrotoxicosis*
-trophy, troph/o: nourishment, growth; *hypertrophy*

Abbreviations

AC: adrenal cortex
ACTH: adrenocorticotropic hormone
ADH: antidiuretic hormone
CAH: congenital adrenal hyperplasia
DI: diabetes insipidus
DKA: diabetic ketoacidosis
DM: diabetes mellitus
FSH: follicle-stimulating hormone
GH: growth hormone
HCG: human chorionic gonadotropin
HGF: human growth factor

ICSH: interstitial cell-stimulating hormone
IDDM: insulin-dependent diabetes mellitus
IGT: impaired glucose tolerance
JOD: juvenile-onset diabetes
LH: luteinizing hormone
MEA: multiple endocrine adenomatosis
MEN: multiple endocrine neoplasia
MSH: melanocyte-stimulating hormone
NIDDM: non-insulin-dependent diabetes mellitus
OXT: oxytocin
PRL: prolactin
PTH: parathyroid hormone
SIADH: syndrome of inappropriate secretion of ADH
STH: somatotropic hormone
T_3: triiodothyronine
T_4: thyroxine
TFT: thyroid function test
TSH: thyroid-stimulating hormone

Integumentary System
- **Skin**
  - Layers
    - Epidermis
    - Dermis/corium
    - Subcutaneous/hypodermis
- **Hair**
  - Components
    - Shaft
    - Root
    - Bulb
  - Cycle: Growth/resting
- **Glands**
  - Sebaceous/oil: Sebum
  - Sudoriferous/sweat
    - Apocrine
    - Eccrine
- **Nails**
  - Components
    - Free edge
    - Nail body
    - Nail root

Terms

acanth/o: thorny, spiny; *acanthoma*
actin/o: ray, radiation; *actinodermatitis*
brom/o: bromine-containing compound, odor; *bromoderma*

caus/o, cauter/o: burn, burning; *causalgia*

-chroia: skin coloration; *xanthochroia*

chrom/o: color; *chromomycosis*

chrys/o: gold; *chrysiasis*

cutane/o: skin; *subcutaneous*

derm/o, dermat/o: skin; *dermatopathy*

erythem/o: flushed, redness; *erythema*

eschar/o: scab; *escharotomy*

graph/o: writing; *graphesthesia*

hidr/o: sweat; *hyperhidrosis*

ichthy/o: fish; *ichthyosis*

iod/o: iodine; *iododerma*

kerat/o: horny tissue, cornea; *keratolysis*

koil/o: hollow, concave, depressed; *koilonychia*

lepid/o: flakes, scales; *lepidosis*

lepr/o: leprosy; *leproma*

onych/o: nail; *onychomycosis*

pachy-: thick; *pachydermatocele*

papul/o: papule, pimple; *papulopustular*

perspir/o: breathe through, sweat; *perspiration*

phyt/o: plant; *phytophotodermatitis*

pil/o: hair; *pilomotor*

prurit/o: itching; *pruritogenic*

pseudo-: false; *pseudochromhidrosis*

psor/o: itching; *psoriasis*

py/o: pus; *pyodermatitis*

rhytid/o: wrinkle; *rhytidectomy*

seb/o: sebum; *seborrhea*

steat/o: fat; *steatocryptosis*

sud/o: sweat; *sudokeratosis*

trich/o: hair; *hypertrichosis*

ul/o: scar, scarring; *uloid*

ungu/o: nail; *subungual*

verruc/i: wart; *verrucosis*

xer/o: dry; *xeroderma*

Abbreviations

BMK: birthmark

Bx: biopsy

decub: decubitus

DLE: discoid lupus erythematosus

DU: decubitus ulcer

EAHF: eczema, asthma, and hay fever

EDR: electrodermal response

EGF: epidermal growth factor

HD: Hansen disease (leprosy)

ID: intradermal

LE: lupus erythematosus

MM: malignant melanoma, multiple myeloma

PSS: progressive systemic sclerosis (scleroderma)

PUVA: psoralen + ultraviolet A

SD: skin dose

SED: skin erythema dose

SG: skin graft

Ski, Sk: skin

SLE: systemic lupus erythematosus

SPF: skin protection factor

sq: squamous

SQ, SC, subq, subcu, subcut: subcutaneous

STSG: split-thickness skin graft

TEN: toxic epidermal necrolysis

TSF: triceps skinfold thickness

UV: ultraviolet

XP, XDP: xeroderma pigmentosum

Respiratory System

- **Upper respiratory tract**
  - Nose: Nasal cavity, paranasal sinuses
  - Pharynx: Nasopharynx, oro-pharynx, laryngopharynx
- **Lower respiratory tract**
  - Larynx: Vocal cords
  - Trachea: C-shaped rings of cartilage
  - Bronchi
    - Right and left bronchus
    - Bronchioles: Alveoli
  - Lungs
    - Lobes: Right (3) and left (2)
    - Pleura
- Pulmonary ventilation
  - Inspiration and expiration
  - Diaphragm

Terms

alveol/o: alveolus; *alveolitis*

aspir/o, aspirat/o: inhaling, removal; *aspiration*

blenn/o: mucus; *blennothorax*

bronch/o: bronchus; *bronchorrhagia*

bronchiol/o: bronchiole; *bronchiolectasis*

-capnia, capn/o: carbon dioxide; *hypercapnia*

coni/o: dust; *coniofibrosis*

epiglott/o: epiglottis; *epiglottitis*

lal/o, -lalia: speech, babble; *laliatry*

lampr/o: clear; *lamprophonia*

laryng/o: larynx; *laryngoxerosis*

lept/o: slender, thin, delicate; *leptophonia*

lob/o: lobe; *lobectomy*

mediastin/o: mediastinum; *mediastinoscopy*

mogi-: difficult; *mogiphonia*

nas/o: nose; *nasolabial*

osm/o, -osmia: sense of smell, odor, impulse; *anosmia*

osphresi/o, -osphresia: sense of smell, odor; *osphresiometer*

ox/o, -oxia: oxygen; *hypoxia*

-pagus: parts fused; *thoracopagus*

pector/o: chest; *pectoralgia*

phas/o, -phasia: speech; *dysphasia*

phon/o, -phonia: voice, sound; *rhinophonia*

phren/o: diaphragm, mind; *phrenalgia*

pimel/o: fat, fatty; *pimelorthopnea*

pleur/o: pleura; *pleurocholecystitis*

-pnea: to breathe; *hyperpnea*

pneum/o: lung, air; *pneumopexy*

pneumon/o: lung, air; *pneumonomycosis*

-ptosis: prolapse, drooping; *laryngoptosis*

-ptysis: spitting; *hemoptysis*

pulmon/o: lung; *pulmonologist*

respir/o, respirat/o: to breathe, breathing; *respirator*

rhin/o: nose; *rhinolithiasis*

sept/o: partition; *septorhinoplasty*

silic/o: silica, quartz; *silicosis*

sinus/o: cavity, sinus; *sinusotomy*

spir/o: to breathe; *bronchospirometer*

steth/o: chest; *stethoscope*

therm/o: heat; *thermopolypnea*

thorac/o: chest; *thoracoschisis*

trache/o: trachea; *tracheostenosis*

traumat/o: trauma, injury, wound; *traumatopnea*

xen/o: strange, foreign; *xenophonia*

Abbreviations

ABC: airway, breathing, and circulation

ABG: arterial blood gas

AR: artificial respiration

ARD: acute respiratory disease

ARDS: adult respiratory distress syndrome, acute respiratory distress syndrome

ARF: acute respiratory failure

BAC: bronchoalveolar cells

BAL: bronchoalveolar lavage

BPD: bronchopulmonary dysplasia

CF: cystic fibrosis

CNH: central neurogenic hyperventilation

CO_2: carbon dioxide

COLD: chronic obstructive lung disease

COPD: chronic obstructive pulmonary disease

CPAP: continuous positive airway pressure

CPE: chronic pulmonary emphysema

CPR: cardiopulmonary resuscitation

CPT: chest physiotherapy

CRD: chronic respiratory disease

CSR: Cheyne-Stokes respiration

CXR: chest X-ray

DOE: dyspnea on exertion

DPT: diphtheria, pertussis, and tetanus

EIA: exercise-induced asthma

ERV: expiratory reserve volume

FEF: forced expiratory flow

FEV: forced expiratory volume

FRC: functional residual capacity

FVC: forced vital capacity

HBOT: hyperbaric oxygen therapy

HMD: hyaline membrane disease

IC: inspiratory capacity

IMV: intermittent mandatory ventilation

IPPB: intermittent positive pressure breathing

IRDS: infant respiratory distress syndrome

IRV: inspiratory reserve volume

LRI: lower respiratory infection

LTB: laryngotracheobronchitis

MBC: maximum breathing capacity

MV: minute volume

MVV: maximal voluntary ventilation

NSCLC: non-small-cell lung cancer

O_2: oxygen

$PaCO_2$: partial pressure of arterial carbon dioxide

PaO_2: partial pressure of arterial oxygen

PCO_2: partial pressure of CO_2

PE: pulmonary embolism

PEEP: positive end-expiratory pressure

PFT: pulmonary function test

PND: paroxysmal nocturnal dyspnea
PO$_2$: partial pressure of O$_2$
PPD: purified protein derivative (TB test)
PPH: primary pulmonary hypertension
PTX, pnx, Px: pneumothorax
PuD, PD: pulmonary disease
R, resp: respiration
RD: respiratory disease
RDS: respiratory distress syndrome
RM: respiratory movement
RQ: respiratory quotient
RR: respiratory rate, regular respirations
RT: respiratory therapy
RV: residual volume
SCLC: small-cell lung cancer
SIDS: sudden infant death syndrome
SOB: shortness of breath
T&A: tonsillectomy and adenoidectomy
TB: tuberculosis
TBT: tracheobronchial tree
TCDB: turn, cough, and deep breathe
TLC: total lung capacity
TV: tidal volume
UAO: upper airway obstruction
URI: upper respiratory infection
VC: vital capacity
VO$_2$: oxygen consumption
V/Q: ventilation-perfusion ratio

Muscular System
- **Characteristics**
  - Excitability
  - Contractility
  - Elasticity
  - Extensibility
- **Types**
  - Skeletal
    - Voluntary/striated
    - Movement
    - Attached to the skeleton
  - Smooth
    - Involuntary/nonstriated
    - Located in walls of hollow organs
  - Cardiac
    - Involuntary/striated
    - Found in the heart

Terms

-asthenia, asthen/o: weakness; *myasthenia*
aux/o: growth, acceleration; *auxotonic*

-chalasia: relaxation; *achalasia*
erg/o: work; *ergometry*
fasci/o: fascia; *fasciodesis*
fibr/o: fiber, fibrous; *fibromyoma*
flex/o: bend; *flexor*
idi/o: distinctive; *idiomuscular*
kinesi/o, -kinesia, -kinetic: movement; *kinesioneurosis*
lei/o: smooth; *leiomyoma*
ligament/o: ligament; *ligamentopexy*
-lysis: dissolution, breakdown; *myolysis*
muscul/o: muscle; *musculoskeletal*
my/o, myos/o: muscle; *myorrhexis*
pale/o: old; *paleokinetic*
palin-, pali-: recurrence, repetition; *palikinesia*
pyg/o: buttocks; *pygalgia*
rhabd/o: rod; *rhabdoid*
rhabdomy/o: striated/skeletal muscle; *rhabdomyolysis*
rot/o, rotat/o: to turn, to revolve; *rotator*
-stasis: standing still, standing; *myostasis*
sthen/o, -sthenia: strength; *sthenometry*
-stroma: supporting tissue of an organ; *myostroma*
syndesm/o: ligament, connective tissue; *syndesmectopia*
ten/o: tendon; *tenorrhaphy*
tenont/o: tendon; *tenontography*
-therapy, therapeut/o: treatment; *kinesiotherapy*
ton/o: tone, tension; *myatonia*

Abbreviations

abd: abduction
ACL: anterior cruciate ligament
add: adduction
ADL: activities of daily living
ART: active resistance training
BMD: Becker muscular dystrophy
CTS: carpal tunnel syndrome
DMD: Duchenne muscular dystrophy
DTR: deep tendon reflex
EMG: electromyography
EMS: electric muscle stimulator
EOM: extraocular muscles
IM: intramuscular
Lig, L: ligament
m: muscle
MAMC: midarm muscle circumference

MD: muscular dystrophy
MG: myasthenia gravis
MH: malignant hyperthermia
mm: muscles
MN: myoneural
MS: musculoskeletal, muscle strength
musc: muscular, muscle
MVIC: maximum voluntary isometric contraction
NM: neuromuscular
PPMA: postpoliomyelitis muscular atrophy
PRE: progressive resistive exercise
RICE: rest, ice, compression, and elevation
RSI: repetitive stress injuries

Special Senses: Eye & Ear
- **Eye**
  - Layers/tunics
    - Fibrous
    - Sclera
    - Cornea
    - Vascular
    - Choroid
    - Ciliary body
    - Iris
    - Nervous: Retina
  - Associated structures
    - Eyebrows
    - Eyelids
    - Lacrimal apparatus
    - Conjunctiva
    - Eyelashes
- **Ear**
  - External
    - Auricle
    - External auditory canal
    - Tympanic membrane (eardrum)
  - Middle
    - Auditory (eustachian tube)
    - Auditory ossicles: Malleus, incus, and stapes
  - Inner
    - Bony labyrinth; semicircular canals, vestibule, cochlea

Terms

acous/o: hearing; *acousma*
acoust/o: hearing, sound; *acoustics*
ambly/o: dim, dull; *amblyoscope*
audi/o, audit/o: hearing; *audiometer*
aur/o, auricul/o: ear; *auriculotemporal*
blephar/o: eyelid; *blepharorrhaphy*

cochle/o: cochlea; *cochleitis*
conjunctiv/o: conjunctiva; *conjunctivitis*
cor/o: pupil; *corectasia*
corne/o: cornea; *corneosclera*
-cusis: hearing; *presbycusis*
cycl/o: ciliary body, circular; *cyclodialysis*
dacry/o: tear; *dacryoadenectomy*
dipl/o: double; *diploscope*
hygr/o: moisture; *hygroblepharic*
ir/o, irid/o: iris; *iridemia*
kerat/o: cornea, horny tissue; *keratomalacia*
lacrim/o: tear, lacrimal duct; *lacrimotomy*
logad/o: whites of the eyes; *logadectomy*
myring/o: eardrum; *myringomycosis*
ocul/o: eye; *oculonasal*
ophry/o: eyebrow; *ophryitis*
ophthalm/o: eye; *ophthalmodynia*
-opia, -opsia, -opsy: vision; *heteropsia*
opt/o: eye, vision; *optometer*
ot/o: ear; *otopyorrhea*
palpebr/o: eyelid; *palpebritis*
phac/o: lens; *phacocele*
phak/o: lens; *phakoma*
phot/o: light; *photophobia*
platy-: broad, flat; *platycoria*
-pterygium: abnormality of the conjunctiva; *pimelopterygium*
pupill/o: pupil; *pupillatonia*
retin/o: retina; *retinotoxic*
scler/o: sclera; *sclerectasia*
scot/o: darkness; *scotopia*
son/o: sound; *sonometer*
staped/o: stapes; *stapedectomy*
stich/o, -stichia: rows; *polystichia*
stigmat/o: mark, point; *astigmatism*
-tropia: to turn; *anatropia*
tympan/o: eardrum; *tympanosclerosis*
uve/o: uvea; *uveoplasty*
vitre/o: glassy, vitreous body; *vitreocapsulitis*

Abbreviations: Ear

AC: air conduction
AD: right ear
AOM: acute otitis media
AS: left ear
AU: both ears
CAPD: central auditory processing disorder

dB: decibel
EE: eye and ear
ENT: ear, nose, and throat
ET: eustachian tube
HD: hearing distance
HL: hearing level, hearing loss
OM: otitis media
ORL: otorhinolaryngology
SOM: serous otitis media
TM: tympanic membrane
VRA: visual reinforcement audiometry

Abbreviations: Eye

acc: accommodation
ARMD: age-related macular degeneration
AS, Ast, Astigm: astigmatism
DV: distance vision
dv: double vision
E: eye
ECCE: extracapsular cataract extraction
EENT: eye, ear, nose, and throat
EM: emmetropia
ENG: electronystagmography
EOM: extraocular movement
ERG: electroretinography
ET: esotropia
ICCE: intracapsular cataract extraction
IOL: intraocular lens
IOP: intraocular pressure
L&A: light and accommodation
L&D: light and distance
LE: left eye
M, My: myopia
NREM: nonrapid eye movement
NV: near vision
OD: right eye
OS: left eye
OU: both eyes
PD: [inter]pupillary distance
PERRLA: pupils equal, round, and reactive to light and accommodation
RE: right eye
REM: rapid eye movement
RK: radial keratotomy
SMD: senile macular degeneration
VA: visual acuity
VF: visual field
XT: exotropia

Lymphatic & Immune System

- **Lymphatic System**
  - Lymph
    - Clear, watery fluid
    - Formed from interstitial fluid
  - Lymphatic vessels: Valves
  - Lymphatic organs
    - Tonsils: Palatine, pharyngeal, lingual
    - Lymph nodes: Concentration of nodes; inguinal, axillary, cervical
    - Spleen
    - Thymus
- **Immune system**
  - Nonspecific response: Skin, inflammation, phagocytosis
  - Specific response
    - Acquired immunity: Natural (active and passive) and artificial (active and passive)
    - Antibody-mediated immunity
    - Cell-mediated immunity

Terms

adenoid/o: adenoids; *adenoidectomy*
allo-: other, different; *allotoxin*
auto-: self; *autoantitoxin*
axill/o: armpit; *axillary*
-edema: swelling; *lymphedema*
-emphraxis: stoppage, obstruction; *splenemphraxis*
immun/o: protection, immune; *immunogenic*
inguin/o: groin; *inguinodynia*
lien/o: spleen; *lienomalacia*
lymph/o: lymph; *lymphangiophlebitis*
nod/o: knot; *nodular*
-penia: deficiency; *lymphocytopenia*
peri-: around; *perilymphangitis*
-phylaxis: protection; *anaphylaxis*
ple/o: more; *pleocytosis*
sarc/o: flesh; *lymphosarcoma*
-sepsis: putrefaction; *antisepsis*
splen/o: spleen; *splenectasis*
tetan/o: tetanus; *tetanophilic*
thym/o: thymus; *thymectomy*
tonsill/o: tonsils; *tonsillolith*
top/o: particular place or area; *splenectopy*
vaccin/o: vaccine; *vaccinogenous*

Abbreviations

Ab: antibody
ADC: AIDS-dementia complex
Ag: antigen
AIDS: acquired immunodeficiency syndrome
ANA: antinuclear antibodies
APLS: antiphospholipid syndrome
ARC: AIDS-related complex
ARV: AIDS-related virus
EBV: Epstein-Barr virus
ELISA: enzyme-linked immunosorbent assay
GVHD: graft-versus-host disease
HD: Hodgkin disease
HIV: human immunodeficiency virus
Ig: immunoglobulin
IM: infectious mononucleosis
IT: immunotherapy
KS: Kaposi sarcoma
LAK: lymphokine-activated killer cells
LE: lupus erythematosus
MAD: multiple autoimmune disorder
NHL: non-Hodgkin lymphoma
NK: natural killer (cells)
OPV: oral poliovirus vaccine
PSS: progressive systemic sclerosis (scleroderma)
SCID: severe combined immunodeficiency disease
SLE: systemic lupus erythematosus
SS: Sjögren syndrome
TAT: tetanus antitoxin
TLI: total lymphoid irradiation
vacc: vaccination

GETTING A JOB
IN THE FIELD

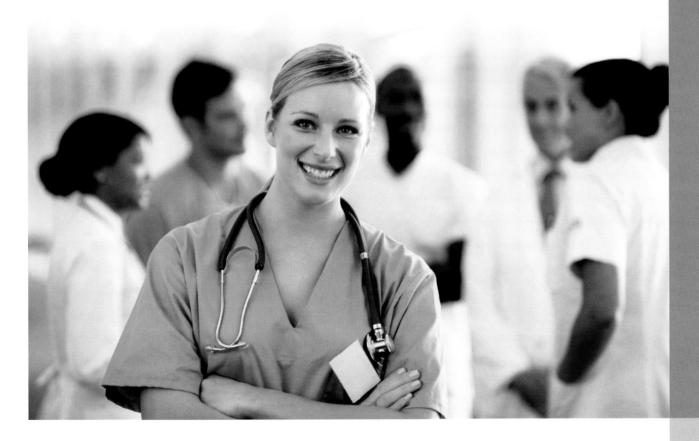

Introduction

The task of finding a job in the nursing field should begin while you are still in nursing school. The best way to ensure that you have a job after graduation is to begin working in a hospital as a student. Many hospitals hire nursing students to work as patient care technicians (PCTs), so look on-line and in the newspaper for job openings at your local hospitals. Some hospitals will require you to become a certified nursing assistant (CNA) before you can be hired. Ask your nursing instructors about CNA classes in your area.

Once you have secured a job as a PCT, let the nurses on your unit know that you are interested in watching and assisting with nursing procedures when time permits. Seek out opportunities to observe or help with any of the following:

- Intravenous (IV) insertion
- IV medication administration
- Injections
- Oxygen therapy
- Tube feedings
- Dressing changes
- Catheter insertion or removal
- Nasogastric tube insertion or removal

The more experience you get as a nursing student, the better your chances of being hired by the hospital after graduation.

Becoming a Specialty Nurse

If you know while in nursing school that you may want to specialize after graduation, volunteer for the float pool while working as a PCT. Let the person in charge of scheduling know that you are interested in a specific field (e.g., pediatrics or obstetrics) and would like to be assigned to that unit when possible. Then seek out opportunities to learn from the nurses on that unit. The nursing float pool is also a good way to break into specialty nursing if you decide after graduation that you would prefer to specialize.

Another thing you can do to help break into specialty nursing is to seek additional educational opportunities in the field. Ask the hospital where you work if they have any internship programs, and attend continuing education programs in the field in which you wish to specialize.

Trouble finding a job? Consider a volunteer position with the Red Cross, Easter Seals, United Cerebral Palsy, or the American Cancer Society. A door may open.

Alternative Career Options

In addition to traditional nursing, there are a lot of career opportunities for nurses.

Agency Nursing

Agency nurses work for organizations that provide workers to cover shifts when hospitals are shorthanded. You will need at least 2 years of experience as a medical-surgical nurse (or other specialty nurse) to quality for most agency jobs.

Agency nursing does have some advantages. For example, you can choose your own hours. The agency will let you know what shifts are available, and you can choose which ones you would like to cover. The downside to agency nursing is that hospitals sometimes schedule nurses in advance in case someone calls in sick. If everyone shows, your shift can be cancelled at the last minute. Nursing agencies also may not provide benefits, such as health insurance.

To find a job as an agency nurse, do an online search for nursing agencies in your city.

Travel Nursing

Travel nurses travel around the country working for periods of time in areas of need. When you finish one job, you move on to another. You will need at least 2 years of experience as a medical-surgical nurse (or other specialty nurse) to quality for most travel nursing jobs.

One advantage of travel nursing is that you get to choose which assignments you want to accept, so you can go where it is warm in the winter and cool in the summer. Housing is also provided free of charge, although you may have to share with a roommate. Travel nursing may be a good choice if you have not yet started a family or if your children are grown. It might not be your best option if you have small children or if you are not fond of change.

To find a job as a travel nurse, do an online search for "travel nursing."

Hospital Administration

Hospital administrators oversee the hospital's operations. The job may include a variety of tasks, such as policy development and oversight, budgeting and financial management, acting as liaison between the hospital board and the medical staff or hospital staff, recruiting and training, and more. Many larger hospitals have more than one administrator.

Most hospital administrators have advanced degrees in health care administration, business administration, public health, or public administration. How many years of experience you will need to become a hospital administrator will depend on the hospital. Other requirements will vary by facility.

> Challenged by a disability? Learn your rights under the Americans with Disabilities Act, and get connected with other nurses with similar challenges. Do not give up your career!

As a hospital administrator, you will likely work daytime hours, Monday through Friday. But because of the job's high level of responsibility, you may find yourself frequently on call for emergencies.

To find a job as a hospital administrator, keep an eye on the career section of your hospital's website. You can also look for hospital administration jobs on online job sites and in your local newspaper.

Nursing Home Administration

Nursing homes also need administrators. Nursing home administrators have responsibilities that are similar to those of a hospital administrator, including policy development and oversight, budgeting and financial management, acting as liaison between the board and the medical staff or nursing home staff, and recruiting and training.

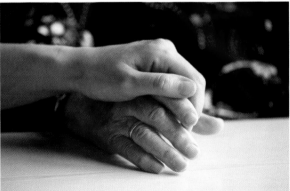

Many nursing home administrators have advanced degrees in health care administration, business administration, public health, or public administration. How many years of experience you will need to become a nursing home administrator will depend on the facility. Other requirements will also vary by facility.

As a nursing home administrator, you will likely work daytime hours, Monday through Friday. But because of the job's high level of responsibility, you may find yourself frequently on call for emergencies.

To find a job as a nursing home administrator, keep an eye on the career section of a nursing home's website. You can also look for nursing home administration jobs on online job sites and in your local newspaper.

Quality Improvement Specialist

Health care quality improvement specialists are responsible for collecting and analyzing organizational data and using that data to improve policies or processes that will ultimately lead to better patient care. Some quality improvement specialists are also responsible for regulatory compliance.

Most quality improvement specialists have advanced degrees in health care administration, business administration, public health, or public administration. How many years of clinical experience you will need to become a quality improvement specialist will depend on the organization. Other requirements will vary by facility.

Quality improvement specialists normally work daytime hours, Monday through Friday, which may be an advantage if you want "regular" hours. A disadvantage of this job is that you will no longer be involved in direct patient care, so you will not be using your clinical skills on a daily basis.

Before applying for a job as a quality improvement specialist, you will need to gain some experience in health care quality. One way to get this experience is to volunteer to serve on the organization's quality improvement committee. You may also want to take some quality improvement continuing education courses.

To find a job as a quality improvement specialist, keep an eye on the career section of your employer's website. You can also look for jobs on online job sites and in your local newspaper.

Risk Management

A risk manager's job is to minimize the organization's risk of patient harm, medical liability, and financial loss. Risk managers are also responsible for responding when adverse events do occur.

Most risk managers have advanced degrees in health care administration, business administration, public health, or public administration. How many years of clinical experience you will need to become a risk manager will depend on the organization. Other requirements will vary by facility.

Risk managers normally work daytime hours, Monday through Friday, although you will likely be on call in emergencies. An advantage of this job is the somewhat "regular" hours. A disadvantage of this job is that you will no longer be involved in direct patient care, so you will not be using your clinical skills on a daily basis.

Before applying for a job as a risk manager, you will need to gain some experience in risk management. One way to get this experience is to volunteer to serve on the organization's risk management committee. You may also want to take some risk management continuing education courses.

To find a job as a risk manager, keep an eye on the career section of your employer's website. You can also look for jobs on online job sites and in your local newspaper.

Vision can change over time. Presbyopia, or "long-arm syndrome," is common in older patients and nurses. Your eyes should be examined regularly.

Other Management Opportunities

Before becoming a freelance medical writer, I was employed by the American Academy of Family Physicians, where I helped physicians with the business aspects of running a medical practice. There were three other nurses in my department. One was an assistant division director, and the other two worked to help physicians with their office quality improvement efforts. There were also nurses working in other divisions, such as continuing medical education and medical education (working with medical students and residents).

There are a lot of health care–related organizations that could benefit from having employees with clinical backgrounds. So if you are looking for a new career opportunity, start by looking for health care management jobs on online job sites. You can also try doing an online search for medical specialty societies or medical associations in your city to see what organizations pop up. Then go to their websites and look for a "Careers" page.

WOUND HEALING

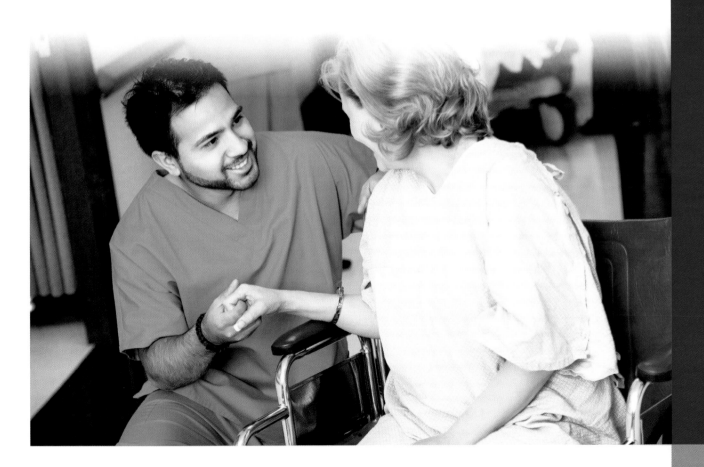

Introduction

There are three types of wound healing:
- **Primary intention:** Minimal tissue loss and edges that are well approximated (closed); healing occurs with minimal granulation tissue and minimal scarring.
- **Secondary intention:** Extensive tissue loss or edges that cannot be approximated; repair time is longer as granulation tissue gradually fills in the deficit; tissue replacement and scarring are greater, and the susceptibility to infection is increased.
- **Tertiary intention:** Delayed closure; can be caused by poor circulation or infection. Suturing of the wound is delayed until the problem resolves and more favorable conditions exist for wound healing.

Wound healing is a three-phase process:
1. Defensive phase
2. Reconstructive phase
3. Maturation phase

Defensive (Inflammatory) Phase

The defensive phase of wound healing occurs immediately after injury and lasts 3–4 days; hemostasis and inflammation are the major events.
- **Hemostasis:** The cessation of bleeding.
  - Blood vessels constrict.
  - Platelets, activated by the injury, aggregate to form a platelet plug and stop the bleeding.
  - Activation of the clotting cascade leads to the formation of fibrin and a fibrinous meshwork, which traps platelets and other cells.
  - Fibrin clot formation provides initial wound closure and prevents excessive loss of blood and body fluids.
- **Inflammation:** The body's defensive adaptation to tissue injury; involves both vascular and cellular responses.
  - Tissue injury stimulates the release of chemical mediators, such as histamine (from mast cells), serotonin (from platelets), complement, and kinins; all of these are vasoactive substances that cause the blood vessels to dilate and become more permeable, resulting in increased blood flow, which carries nutrients and oxygen essential to wound healing.
    - Increased blood flow transports leukocytes, or white blood cells, to the area to participate in phagocytosis (the envelopment and disposal of microorganisms).
    - Increased blood supply also removes dead cells, bacteria, and exudates (material and cells discharged from the blood vessels).
  - Inflammation results in the area appearing red, edematous (swollen), and warm to the touch, with varying amounts of exudates present.

Reconstructive (Proliferative) Phase

The reconstructive phase of wound healing begins on day 3 or 4 following the injury and lasts 2–3 weeks. The reconstructive phase consists of collagen deposition, angiogenesis, granulation, and wound contraction.

- **Collagen deposition:** The introduction of the material of tissue repair.
  - Connective tissue contains fibroblasts, which migrate into the wound as a result of cellular mediators.
  - Fibroblasts secrete collagen.
  - Initially, collagen is gel-like; however, over months of healing time, it forms collagen fibrils and adds tensile strength to the wound.
  - As the wounded tissues become stronger, the risk of wound separation or rupture decreases.
  - A properly healing wound can resist normal stress, such as tension or twisting, after 15–20 days.
- **Angiogenesis:** The formation of new blood vessels.
  - With injury, the endothelial cells in the existing vessels produce enzymes that break down the basement membrane; as a result, new vessels form and grow across the wound to increase blood flow.
- **Granulation:** The development of tissue.
  - Granulation tissue (new tissue) grows inward from the surrounding healthy connective tissue.
  - Granulation tissue, which is red and translucent with a granular appearance, is filled with new capillaries that are fragile and bleed easily.
- **Wound contraction:** The process of wound closure; contraction is noticeable 6–12 days after injury.
  - The edges of the wound are drawn together by the action of myofibroblasts, which are specialized cells that contain bundles of parallel fibers in the cytoplasm.
  - These myofibroblasts bridge across a wound and then contract to pull the wound closed.

Maturation Phase

The final stage of wound healing begins on approx. day 21 and can continue for up to 2 years, depending on the depth of the wound; scar tissue is remodeled by collagen deposition, lysis (disintegration), and debridement (removal, usually surgical) of wound edges.

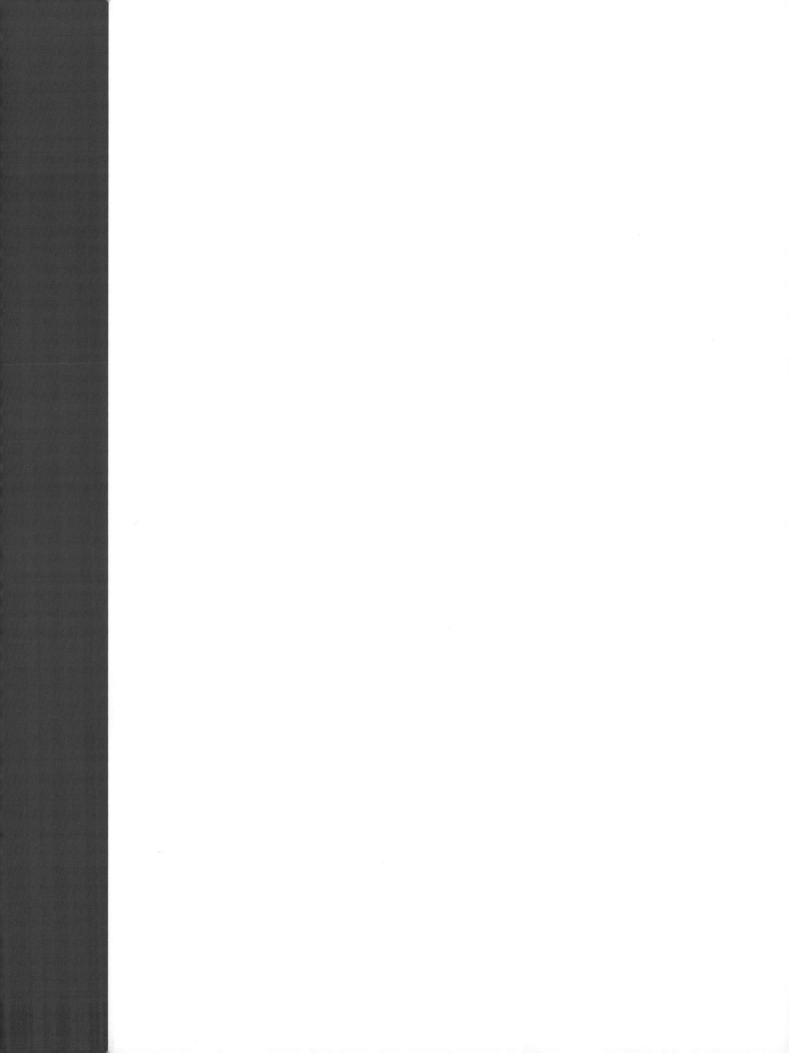

MATH
REVIEW

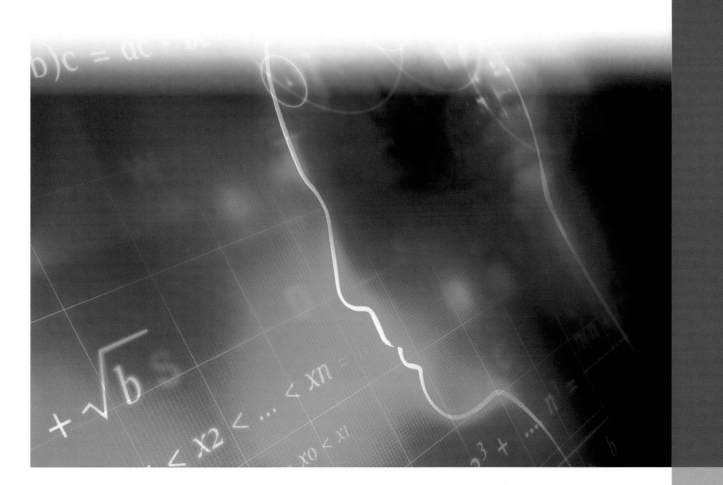

Symbols

+	plus
–	minus
×	multiplied by (times)
/, ÷	divided by
±	plus or minus
<	less than
>	greater than
≤	less than or equal to
≥	greater than or equal to
=	equal to
≠	not equal to

Addition

Addition is the process of adding, or uniting, two or more numbers, which are called **addends**. The result of adding two or more numbers is called the **sum**.

Example

Solve $1,502 + 326 + 54$.

1. Align the numbers:

$$
\begin{array}{r}
1,502 \\
326 \\
+54 \\
\hline
\end{array}
$$

Hint: When adding numbers, align them in a column so that the right sides line up. This will ensure the place values are aligned starting with the ones column and moving to the tens, hundreds, thousands, ten thousands, etc.

2. Start with the rightmost column (the ones), and add: $2 + 6 + 4 = 12$, which is more than 9, the maximum number for this column. Write a 2 in the answer's ones column, and carry the 1 to the next column, the tens.
3. Add the numbers in the middle column: $0 + 2 + 5 + 1 = 8$. Write an 8 in the answer's tens column, and move to the next column, the hundreds.
4. Add the numbers in the third column: $5 + 3 = 8$. Write an 8 in the answer's hundreds column, and move to the next column, the thousands.
5. There is only one number in the thousands column: 1. Write a 1 in the answer's thousands column to show your complete answer: **1,882**.

$$
\begin{array}{r}
\overset{1}{1,5}02 \\
326 \\
+54 \\
\hline
1,882
\end{array}
$$

Subtraction

Subtraction is the process of subtracting, or taking away, one or more numbers from another number. The number from which other numbers are being taken away is called the **minuend**. The number being subtracted is called the **subtrahend**. The result of subtracting is called the **difference**.

Example

Solve 842 − 96.

1. Align the numbers:

$$842$$
$$-96$$

2. Start with the rightmost column (the ones), and subtract: 2 − 6. Since 6 is greater than 2, you must borrow from the next column (the tens). Once you borrow a 10, the first number in the ones column becomes 12 (from 2 + 10). Now subtract: 12 − 6 = 6. Write a 6 in the answer's ones column, and subtract the borrowed 1 from the 4 in the next column, the tens, which becomes 3.

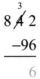

$$8\overset{3}{\cancel{4}}2$$
$$-96$$
$$6$$

3. Subtract the numbers in the middle column: 3 − 9. Again, since 9 is greater than 3, you must borrow from the next column (the hundreds). Once you borrow a 10, the first number in the middle column becomes 13. Now subtract: 13 − 9 = 4. Write a 4 in the answer's tens column, and subtract the borrowed 1 from the next column, the hundreds, which becomes 7.

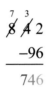

$$\overset{7}{\cancel{8}}\overset{3}{\cancel{4}}2$$
$$-96$$
$$746$$

4. There is only one number in the hundreds column: 7. Write a 7 in the answer's hundreds column to show your complete answer: **746**.

> **Hint:** When subtracting numbers, make sure the greater number is on top. Align the numbers in a column so that the right sides line up. This will ensure the place values are aligned starting with the ones column and moving to the tens, hundreds, thousands, ten thousands, etc.

Multiplication

Multiplication is the process of multiplying two or more numbers together. The numbers being multiplied are each called **factors**. The result of multiplying is called the **product**. Multiplication is the same as repeated addition; therefore, 3 × 4 is like adding four groups of 3 (or 3 + 3 + 3 + 3).

> **Hint:** It helps to memorize the multiplication table or all multiplication factors from 0 to 12.

x	0	1	2	3	4	5	6	7	8	9	10	11	12
0	0	0	0	0	0	0	0	0	0	0	0	0	0
1	0	1	2	3	4	5	6	7	8	9	10	11	12
2	0	2	4	6	8	10	12	14	16	18	20	22	24
3	0	3	6	9	12	15	18	21	24	27	30	33	36
4	0	4	8	12	16	20	24	28	32	36	40	44	48
5	0	5	10	15	20	25	30	35	40	45	50	55	60
6	0	6	12	18	24	30	36	42	48	54	60	66	72
7	0	7	14	21	28	35	42	49	56	63	70	77	84
8	0	8	16	24	32	40	48	56	64	72	80	88	96
9	0	9	18	27	36	45	54	63	72	81	90	99	108
10	0	10	20	30	40	50	60	70	80	90	100	110	120
11	0	11	22	33	44	55	66	77	88	99	110	121	132
12	0	12	24	36	48	60	72	84	96	108	120	132	144

> **Hint:** For numbers with three or more digits, always align the numbers in a column so that the right sides line up, and then multiply each digit in the top number by each digit in the bottom number.

Example

Solve 247×36.

1. Align the numbers:

$$\begin{array}{r} 247 \\ \times 36 \\ \hline \end{array}$$

2. Start with the rightmost column (the ones), and multiply: $6 \times 7 = 42$, which is more than 9, the maximum number for this column. Write a 2 in the answer's ones column, and carry the 4 to the next column, the tens.

3. Multiply 6 by the digit in the first number's tens place (4): $6 \times 4 = 24$, then add the carried 4: $24 + 4 = 28$, which is more than 9, the maximum number for this column. Write an 8 in the answer's tens column, and carry the 2 to the next column, the hundreds.

4. Multiply 6 by the digit in the first number's hundreds place (2): $6 \times 2 = 12$, then add the carried 2: $12 + 2 = 14$. Since there are no more numbers in a higher place value, write 14 in the answer. The first *partial product* is 1,482.

$$\begin{array}{r} {}^{2\;4}247 \\ \times 36 \\ \hline 1,482 \end{array}$$

5. To start the next digit, 3, write a 0 in the ones column of the next line of the answer.

6. Multiply 3 by the digit in the first number's ones place (7): $3 \times 7 = 21$, which is more than 9, the maximum number for this column. Write a 1 in the answer's tens column, and carry the 2 to the next column, the tens.

7. Multiply 3 by the digit in the first number's tens place (4): $3 \times 4 = 12$, then add the carried 2: $12 + 2 = 14$, which is more than 9, the maximum number for this column. Write a 4 in the answer's hundreds column, and carry the 1 to the next column, the hundreds.

8. Multiply 3 by the digit in the first number's hundreds place (2): $3 \times 2 = 6$, then add the carried 1: $6 + 1 = 7$. Since there are no more numbers in a higher place value, write a 7 in the answer. The second *partial product* is 7,410.

$$\begin{array}{r} {}^{1\;2}247 \\ \times 36 \\ \hline 1,482 \\ 7,410 \end{array}$$

9. To find the overall product, add the two partial products to get **8,892**.

$$\begin{array}{r} 1,482 \\ +7,410 \\ \hline 8,892 \end{array}$$

Division

Division is the process of finding how many times one number goes into another number. The number being divided is called the **dividend**. The number by which it is divided is called the **divisor**. The result of division is called the **quotient**.

Example

Solve 682 ÷ 14.

1. Write the problem in long-division format: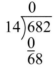

2. The first number of the dividend, 6, cannot be divided by 14, since 14 is greater than 6. Write a 0 on top in the hundreds place, write a 0 under the 6, find the difference between 6 and 0, and bring the next place value down.

$$
\begin{array}{r}
0 \\
14\overline{)682} \\
\underline{0} \\
68
\end{array}
$$

> **Hint:** Division problems are often written with the division symbol (÷), but to solve them, it is best to write them in the long-division format, with a ⌐. Also remember that division problems may not result in whole-number answers.

3. Since the number of times that 14 goes into 68 is not a whole number, you must use the greatest whole number of times it does go in (4). Write that number above the 8, write the product of 4 and 14 (56) beneath the 68, find the difference between those two, and bring the next place value down.

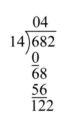

4. Since the number of times that 14 goes into 122 is not a whole number, you must use the greatest whole number of times it does go in (8). Write that number above the 2, write the product of 8 and 14 (112) beneath the 122, and find the difference between those two.

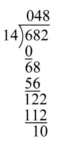

5. Since 14, the divisor, is greater than 10, this is as far as you can go. This means that 682 ÷ 14 = **48 with a remainder of 10**.

Positive & Negative Numbers

- **Positive numbers** are greater than 0 (i.e., to the right of 0 on a number line) and get greater as you move farther away from 0. They *may* be written with or without a positive (+) sign (e.g., 5 or +5).
- **Negative numbers** are less than 0 (i.e., to the left of 0 on a number line) and get lesser as you move farther away from 0. They *must* be written with a negative (–) sign (e.g., –5).

Rules for Addition

- The sum of two positive numbers is a positive number:
  $3 + 4 = 7$
- The sum of two negative numbers is a negative number:
  $-2 + -6 = -8$
- The sum of one positive number and one negative number may be positive or negative, depending on which number's absolute value is greater. Remember that adding a negative number is the same as subtracting that number:
  $9 + (-2) = 9 - 2 = 7$
  $-9 + 2 = 2 - 9 = -7$

Rules for Subtraction

- Think of subtraction as addition of the opposite. So, first change the subtraction sign to an addition sign, then write the opposite of the original number being subtracted, and solve as usual.
  $3 - 8 = 3 + (-8) = -5$
  $5 - (-2) = 5 + 2 = 7$

Rules for Multiplication

- The product of two positive numbers is a positive number:
  $3 \times 6 = 18$
- The product of two negative numbers is a positive number:
  $(-2) \times (-5) = 10$
- The product of one positive number and one negative number is a negative number:
  $4 \times (-7) = -28$

Rules for Division

- The quotient of two positive numbers is a positive number:
  $9 \div 3 = 3$
- The quotient of two negative numbers is a positive number:
  $(-20) \div (-4) = 5$
- The quotient of one positive number and one negative number is a negative number:
  $42 \div (-7) = -6$
  $(-32) \div 4 = -8$

Hint: Remember to use the rules for multiplying negative and positive numbers if negative numbers are included in the expression.

Distributive Property

The **distributive property** is a rule used in multiplication that states $a(b + c) = ab + ac$ and $a(b - c) = ab - ac$; in other words, the first term outside the parentheses must be distributed to, or multiplied by, each term inside the parentheses.
  $5(x - y + 3) = 5x - 5y + 15$
  $-8(-x + 3y + 7) = 8x - 24y - 56$

Fractions

- Fractions represent parts of a whole; they are another way of showing division.
- The top number is called the **numerator**, and the bottom number is called the **denominator**.
- There are three types of fractions:

  - **Proper fractions:** The numerator is less than the denominator: $\dfrac{3}{10}$

  - **Improper fractions:** The numerator is greater than or equal to the denominator: $\dfrac{7}{5}$

  - **Mixed numbers:** Contain a whole number and a fraction part: $1\dfrac{1}{3}$

- Putting a fraction in **lowest terms** (also called **reducing** a fraction or writing it in **reduced form**) means reducing the fraction so that the only **common factor** between the numerator and the denominator is 1.

> Fractions that have the same value (e.g., a fraction and that same fraction in lowest terms) are called **equivalent fractions**.

Example

Reduce $\dfrac{6}{10}$.

The numerator and denominator have a common factor of 2, so divide each by 2 to put it in lowest terms: $\dfrac{3}{5}$. Now their only common factor is 1, so this is lowest terms.

Finding the Least Common Denominator (LCD)

The **LCD** is the smallest number into which two or more denominators will divide evenly. This number is useful for performing operations (especially addition and subtraction) with fractions.

Example

Given the fractions $\dfrac{3}{5}$ and $\dfrac{1}{4}$, what is the LCD?

1. Think about the smallest number that is divisible by both 5 and 4. In this case, it is 5 × 4, or 20.
2. Multiply each of the numerators and denominators by whatever is needed to make each denominator equal to 20.

$$\frac{3}{5} \times \frac{4}{4} = \frac{12}{20} \text{ and } \frac{1}{4} \times \frac{5}{5} = \frac{5}{20}$$

3. The LCD is **20**.

Adding Fractions

- If the fractions have the **same denominator**:
  1. Add the numerators. The denominator stays the same.
  2. Write the fraction in reduced form if necessary.

Example

Solve $\dfrac{1}{9} + \dfrac{5}{9}$.

$$\dfrac{1+5}{9} = \dfrac{6}{9}$$

Since the numerator and denominator are both divisible by 3, reduce the fraction: $\dfrac{6}{9} = \dfrac{2}{3}$.

- If the fractions have **different denominators**:
  1. Find the LCD, and use it to write equivalent fractions for each fraction.
  2. Add the numerators. The denominator stays the same.
  3. Write the fraction in reduced form if necessary.

Example

Solve $\dfrac{2}{3} + \dfrac{3}{4}$.

The LCD is 12, so rewrite equivalent fractions with a denominator of 12:

$\dfrac{2}{3} \times \dfrac{4}{4} = \dfrac{8}{12}$; $\dfrac{3}{4} \times \dfrac{3}{3} = \dfrac{9}{12}$. Then add the numerators: $\dfrac{8+9}{12} = \dfrac{17}{12}$. Reduce the fraction by writing it as a mixed number: $\dfrac{17}{12} = 1\dfrac{5}{12}$.

Subtracting Fractions

- If the fractions have the **same denominator**:
  1. Subtract the numerators. The denominator stays the same.
  2. Write the fraction in reduced form if necessary.

Example

Solve $\dfrac{6}{17} - \dfrac{4}{17}$.

$$\dfrac{6-4}{17} = \dfrac{2}{17}$$

Since the greatest common factor of the numerator and denominator is 1, the fraction is already in reduced form.

- If the fractions have **different denominators**:
  1. Find the LCD, and use it to write equivalent fractions for each fraction.
  2. Subtract the numerators. The denominator stays the same.
  3. Write the fraction in reduced form if necessary.

Example

Solve $\dfrac{2}{3} - \dfrac{3}{5}$.

The LCD is 15, so rewrite equivalent fractions with a denominator of 15:

$\dfrac{2}{3} \times \dfrac{5}{5} = \dfrac{10}{15}$; $\dfrac{3}{5} \times \dfrac{3}{3} = \dfrac{9}{15}$. Then subtract the numerators: $\dfrac{10-9}{15} = \dfrac{1}{15}$.

Since the greatest common factor of the numerator and denominator is 1, the fraction is already in reduced form.

Multiplying Fractions
1. Write all numbers (even whole numbers and mixed numbers) in fraction form.
2. Multiply the numerators, and then multiply the denominators.
3. Write the results in fraction form, and then write the fraction in reduced form.

Example

Solve $\dfrac{1}{4} \times 2\dfrac{2}{5}$.

First, write all numbers in fraction form: $\dfrac{1}{4} \times \dfrac{12}{5}$. Multiply the numerators ($1 \times 12 = 12$), and then multiply the denominators ($4 \times 5 = 20$). Write the results in fraction form: $\dfrac{12}{20}$, and finally, reduce. Since each number is divisible by 4, divide each by 4 to

reduce: $\dfrac{12}{20} = \dfrac{3}{5}$.

Dividing Fractions
1. Write all numbers (even whole numbers and mixed numbers) in fraction form.
2. Change the division sign to a multiplication sign.
3. Write the **reciprocal** of the second fraction (reciprocals are found by inverting, or flipping, a fraction so that the numerator is on the bottom and the denominator is on the top).
4. Multiply the numerators, and then multiply the denominators.
5. Write the results in fraction form, and then write the fraction in reduced form.

Example

Solve $\dfrac{3}{7} \div \dfrac{1}{4}$.

The numbers are both already in fraction form, so change the division sign to a multiplication sign and write the reciprocal of the second fraction: $\dfrac{3}{7} \times \dfrac{4}{1}$.
Multiply the numerators ($3 \times 4 = 12$), and then multiply the denominators ($7 \times 1 = 7$).
Write the results in fraction form, $\dfrac{12}{7}$, or as a mixed number, $1\dfrac{5}{7}$.

Converting Fractions to Decimals
1. Write all numbers (even whole numbers or mixed numbers) in fraction form.
2. Divide the numerator by the denominator, and add a zero in front of the decimal point if necessary.

Example

Convert $1\dfrac{3}{10}$ to a decimal.

Write the mixed number in fraction form: $\dfrac{13}{10}$. Then divide 13 by 10 to get 1.3. Since there is already a number to the left of the decimal point, there is no need to write a zero in front of it.

Converting Fractions to Percentages
1. Convert the fraction to a decimal (as explained previously).
2. Round the decimal to the nearest hundredth.
3. Multiply by 100 and add the percent sign (%).

Example

Convert $\dfrac{5}{8}$ to a percentage.

Since the number is already in fraction form, divide 5 by 8 to get 0.625. Then round to the nearest hundredth: 0.63. Multiply by 100 and add the percent sign to get 63%.

Decimals

- Decimals, like fractions, represent parts of a whole. Decimal numbers may contain a **whole number part** (to the left of the decimal point) and a **fractional part** (to the right of the decimal point).
- Each number to the right of the decimal point represents a different **place value**, similar to numbers to the left of the decimal point.

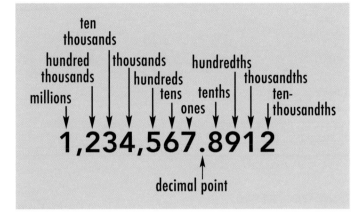

Generally, decimals that are less than 1 should always have a zero to the left of the decimal point but "trailing zeros" (i.e., zeros that come after digits on the right) should not be included (e.g., 0.65, not .65, but 1.7, not 1.70).

Rounding Decimals

Rounding is a way of estimating numbers, or describing their approximate value. Numbers can be rounded to any decimal place.

1. Determine the place value to which you are rounding.
2. Look to the right of that number. If the number is less than 5, the number to which you are rounding stays the same. If the number is greater than or equal to 5, add 1 to the number you are rounding. In either case, drop the numbers to the right.

Example

Round 3.4762 to the nearest hundredth.
The value in the hundredths place is 7, and the number to its right is 6. Since 6 is greater than 5, that means you must add 1 to the number you are rounding ($7 + 1 = 8$), so the answer is **3.48**.

Adding Decimals

1. Line up the decimal points in a column so that the place values are aligned vertically.
2. For any missing place value digits in either decimal, add zeros as placeholders.
3. Add normally as you would with whole numbers.

Example

Solve $3.2 + 5.47$.

1. Line up the numbers so that the decimal points are aligned vertically:

$$3.2$$
$$+5.47$$

2. Add a 0 in the hundredths place of the top number as a placeholder:

$$
\begin{array}{r}
3.20 \\
+5.47 \\
\end{array}
$$

3. Add:

$$
\begin{array}{r}
3.20 \\
+5.47 \\
\hline
8.67 \\
\end{array}
$$

The answer is **8.67**.

Subtracting Decimals

1. Line up the decimal points in a column so that the place values are aligned vertically.
2. For any missing place value digits in either number, add zeros as placeholders.
3. Subtract normally as you would with whole numbers.

Example

Solve 16.371 – 9.24.

1. Line up the numbers so that the decimal points are aligned vertically:

$$
\begin{array}{r}
16.371 \\
-9.24 \\
\end{array}
$$

2. Add a 0 in the thousandths place of the bottom number as a placeholder:

$$
\begin{array}{r}
16.371 \\
-9.240 \\
\end{array}
$$

3. Subtract:

$$
\begin{array}{r}
16.371 \\
-9.240 \\
\hline
7.131 \\
\end{array}
$$

The answer is **7.131**.

Multiplying Decimals

1. Line up the numbers in a column so that the right sides of both numbers are aligned vertically. Make sure the longest number (with the most place values) is on top.
2. Multiply normally as you would with whole numbers.
3. Determine the correct number of decimal places by adding the number of decimal places in each factor. Then, starting from the right of the product, count to the left as many places as necessary, and insert the decimal point.

Example

Solve 1.924×0.7.

1. Line up the numbers so that they are aligned on the right side and the longest number is on top:

$$
\begin{array}{r}
1.924 \\
\times 0.7 \\
\end{array}
$$

2. Multiply:

$$
\begin{array}{r}
1.924 \\
\times 0.7 \\
\hline
13468 \\
00000 \\
\hline
13468 \\
\end{array}
$$

3. Count the number of decimal places in each factor. There are three in 1.924, and there is one in 0.7. Starting from the right, count four decimal places, and insert the decimal point, which gives the final answer: **1.3468**.

Dividing Decimals

1. Change the divisor to a whole number by moving the decimal point to the right (which is equivalent to multiplying by powers of ten).
2. Move the decimal point in the dividend the same number of places you moved the decimal point in the divisor, and add zeros if necessary.
3. Put the decimal point in the quotient right above the decimal point in the dividend.
4. Divide normally as you would with whole numbers, adding zeros to the end of the dividend as needed.
5. If necessary, fill in zeros in the quotient to get to the decimal point.
6. Round to the desired place value if necessary.

Example

Solve $16.731 \div 2.84$. Round the answer to the nearest hundredth.

1. Rewrite the division problem in long-division format: $2.84 \overline{)16.731}$

2. Change the divisor to a whole number: $284\overline{)16.731}$

3. Since the decimal point was moved two places to the right in the divisor, do the same to the dividend, and put the decimal point in the same spot above the dividend: $284\overline{)1673.1}$

4. Divide normally, adding zeros to the end of the dividend as needed:

$$
\begin{array}{r}
5.891 \\
284\overline{)1673.100} \\
1420 \\
\hline
2531 \\
2272 \\
\hline
2590 \\
2556 \\
\hline
340 \\
284 \\
\hline
56
\end{array}
$$

5. Since you need to round only to the hundredths place, you can stop here. Since the digit to the right of the hundredths place is less than 5, the hundredths place will stay the same when rounding, making the answer **5.89**.

Converting Decimals to Fractions
1. Remove the decimal point from the number, and make the resulting number the numerator.
2. Make the denominator whatever power of ten is indicated by the last digit in the number.
3. Reduce to lowest terms.

Example
Convert 0.275 to a fraction.

1. Set 275 as the numerator. The denominator is 1,000 because the last digit in the decimal is in the thousandths place: $\dfrac{275}{1,000}$
2. Reduce to lowest terms: $\dfrac{11}{40}$

Converting Decimals to Percentages
1. Round the decimal to the nearest hundredth.
2. Multiply by 100 and add the percent sign (%).

Example
Convert 0.2483 to a percentage.
1. Round to the nearest hundredth: 0.25
2. Multiply by 100 and add the percent sign: 25%

Percentages

- Percentages are used to represent relationships between numbers. A percentage, like a fraction or decimal, is another way of expressing parts of a whole.
- Percentages represent the number of parts out of a total of 100.

Converting Percentages to Fractions

1. Take away the percent sign, and set that number as the numerator. Then set 100 as the denominator.
2. Reduce to lowest terms.

Example

Write 48% as a fraction.

1. Remove the percent sign, and set the number as the numerator with 100 as the denominator: $\dfrac{48}{100}$
2. Reduce to lowest terms: $\dfrac{48}{100} = \dfrac{12}{25}$

Converting Percentages to Decimals

1. Take away the percent sign and divide by 100.
2. Alternatively, take away the percent sign and move the decimal point two places to the left.

Example

Write 37% as a decimal.

Using the "divide by 100" method, take away the percent sign and divide 37 by 100: 37 ÷ 100 = 0.37. Alternately, using the decimal-point method (37.0), move the decimal point two places to the left to get .37 and add the zero to the left of the decimal point: 0.37.

Ratios, Proportions & Rates

Ratios

- Ratios are the same as fractions. They show the relationship of a part to the whole.
- Ratios are written using colons (:). When you read a ratio, you say "to" or "is to" when you see the colon: 1:3 ("1 to 3" or "1 is to 3") is the same as $\dfrac{1}{3}$.

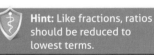

Hint: Like fractions, ratios should be reduced to lowest terms.

Proportions

- Proportions are used to compare ratios or fractions that are equal. Proportions may be written in several ways: as fractions with an equals sign, such as $\dfrac{2}{4} = \dfrac{1}{2}$; as ratios with a colon and an equals sign in the middle (e.g., 2:4 = 1:2); or as ratios with colons and a double colon in the middle, which means the same thing as an equals sign (e.g., 2:4::1:2).
- The **means and extremes method** is a way to check if ratios are proportional. The two middle numbers of the ratio are the means, and the two outer numbers are the

extremes. If you multiply the means and then multiply the extremes, the two results should be equal. If they are not equal, the ratios are not proportional.

- **Solving for x in proportions:** If there is an unknown in a proportion, the variable x is often used and can be solved for using the means and extremes method.

Example
Use the means and extremes method to determine if 1:6 and 3:18 are proportional.
1. Multiply the means: $6 \times 3 = 18$.
2. Multiply the extremes: $1 \times 18 = 18$.
3. Since the two products are equal, the two ratios are proportional.

Example
Solve for x in the following proportion: 4:12::x:9
1. Multiply the means: $12 \times x = 12x$.
2. Multiply the extremes: $4 \times 9 = 36$.
3. Set the two equal to one another: $12x = 36$.
4. Solve by dividing both sides by 12: $x = 3$.

Rates
- Rates are special kinds of ratios that compare two numbers using units. The words "per" and "for" often indicate a rate (e.g., 3 limes for \$1; 24 miles per gallon). Rates are often used in costs, speeds, etc.
- To solve rate problems involving an unknown, it is often useful to use proportions. Break the word problem into numbers, and set it up like an equation.

Example
A store sells a 5-pound bag of potatoes for \$7.99. How much do potatoes cost per pound?

1. Set up the known part of the equation: 5 pounds of potatoes cost \$7.99, so write 5:7.99 or $\dfrac{5}{7.99}$.

2. You want to know how much 1 pound costs. You know the weight, or the first number in the second part of the equation (1), and the second number is unknown, so use x to represent it: 1:x, or $\dfrac{1}{x}$.

3. Now set up the proportion: 5:7.99::1:x, or $\dfrac{5}{7.99} = \dfrac{1}{x}$.

4. Solve for x using the means and extremes method: $7.99 \times 1 = 7.99$; and $5 \times x = 5x$.
5. Set the two equal to one another: $7.99 = 5x$.
6. Solve by dividing both sides by 5: $x = 1.598$.
7. Since we are dealing with money, round to the nearest hundredth: $x =$ **\$1.60 per pound**.

PERIODIC TABLE
OF ELEMENTS

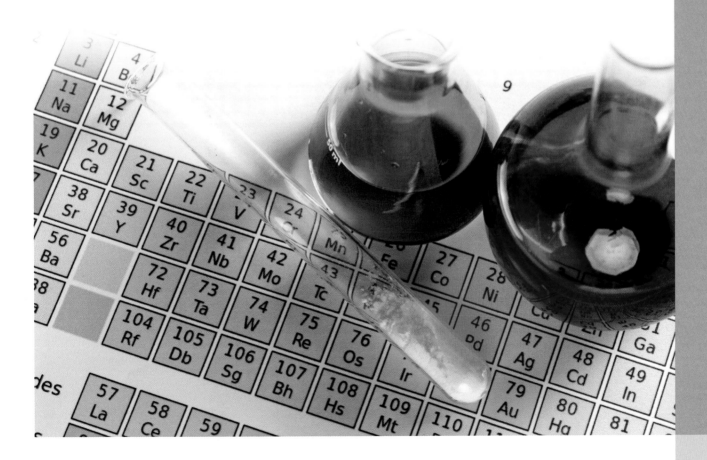

Periodic Table of the Elements

Legend:
- atomic number
- **Symbol**
- name
- standard atomic weight

1	2	3	4	5	6	7	8	9	10	11	12	13	14	15	16	17	18
1 **H** hydrogen [1.007; 1.009]																	2 **He** helium 4.003
3 **Li** lithium [6.938; 6.997]	4 **Be** beryllium 9.012											5 **B** boron [10.80; 10.83]	6 **C** carbon [12.00; 12.02]	7 **N** nitrogen [14.00; 14.01]	8 **O** oxygen [15.99; 16.00]	9 **F** fluorine 19.00	10 **Ne** neon 20.18
11 **Na** sodium 22.99	12 **Mg** magnesium 24.31											13 **Al** aluminum 26.98	14 **Si** silicon [28.08; 28.09]	15 **P** phosphorus 30.97	16 **S** sulfur [32.05; 32.08]	17 **Cl** chlorine [35.44; 35.46]	18 **Ar** argon 39.95
19 **K** potassium 39.10	20 **Ca** calcium 40.08	21 **Sc** scandium 44.96	22 **Ti** titanium 47.87	23 **V** vanadium 50.94	24 **Cr** chromium 52.00	25 **Mn** manganese 54.94	26 **Fe** iron 55.85	27 **Co** cobalt 58.93	28 **Ni** nickel 58.69	29 **Cu** copper 63.55	30 **Zn** zinc 65.38(2)	31 **Ga** gallium 69.72	32 **Ge** germanium 72.63	33 **As** arsenic 74.92	34 **Se** selenium 78.96(3)	35 **Br** bromine 79.90	36 **Kr** krypton 83.80
37 **Rb** rubidium 85.47	38 **Sr** strontium 87.62	39 **Y** yttrium 88.91	40 **Zr** zirconium 91.22	41 **Nb** niobium 92.91	42 **Mo** molybdenum 95.96(2)	43 **Tc** technetium	44 **Ru** ruthenium 101.1	45 **Rh** rhodium 102.9	46 **Pd** palladium 106.4	47 **Ag** silver 107.9	48 **Cd** cadmium 112.4	49 **In** indium 114.8	50 **Sn** tin 118.7	51 **Sb** antimony 121.8	52 **Te** tellurium 127.6	53 **I** iodine 126.9	54 **Xe** xenon 131.3
55 **Cs** cesium 132.9	56 **Ba** barium 137.3	57–71 lanthanides	72 **Hf** hafnium 178.5	73 **Ta** tantalum 180.9	74 **W** tungsten 183.8	75 **Re** rhenium 186.2	76 **Os** osmium 190.2	77 **Ir** iridium 192.2	78 **Pt** platinum 195.1	79 **Au** gold 197.0	80 **Hg** mercury 200.6	81 **Tl** thallium [204.3; 204.4]	82 **Pb** lead 207.2	83 **Bi** bismuth 209.0	84 **Po** polonium	85 **At** astatine	86 **Rn** radon
87 **Fr** francium	88 **Ra** radium	89–103 actinides	104 **Rf** rutherfordium	105 **Db** dubnium	106 **Sg** seaborgium	107 **Bh** bohrium	108 **Hs** hassium	109 **Mt** meitnerium	110 **Ds** darmstadtium	111 **Rg** roentgenium	112 **Cn** copernicium		114 **Fl** flerovium		116 **Lv** livermorium		

Lanthanides

57 **La** lanthanum 138.9	58 **Ce** cerium 140.1	59 **Pr** praseodymium 140.9	60 **Nd** neodymium 144.2	61 **Pm** promethium	62 **Sm** samarium 150.4	63 **Eu** europium 152.0	64 **Gd** gadolinium 157.3	65 **Tb** terbium 158.9	66 **Dy** dysprosium 162.5	67 **Ho** holmium 164.9	68 **Er** erbium 167.3	69 **Tm** thulium 168.9	70 **Yb** ytterbium 173.1	71 **Lu** lutetium 175.0

Actinides

89 **Ac** actinium	90 **Th** thorium 232.0	91 **Pa** protactinium 231.0	92 **U** uranium 238.0	93 **Np** neptunium	94 **Pu** plutonium	95 **Am** americium	96 **Cm** curium	97 **Bk** berkelium	98 **Cf** californium	99 **Es** einsteinium	100 **Fm** fermium	101 **Md** mendelevium	102 **No** nobelium	103 **Lr** lawrencium

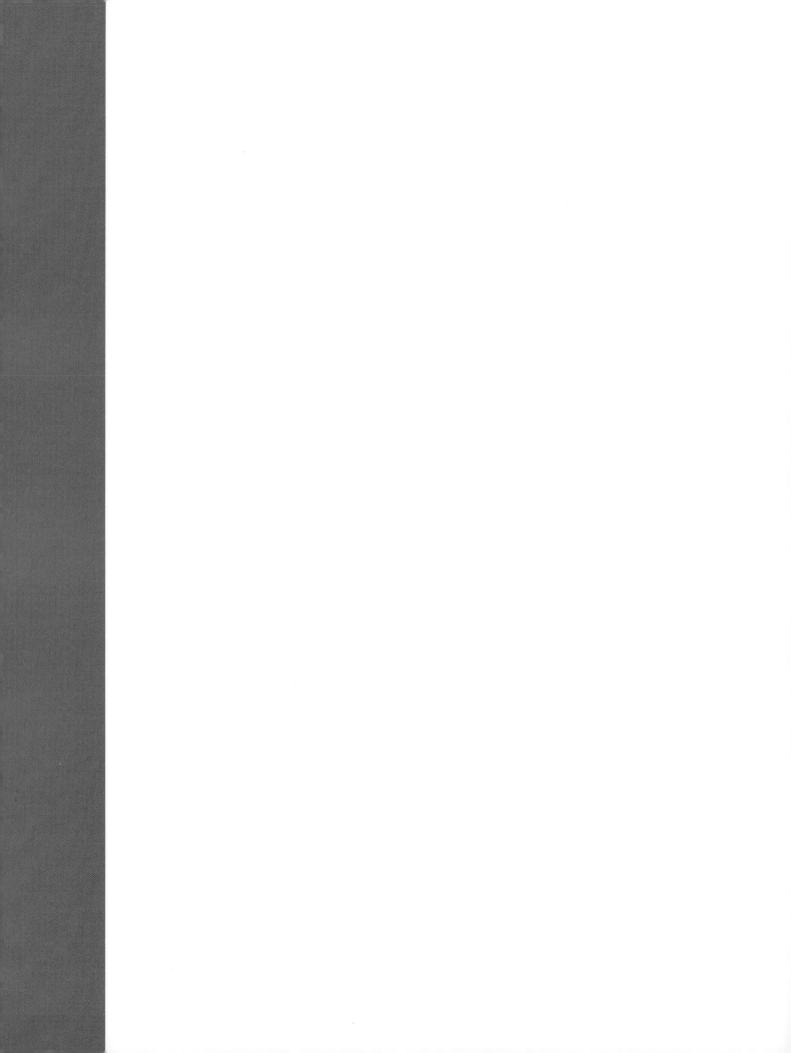

NCLEX-RN
STUDY GUIDE

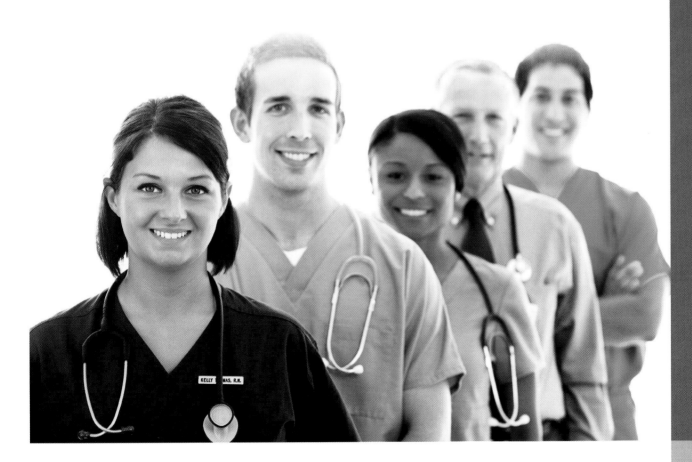

Components of the Nursing Process

- **Assessment:** The physical, psychosocial, and spiritual needs of a patient are investigated through the collection of subjective and objective data.
- **Analysis (a.k.a. diagnosis):** The data collected during the assessment phase are analyzed to determine the plan of care.
- **Planning:** The data from the assessment and analysis phases are used to develop measurable goals and outcomes (i.e., nursing interventions).
- **Implementation:** The nursing interventions are put into practice.
- **Evaluation:** The outcomes of the nursing interventions are measured.

Assessment Techniques

Inspection

Inspection is the careful examination of the patient as a whole, as well as of each body system, using the visual, auditory, and olfactory senses to gather information. Inspection:
- Looks at the color, shape, symmetry, and position of body parts
- Should be purposeful and systematic; body parts should be compared bilaterally throughout the entire examination
- Requires good lighting to visually inspect the body without distortion or shadows

Palpation

Palpation is the technique of using touch to gather information about the temperature, turgor, texture, moisture, size, shape, consistency, location, and tenderness of an organ or body part.
- Palpation can be **light** (using inward pressure to depress the skin and underlying structures approx. ½ inch) or **deep** (using inward pressure to depress the skin and underlying structures approx. 1 inch).
- The patient should be provided with privacy, and the nurse should have warm hands and short fingernails. Any areas of tenderness should be palpated last.
- During palpation, make sure you assess:
  - Consistency of tissues
  - Alignment and intactness of structures
  - Symmetry of body parts or movements
  - Transmission of fine vibrations

Percussion

Percussion is the art of striking one object with another to create sound to assess the location, size, and density of underlying tissues. The sound changes as you move from one area to the next. Percussion is done with the middle finger of the dominant hand tapping on the middle finger of the nondominant hand while the nondominant palm is on the body.
- The nondominant hand is placed on the area to be percussed, with fingers slightly separated.
- The dominant hand is used to deliver the striking force by exerting a sharp downward wrist movement so that the tip of the middle finger of the dominant hand strikes the joint of the middle finger on the nondominant hand.
- There are five types of percussion sounds:
  - **Tympany:** Loud; drumlike sound
  - **Resonance:** Moderate to loud; low-pitched, hollow sound
  - **Hyperresonance:** Very loud; low-pitched, booming sound
  - **Flatness:** Soft; high-pitched, flat sound
  - **Dullness:** Soft to moderate; high-pitched, thud-like sound

Percussion Sounds & Potential Causes

Percussion Sound	Where Normally Heard	Potential Cause
Tympany	Abdomen	Normal
Resonance	Chest	Healthy lungs
Hyperresonance	Chest	Chronic obstructive pulmonary disease, asthma, pneumothorax
Flatness	Solid areas	Muscle or bone, severe pneumonia
Dullness	Liver or heart	Organs, pneumonia, tumor, pleural effusion

Auscultation

Auscultation is the act of listening to sounds produced by the body using a stethoscope. Auscultation is performed for the purposes of examining the circulatory system, respiratory system, and gastrointestinal (GI) system.

- Sounds must be isolated for proper identification and evaluation.
- The stethoscope has a diaphragm, which detects high-pitched sounds best, and a bell, which detects low-pitched sounds best.
- Four characteristics of sounds should be noted:
  - Pitch
  - Loudness
  - Quality
  - Duration

> Auscultation is a skill that requires substantial clinical experience, a fine stethoscope, and good listening skills. High-pitched tones are best heard with the diaphragm of the stethoscope; low-pitched tones are best heard with the bell of the stethoscope.

Basic Head-to-Toe Assessment

- **General:** Assess general appearance and behavior, posture, gait, hygiene, speech, mental status, height and weight, hearing and visual acuity, vital signs, and nutrition.
- **Head and neck:** Assess skull size, shape, and symmetry; hair; and scalp. Palpate for masses on scalp, ears, face, throat, and neck. Palpate sinuses for tenderness and masses. Inspect sclera and conjunctiva. Assess pupil response (use **PERRLA**: **p**upils **e**qual, **r**ound, **r**eactive to **l**ight and **a**ccommodation). Test convergence (as eyes shift from a far object to a near object, pupils constrict), confrontation (extent of peripheral field), and corneal reflex. Inspect and palpate teeth and gums. Test rise of uvula and gag reflex. Assess sense of smell and taste. Check range of motion (ROM) in neck and shoulders. Palpate lymph nodes for tenderness and swelling, trachea for symmetry, and thyroid for masses.
- **Upper extremities:** Inspect skin, test capillary refill, palpate peripheral pulses, rate muscle strength, assess ROM, and check deep tendon reflexes.
- **Posterior thorax:** Inspect spine for alignment, assess anteroposterior to lateral diameter, assess thoracic expansion, palpate for tactile fremitus, auscultate breath sounds, and perform blunt percussion over costovertebral angles for tenderness.
- **Anterior thorax:** Observe respiratory pattern, palpate respiratory excursion, auscultate breath sounds, auscultate heart sounds, inspect jugular veins, and perform breast examination.
- **Abdomen:** Auscultate for bowel sounds, percuss for masses and tenderness, percuss the liver, and palpate the kidneys and spleen.
- **Lower extremities:** Inspect skin, palpate peripheral pulses, assess for Homans sign, inspect and palpate joints for swelling, assess for pedal and ankle edema, and assess ROM.

Systems Assessment

Integumentary

- Inspect skin for color, texture, tone, and lesions. Palpate with the back of the hand for temperature, moisture, and texture. Note any abnormal findings (shiny skin on lower extremities, mole with irregular borders, lesions, masses, bruising, jaundice, high or low temperature).
- Inspect hair for distribution and for presence of head lice.
- Inspect scalp for lesions.
- Inspect nails for color, contour, texture, symmetry, and capillary refill. Note any abnormal findings (white spots, pitting, ridges, clubbing, cyanosis, slow capillary refill).

Cardiovascular

- Record blood pressure (BP).
- Auscultate the carotid arteries using the bell of the stethoscope.
- Listen for carotid bruits (blowing or rushing sounds).
- Listen to heart sounds. Note any abnormal findings (murmurs, gallops, clicks, rubs).
- Palpate pulses (carotid, radial, brachial, femoral, popliteal, posterior tibial, dorsalis pedis).
- Assess feet for vascularity (warmth, capillary refill, elevation pallor, dependent rubor).

Respiratory

- Inspect skin color; observe level of consciousness.
- Look for signs of respiratory distress (cyanosis, pursed-lip breathing, accessory muscle use, nasal flaring, retractions).
- Evaluate rate, depth, and rhythm of breathing.
- Palpate for tracheal deviation, crepitus, tactile fremitus, and equal thoracic expansion.
- Percuss beginning at the apex of the left lung; listen for resonance (normal), hyper-resonance (too much air; may indicate emphysema), and flatness (presence of fluid or solid mass; may indicate pleural effusion, pneumonia, or tumor).
- Listen to breath sounds. Note any abnormal sounds (adventitious sounds, crackles, wheezes, rubs, stridor).

Gastrointestinal (GI)

- Inspect mouth for lesions, irritations, or tumors.
- Check gag reflex.
- Inspect all four quadrants of the abdomen for contour, symmetry, abdominal aorta pulsation, and distention.
- Percuss all four quadrants (**Note:** Do not percuss if an abdominal aortic aneurysm is suspected.); listen to bowel sounds for frequency and classification (e.g., hypoactive, normal, or hyperactive). Note any abnormal bowel sounds (bruits, venous hums, friction rubs).
- Palpate by quadrant, noting any guarding, rigidity, tenderness, or masses.

Genitourinary (GU)

- Assess urinary intake and output.
- Ask about potentially abnormal urinary symptoms (urgency, pain with urination, pelvic pain, back pain, nocturia, dysuria, incontinence, blood in urine, difficulty in starting or stopping urinary stream, pain in testicles, leaking or feeling of full bladder after voiding).
- Inspect genitalia for discharge, lesions, swelling, warts, bumps, blisters, and redness.

- Ask about pain during intercourse, history of sexually transmitted diseases, and menstrual history (menarche, regularity, duration, flow, dysmenorrhea, menopause).

Musculoskeletal

- Inspect each extremity bilaterally for symmetry.
- Inspect each joint for size, contour, masses, and deformities.
- Palpate each extremity for edema.
- Perform ROM tests of the extremities bilaterally (shoulders, elbows, wrists, fingers, hips, knees, ankles, toes).
- Test ROM of the spine by asking the patient to bend forward and touch his or her toes.

Types of Musculoskeletal Pain

- **Bone pain:**
  - Is deep, aching, and constant
  - Is unrelated to movement unless fracture is present
- **Muscle pain:**
  - May be related to posture or occur with movement
  - May be accompanied by tremors, twitches, or weakness
  - May produce referred pain
- **Joint pain:**
  - Is tender to palpation
  - May produce referred pain
  - May produce distal pain because of nerve root irritation
  - Is worse with movement and worsens throughout the day

Neurologic

- Inspect gait and balance.
- Assess recent and remote memory.
- Test cerebellar functions by finger-to-nose test for upper extremities and running each heel down the opposite shin for lower extremities.
- Test the Babinski reflex: the big toe bends back toward the top of the foot and the other toes fan out when the sole of the foot is firmly stroked.
- Assess mental status (appearance, attitude, behavior, mood and affect, speech, thought process, thought content, perception, cognition, insight, judgment).
- Assess cranial nerves (olfactory, optic, oculomotor, trochlear, trigeminal, abducens, facial, acoustic, glossopharyngeal, vagus, spinal accessory, hypoglossal).
- Assess reflexes bilaterally (biceps, triceps, brachioradialis, patellar, Achilles).
- Assess motor skills (bilateral muscle strength, balance, coordination).
- Assess sensory perception bilaterally (use different stimuli, such as a cotton ball for light touch and fingertips for pressure).

Cranial Nerve (CN) Assessment

- **CN I (olfactory):** Use easily identifiable substances (e.g., coffee, orange, soap, toothpaste) to assess unilateral sense of smell.
- **CN II (optic):** Check visual acuity; check near vision by having the patient read newspaper print and far vision with a Snellen chart.
- **CN III (oculomotor):** Assess pupil size and light reflex.
- **CN IV (trochlear) and CN VI (abducens):** Check eye movement by having the patient turn eyes downward, temporally, and nasally.
- **CN V (trigeminal):** Assess motor function by palpating jaw and temples while having the patient clench teeth; assess sensory function by touching a cotton ball to areas of the face.
- **CN VII (facial):** Check symmetry and mobility of face by having the patient frown, close eyes, lift eyebrows, and puff out cheeks; check the patient's ability to identify tastes (e.g., sugar, salt, lemon).

- **CN VIII (acoustic):** Check hearing acuity.
- **CN IX (glossopharyngeal) and CN X (vagus):** Evaluate movement of uvula and soft palate; also check gag reflex.
- **CN XI (spinal accessory):** Check movement of head and neck.
- **CN XII (hypoglossal):** Assess tongue control.

Psychosocial

- Perform mental status examination (appearance, attitude, behavior, mood, affect, speech, thought process, thought content, perception, cognition, insight, judgment).
- Assess home environment (family structure, interactions, support systems, safety).
- Assess community environment (recreational activities, transportation, safety).
- Perform spiritual assessment (religious affiliations, spiritual beliefs).

Pregnancy, Labor & Delivery, Postpartum Care

Definitions

- **Perinatal period:** From before birth through day 28 after birth
  - **Prematurity:** Birth prior to completion of 37 weeks' gestation
  - **Low birth weight (LBW):** Baby born weighing less than 2500 grams (5 lb, 8 oz)
  - **Full term:** Gestation weeks 38–40 (266–280 days)
- **Prenatal periods**
  - **Embryonic period:** Gestation weeks 2–8
  - **Fetal period:** Gestation week 9 through delivery
- **Postpartum period:** First 6 weeks after childbirth
  - **Puerperium period:** From the end of labor until the uterus returns to normal size (typically 3–6 weeks)

Nursing Care during Labor

- Monitor fetal heart rate by auscultation or external fetal monitor. (Optimal is 120–160 beats per minute [bpm].)
- Monitor mother's vital signs.
- Assess frequency, duration, and intensity of contractions by palpating uterine fundus.
- Perform vaginal examination; assess:
  - Dilation (use index and middle fingers to measure the size of the opening)
  - Effacement (thinning and shortening of the cervix)
  - Membrane status (ruptured or intact)
  - Station (the relationship between the baby's presenting part and the mother's ischial spines)
  - Fetal presentation and position (through vaginal examination and Leopold maneuvers)
  - Bloody show (amount and character)

Postpartum Care

Assess:
- **Uterus:** Fundal height, involution
- **Perineum:** Edema, infection, hematoma
- **Lochia:** Color, amount
- **Breasts:** Engorgement
- **Voiding:** Frequency, amount, bladder distention
- **Pain:** Location, intensity, duration

Common Pregnancy Complications

Complication	Symptoms	Potential Causes
Bleeding	Vaginal bleeding	Vaginal bleeding during pregnancy (especially during the first trimester) is common and may not be a sign of a problem; potential problems include miscarriage, premature labor, ectopic pregnancy, placenta previa, and cervical cancer
Gestational hypertension	High BP during pregnancy; usually no symptoms, but may have headache, blurred vision	Unknown
Gestational diabetes	High blood sugar during pregnancy; usually no symptoms, but may have fatigue, increased thirst, increased urination, weight loss	Hormonal changes that lead to progressive impaired glucose intolerance
Eclampsia	Seizures that are not related to a preexisting brain condition; muscle pain; agitation; loss of consciousness	Blood vessel problems, neurological factors, genetics
Ectopic pregnancy	Pregnancy outside the uterus (usually in the fallopian tube); symptoms may include vaginal bleeding, abdominal or pelvic pain	Damage to the fallopian tube caused by previous infection, endometriosis, or pelvic surgery
Preterm labor	Labor before 37 weeks; symptoms may include abdominal cramping, pressure in the abdomen or pelvis, contractions, vaginal bleeding, lower back pain	Smoking, drug abuse, multiple pregnancy (more than one fetus), infection, hypertension, diabetes
Placenta previa	Placenta covering the cervix; symptoms may include cramps, vaginal bleeding in the second or third trimester	Abnormal shape or size of uterus; multiple pregnancy (more than one fetus); uterine scarring from previous pregnancies, C-section, or surgery
Preeclampsia	Hypertension and proteinuria after the 20th week of pregnancy; symptoms may include edema, sudden weight gain, pain in the right upper quadrant, decreased urine output, nausea and vomiting, headaches, vision problems	Autoimmune disorders, poor nutrition, blood vessel damage

Newborn Assessment

- APGAR score
- Weight
- Measurement
- Vital signs
  - **BP:** 65–85/45–55 mm Hg
  - **Pulse:** 120–160 bpm
  - **Respiratory rate:** 30–50 breaths per minute
  - **Temperature:** 98.6°F–99.8°F (37°C–37.7°C)
- General appearance
- Skin
- Head and neck (appearance, shape, fontanels)
- Breath sounds
- Heart sounds
- GI and GU systems
- Extremities

APGAR Score			
Signs	**0**	**1**	**2**
Activity	No muscle tone	Some muscle tone	Active motion
Pulse	No pulse	<100 bpm	>100 bpm
Grimace (reflex in response to stimulation)	No reaction	Grimace	Grimace and cough, sneeze, or cry
Appearance	Pale blue body and extremities	Pink body, blue extremities	Pink body and extremities
Respiration	No breathing	Slow or irregular breathing	Strong cry

Note: A normal APGAR score is 7–9.

Pediatrics

Human Growth & Development

- **Infancy:** Gains control of eye movements; smiles, coos, grasps objects, rolls over, sits; birth weight doubles.
- **Early childhood:** Walks, talks, identifies common objects, undergoes toilet training.
- **Preschool:** Develops gross motor skills (pedaling, hopping on one foot, kicking, catching a ball) and fine motor skills (drawing, using scissors, dressing self), follows commands.
- **School age:** Has strong motor skills; grammar and pronunciation become normal.
- **Adolescence:** Experiences rapid growth, understands abstract ideas, establishes relationships.
  - **Girls:** Breast development, hair growth (pubic, armpits, arms, legs), menarche.
  - **Boys:** Genital growth, hair growth (pubic, armpits, arms, legs, chest, face); voice changes.

- **Young adulthood:** Experiences minimal physical growth, develops lasting relationships; physical performance, strength, and flexibility peak.
- **Middle adulthood:** Experiences hair loss and graying, develops fine lines and wrinkles; hearing and eyesight decline, menopause occurs (in women).
- **Late adulthood:** Slowing of all major organs and systems.

Erikson's Stages of Psychosocial Development

- **Trust versus mistrust (birth–18 months):** When needs are met, the child develops trust; if the caregiver is unreliable or inconsistent, mistrust develops.
- **Autonomy versus shame and doubt (18 months–3 years):** Successfully conquering new skills leads to a sense of autonomy; a lack of success in learning new skills can lead to shame and doubt.
- **Initiative versus guilt (3–5 years):** The child becomes more assertive in order to feel more in control over his or her environment; if the parents approve of the child's attempts to take the initiative, the child develops a sense of purpose. Disapproval can lead to feelings of guilt.
- **Industry versus inferiority (6–11 years):** The child goes to school and begins to acquire new social and learning skills; failure can lead to feelings of inferiority.
- **Identity versus role confusion (12–18 years):** The adolescent or teen begins to develop a sense of self or identity; failure can lead to confusion or identity crisis.
- **Intimacy versus isolation (19–40 years):** The young adult forms intimate relationships with others; failure can lead to feelings of isolation.
- **Generativity versus stagnation (40–65 years):** Those in middle adulthood need to feel that they are doing something worthwhile that will outlast them; failure may lead to a societal disconnect and shallow relationships.
- **Ego integrity versus despair (65 years old and older):** Older adults need to look back and feel that their lives were well-lived and had meaning; failure can lead to feelings of despair.

Common Childhood Diseases

- **Chickenpox:** A highly contagious virus that is characterized by itchy, fluid-filled blisters on the skin. A vaccine is available for the prevention of chickenpox.
- **Respiratory syncytial virus (RSV):** A respiratory virus that infects the lungs and airways. Symptoms may include runny nose, decreased appetite, coughing, sneezing, fever, and wheezing.
- **Whooping cough (pertussis):** A highly contagious respiratory disease that is characterized by uncontrollable, violent coughing fits followed by a "whooping" sound. A vaccine is available for the prevention of whooping cough.
- **Fifth disease (erythema infectiosum):** A virus that is characterized by a red facial rash that is known as a "slapped cheek" rash. Other symptoms may include runny nose, fever, and headache.
- **Hand, foot, and mouth disease:** A virus that is characterized by blister-like sores in the mouth and a skin rash (usually on the hands and/or feet). Other symptoms may include fever and malaise.
- **Croup:** An infection that is characterized by a "barking cough." Other symptoms may include cold-like symptoms and difficulty breathing.
- **Scarlet fever:** A strep infection that is characterized by a red rash that feels like sandpaper. Other symptoms may include sore throat, fever, chills, vomiting, and abdominal pain.
- **Impetigo:** A skin infection characterized by itchy, pus-filled blisters. Other symptoms may include a rash that spreads with scratching and swollen lymph nodes.

Classifications of Young Patients	
Age	**Classification**
<38 weeks' gestation	Premature or preterm infant
<1 month	Neonate or newborn infant
1 month to 1 year	Infant
1 year to 12 years	Child

Expected Growth Rate for Infants & Children	
Age	**Expected Growth Rate per Year**
1–6 months	18–22 cm
6–12 months	14–18 cm
Second year	11 cm
Third year	8 cm
Fourth year	7 cm
Fifth to tenth years	5–6 cm

Timeline of Childhood Milestones	
Age	**Milestone(s)**
2 months	Smiles at the sound of a familiar voice
3 months	Raises head and chest when lying on stomach, grasps objects, smiles at other people
4 months	Babbles, laughs, tries to imitate sounds
6 months	Rolls from back to stomach

Nursing Care Delivery Models

- **Case method:** A nurse is assigned to provide complete care for a patient or group of patients for a defined time period.
- **Functional:** A variety of caregivers are assigned to perform specific tasks or functions for each patient.
- **Team:** A team that is made up of licensed and unlicensed providers is assigned to deliver care under the direction of a team leader.
- **Primary:** A single nurse has sole responsibility for assessing patient needs, developing a plan of care, and evaluating the patient's response to the plan of care.
- **Case management:** This is an integrated system of care that uses a multidisciplinary team approach in a variety of care settings.

Nursing Ethics

Ethical Principles

- **Autonomy:** A patient has the right to make health care decisions for him- or herself even if the nurse does not agree with those decisions. Exceptions may be made when autonomy interferes with another person's rights, health, or well-being.
- **Justice:** Patients have the right to be treated equally, regardless of race, ethnicity, gender, marital status, sexual orientation, medical diagnosis, social standing, economic level, or religious beliefs.
- **Fidelity:** Nurses should keep commitments to others. Fidelity includes loyalty to agreements and responsibilities accepted as part of the practice of nursing.

- **Beneficence:** It is a nurse's responsibility to do good. Good care requires a holistic approach to patients, which includes attention to their beliefs, feelings, and wishes.
- **Nonmaleficence:** In addition to doing good, nurses should also strive to do no harm. This includes helping determine whether benefits of treatments outweigh the risks.
- **Veracity:** Nurses should tell the truth and not intentionally deceive or mislead patients.
- **Confidentiality:** Privileged information should be kept private. Communications between the nurse and the patient should not be divulged to third parties.

Steps of Ethical Decision Making
1. Collect, analyze, and interpret the data.
2. Bring all the data together in a form that puts the dilemma into a clear and sharp focus.
3. Clearly and succinctly state the dilemma.
4. Identify morally relevant facts.
5. Consider possible courses of action.
6. Analyze the advantages and disadvantages of each course of action.
7. Make the decision.
8. Evaluate the decision and the outcome.

Informed Consent

Informed consent is the process by which a patient makes an informed decision about whether to undergo a medical treatment or procedure. There are four components to the informed consent process:
- **Decision-making capacity:** The person signing the consent form must have the ability to make an informed decision.
- **Disclosure:** During the process of obtaining an informed consent, the nurse should give the patient information about his or her diagnosis, the reason for the treatment or procedure, the potential benefits of the procedure, any potential risks or complications associated with the procedure, any potential risks of not undergoing the procedure, and the risks and benefits of alternative treatments.
- **Comprehension:** The person signing the consent form must have the ability to comprehend the information given during the disclosure.
- **Voluntary participation:** The person signing the consent form must consent voluntarily, without coercion.

Risk Reduction

Preventing Medication Errors
- Follow the **five rights of medication administration**: right patient, right dose, right route, right time, and right medication.
- Read back and spell back verbal or telephone orders.
- Use bar code scanning if available.
- Use independent double checks for high-alert medications.
- Ask about drug allergies before giving a new medication.
- Provide patient education. Teach patients about their medications, what they are for, what they look like, and when and how they should take them. Have patients demonstrate understanding.

Preventing Communication Errors
- During shift change report, or when a patient transfers from one unit or facility to another, make sure to verbally report the patient's history, current condition, treatment modalities, and recent changes in condition. Allow time for questions.

- When communicating with physicians, use clear, direct statements to describe the situation.
- When communicating with patients:
  - Use simple language; avoid medical jargon.
  - Ask patients to repeat back verbal instructions.
  - Use an interpreter when necessary.
  - Be specific with instructions (e.g., "Check your blood sugar before meals" instead of "Check your blood sugar while fasting").

Preventing Falls
- Clean up spills as soon as they happen.
- Make sure the patient's call light and personal belongings are within reach.
- Make sure the path to the bathroom is clear.
- Provide nonskid footwear.
- Provide adequate lighting.
- Assess fall risk.
- Do not leave at-risk patients unattended.

Preventing Surgical Errors
- **Preoperative verification:** At scheduling, admission, and handoff and before leaving the pre-op area, verify right person, right procedure, and right site.
- **Time-out:** Just before starting the procedure, verify right patient, right surgical procedure, right surgical site, right patient position, and right equipment.

Infection Prevention & Control

Hand Hygiene
Hand hygiene is the single most important aspect of infection prevention and control. The Centers for Disease Control and Prevention (CDC) recommends that hand hygiene be performed:
- Before and after direct patient contact
- Before procedures, such as administering intravenous (IV) medications
- Before and after contact with vascular access
- Before and after dressing changes
- After contact with blood, body fluids, or contaminated surfaces
- After removing gloves

Hand hygiene can be performed with alcohol-based hand rubs or by washing hands with antimicrobial soap.

Standard Precautions
The CDC developed the following standard precautions to protect against the transmission of infection. Under standard precautions, all blood, body fluids, secretions and excretions, broken skin, and mucous membranes should be treated as potentially infectious.
- Perform hand hygiene in the following situations:
  - Before touching a patient, even if gloves will be worn
  - Before exiting the patient care area after touching a patient or the patient's immediate environment
  - After contact with blood, body fluids or excretions, or wound dressings
  - Prior to performing an aseptic task (e.g., accessing a port, preparing an injection)
  - If hands will be moving from a contaminated body site to a clean body site during patient care
  - After glove removal
- Wear gloves when there is a potential for contact with blood, body fluids, mucous membranes, nonintact skin, or contaminated equipment.

- Wear a gown to protect skin and clothing during procedures or activities where contact with blood or body fluids is anticipated.
- Wear a face mask, goggles, or a face shield during any procedure where there may be a potential for splashing.

Contact Precautions

According to the CDC, the following contact precautions should be applied to patients with stool incontinence, draining wounds, uncontrolled secretions, pressure ulcers, ostomy tubes or, bags draining body fluids, or generalized rashes or exanthems:
- Perform hand hygiene before touching the patient and before putting on gloves.
- Wear gloves when touching the patient or the patient's immediate environment or belongings.
- Wear a gown if substantial contact with the patient or patient's environment is anticipated.
- Perform hand hygiene after removal of personal protective equipment (PPE); use soap and water when hands are visibly soiled or after caring for patients with known or suspected infectious diarrhea.

Droplet Precautions

CDC guidelines suggest that the following droplet precautions be applied to patients who are known or suspected to be infected with a pathogen that can be transmitted by droplet route:
- Place the patient in a private room with a closed door as soon as possible.
- Use PPE:
  - Wear a face mask for close contact with the patient.
  - Wear gloves, a gown, and goggles if spraying is likely to occur.
- Perform hand hygiene before and after touching the patient and after contact with respiratory secretions or with contaminated objects or materials; use soap and water when hands are visibly soiled.
- Instruct the patient to wear a face mask when exiting the room, to avoid close contact with other patients, and to practice respiratory hygiene and cough etiquette.

Airborne Precautions

According to the CDC, the following airborne precautions should be applied to patients known or suspected to be infected with a pathogen that can be transmitted by airborne route:
- Place the patient in an airborne infection isolation room.
- Wear a fit-tested N-95 or higher-level disposable respirator mask, if available, when caring for the patient.
- Wear gloves, a gown, and goggles if spraying is likely to occur.
- Perform hand hygiene before and after touching the patient and after contact with respiratory secretions or with contaminated objects or materials; use soap and water when hands are visibly soiled.
- Instruct the patient to wear a face mask when exiting the room, to avoid close contact with other patients, and to practice respiratory hygiene and cough etiquette.

Preventive Care

Health Screenings for Women
- **Mammogram:** Every 2 years starting at age 50
- **Pap test:** Every 3 years starting at age 21
- **Colorectal cancer screening:** As determined by their doctor starting at age 50

Health Screenings for Men
- **Colorectal cancer screening:** As determined by their doctor starting at age 50
- **Prostate cancer screening:** As determined by their doctor starting at age 50

Recommended Immunizations for Birth–6 Years

Birth	1 mo	2 mo	4 mo	6 mo	12 mo	15 mo	18 mo	19–23 mo	2–3 yr	4–6 yr
HepB	HepB			HepB						
		RV	RV	RV						
		DTaP	DTaP	DTaP		DTaP				DTaP
		Hib	Hib	Hib	Hib					
		PCV	PCV	PCV	PCV					
		IPV	IPV	IPV						IPV
				Influenza (yearly)						
					MMR					MMR
					Varicella					Varicella
					HepA					

Key: Shaded boxes indicate the vaccine can be given during shown age range.

Recommended Immunizations for Ages 7–18 Years

7–10 yr	11–12 yr	13–18 yr	
Tdap	Tdap	Tdap	
	HPV (3 doses)	HPV	
MCV4	MCV4 dose 1	MCV4 dose 1	Booster at age 16 yr
Influenza (yearly)			
PCV			
HepA			
HepB			
IPV			
MMR			
Varicella			

Key:
Yellow: These shaded boxes indicate when the vaccine is recommended for all children unless a doctor says the child cannot safely receive the vaccine.
Green: These shaded boxes indicate the vaccine should be given if a child is catching up on missed vaccines.
Purple: These shaded boxes indicate the vaccine is recommended for children with certain health conditions that put them at high risk for serious diseases. Note that healthy children can get the HepA series.

Note: Tdap vaccine is a combination vaccine that is recommended at age 11 or 12 to protect against tetanus, diphtheria, and pertussis. If a child has not received any or all of the DTaP vaccine series or if the parent or guardian does not know if the child has received these shots, the child needs a single dose of Tdap when he or she is 7–10 years old. Check with the child's health care provider to find out if the child needs additional catch-up vaccines.

Recommended Immunizations for Ages 19 Years & Older						
Vaccine	19–21 yr	22–26 yr	27–49 yr	50–59 yr	60–64 yr	≥65 yr
Influenza	1 dose annually					
Td/Tdap	Get Tdap vaccine once, then Td booster vaccine every 10 yr					
Varicella	2 doses					
HPV, female	3 doses					
HPV, male	3 doses	3 doses				
Zoster					1 dose	
MMR	1 or 2 doses					
Pneumococcal (polysaccharide)	1–3 doses					1 dose
Meningococcal	1 or more doses					
HepA	2 doses					
HepB	3 doses					

Key:
Yellow: Boxes this color show that the vaccine is recommended for all adults who have not been vaccinated, unless a doctor or nurse tells the person that he or she cannot safely receive the vaccine or that he or she does not need it.
Purple: Boxes this color show when the vaccine is recommended for adults with certain risks related to their health, job, or lifestyle that put them at higher risk for serious diseases.

Vaccine abbreviation key: DTaP = Diphtheria, pertussis, and tetanus; HepA = Hepatitis A; HepB = Hepatitis B; Hib = *Haemophilus influenzae* type b; HPV = Human papillomavirus; IPV = Polio; MCV4 = Meningococcal conjugate vaccine; MMR = Measles, mumps, rubella; PCV = Pneumococcal conjugate vaccine; RV = Rotavirus; Tdap = Tetanus, diphtheria, and pertussis.

Source: Centers for Disease Control and Prevention, 2013.

Nutrition

Physiologic Basics

- The consumption of nutrients is necessary to support the physiologic activities of digestion, absorption, and metabolism, as well as to maintain homeostasis.
- Nutrients are classified into three groups:
  - **Energy nutrients:** Release energy for maintenance of homeostasis.
  - **Organic nutrients:** Build and maintain body tissues and regulate body processes.
  - **Inorganic nutrients:** Provide a medium for chemical reactions, transport materials, maintain body temperature, promote bone formation, and conduct nerve impulses.

Diet Therapy

- **Nothing by mouth (NPO):** A type of diet ordered to rest the GI tract, either prior to surgery or certain diagnostic procedures or when the source of the patient's nutritional problem is unidentified.
- **Clear-liquid diet:** Consists of liquids that have no residue, such as water, apple juice, and gelatin; dairy products are not allowed.
- **Liquid or full-liquid diet:** Consists of substances that are liquid at room temperature (e.g., ice cream, pudding).
- **Low-residue diet:** Consists of reduced fiber and cellulose; prescribed to decrease GI mucosal irritation; foods to be avoided are raw fruits (except bananas), vegetables, seeds, plant fiber, and whole grains; dairy products are limited to 2 servings per day.

- **Soft diet:** Consists of reduced fiber and cellulose, prescribed to decrease GI mucosal irritation. Foods to be avoided are raw fruits (except bananas), vegetables, seeds, plant fiber, and whole grains; dairy products are limited to 2 servings per day.
- **High-fiber diet:** Consists of foods that are high in fiber or cellulose; used to increase the forward motion of indigestible wastes through the colon.
- **Diabetic diet:** Used to control blood sugar. Consists of smaller portions spread throughout the day and a variety of whole grains, fruits, and vegetables. The timing and amount of carbohydrates to be consumed is determined by a dietitian. Foods that should be limited are foods that are high in sugar, fatty foods, salt, and alcohol.
- **Sodium-restricted diet:** Used with patients who have excess fluid volume, hypertension, heart failure, myocardial infarction, or renal failure; sodium intake may be restricted as follows:
  - **Mild:** 2000–3000 mg (2–3 g)
  - **Moderate:** 1000 mg (1 g)
  - **Strict:** 500 mg (0.5 g)

Parenteral Nutrition
- Provides nutrition through a route outside the alimentary tract.
- Solution is infused directly into the vein to meet daily nutritional needs.
- Total parenteral nutrition (TPN) consists of an IV solution containing dextrose, amino acids, fats, essential fatty acids, vitamins, and minerals.

Enteral Nutrition
- Used for patients with a functional GI tract who will not or cannot eat and therefore are at risk for malnutrition.
- Tube feedings are contraindicated in patients with:
  - Diffuse peritonitis
  - Intestinal obstruction
  - Intractable vomiting
  - Severe diarrhea
- Types of enteral feeding tubes:
  - **Large-bore nasogastric tube:** A tube that is inserted through the nostril and passed into the gastric cavity.
  - **Gastrostomy or percutaneous endoscopic gastrostomy (PEG) tube:** A tube that is inserted directly into the gastric cavity.
  - **Nasointestinal tube:** A tube that is inserted through the nose and passed into the intestines (either the duodenum or the jejunum).
  - **Jejunostomy tube:** A tube that is surgically inserted into the jejunum.
- Types of enteral formulas:
  - **Isotonic:** Contains proteins, fats, and carbohydrates with a high molecular weight and osmolarity equal to that of the body.
  - **Elemental:** Contains monosaccharides and amino acids with minimal triglycerides in hypertonic concentrations.
  - **Fluid restriction formula:** Contains a highly concentrated form of kilocalories.

Exercise

Exercise is a key element in preventing heart disease, diabetes, and some types of cancer. It can also help reduce the symptoms of certain chronic conditions, such as depression, back pain, and arthritis. Most adults should be getting 30 minutes of aerobic exercise at least 5 days a week and 20 minutes of strength training 2–3 days a week.
- **Aerobic exercise** is physical activity that increases the workload of the heart, lungs, and muscles for a sustained period of time. Aerobic exercises include activities such

as walking, running, swimming, bicycling, and aerobics classes. Benefits of aerobic exercise include increased blood flow, improved oxygen consumption, weight loss, increased energy, decreased BP, elevated mood, and blood sugar control.

- **Strength training** (a.k.a. weight training) is a form of exercise that increases muscle mass. Strength training can be done using a weight bench, hand weights, exercises (e.g., push-ups), or exercise machines. Benefits of strength training include pain relief (e.g., from arthritis and back pain), improved balance, bone strengthening, weight loss, elevated mood, and blood sugar control.

Pain Management

Pain Scales

Visual Analog Scale
Ask the patient to put a mark, such as an X, on the scale to show his or her current level of pain.

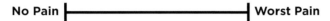

No Pain |—————————————————| Worst Pain

Numerical Scale
Ask the patient to rate his or her pain from 0 (indicating no pain) to 10 (indicating the worst pain possible). The patient may either say the number or circle the number on the scale.

No Pain   0 1 2 3 4 5 6 7 8 9 10   Worst Pain

Faces Scale
This scale may be helpful to a child or an adult with language barriers. Ask the patient to choose the face that best shows the severity of his or her own pain on a scale of 0–10.

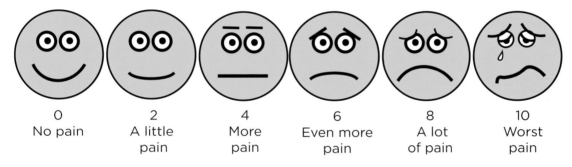

| 0 | 2 | 4 | 6 | 8 | 10 |
| No pain | A little pain | More pain | Even more pain | A lot of pain | Worst pain |

Pain Medications
Pain medications should be given as prescribed. Pain medication is more effective if given before pain becomes severe. When medications are prescribed as needed (PRN), it is important to assess the patient's pain at regular intervals to see if pain medication is needed.

Acute vs. Chronic Pain		
Pain Type	**Physiologic Evidence**	**Behavioral Evidence**
Acute	Increased respirations, increased pulse, increased BP, dilated pupils, diaphoresis	Restlessness, distraction, worry, distress
Chronic	Normal respirations, pulse, BP, pupil size; no diaphoresis	Reduced or no physical activity, depression or despair, feelings of hopelessness

Medication Administration Routes

- **Oral:** Capsule, tablet, or liquid; absorbed in GI tract
- **Intravenous (IV):** Injection into bloodstream via vein
- **Intradermal:** Injection into the dermal layer of the skin
- **Intramuscular (IM):** Injection into muscle; can use large doses; fast systemic action
- **Intrathecal:** Injection into spinal canal; affects spinal fluid
- **Subcutaneous (subcut):** Injection into tissue below dermis
- **Sublingual:** Absorbed under the tongue
- **Rectal or vaginal:** Suppositories or creams; usually for local distribution
- **Inhalation:** Absorbed in lungs; gaseous form; rapid absorption

Considerations across the Life Span

Pregnant or Breast-Feeding Women
- Renal excretion rate and hepatic metabolism are accelerated; consider higher doses.
- Intestinal excretion rate is decreased, which leads to a longer absorption time; consider lower doses.
- Assume that all drugs can enter the fetus via the placenta.
- Consult U.S. Food and Drug Administration risk categories for every drug before administration.
- Gestation weeks 3–8 present the greatest risk of drug-induced malformation of the fetus.
- After delivery, doses should be taken directly after breast-feeding to ensure minimal drug concentration in the breast milk for the next feeding.

Pediatric Patients
- Assume increased drug sensitivity because of immature organ system.
- Infants have irregular gastric patterns; absorption rates may vary.
- Infants and young children have thin skin, which may lead to rapid topical drug absorption.
- An infant's blood-brain barrier is not fully developed, which may lead to increased sensitivity to central nervous system (CNS) drugs and risk of toxicity.
- Neonates absorb IM drugs slower than adults; infants absorb IM drugs faster.
- Infants have reduced protein-binding ability, which can lead to high free concentrations of drugs.
- The liver and kidneys are not fully developed until after 1 year of age; assume reduced hepatic and renal metabolism in infants.
- In children older than 1 year of age, drug metabolism rate is higher than that of adults.
- Children may have unique side effects from certain drugs, including suppressed growth.

Geriatric Patients
- Assume increased drug sensitivity because of deterioration of organ systems.
- Reactions vary greatly based on the individual patient's condition.
- Rate of absorption is generally slowed, which could lead to a delayed therapeutic response.
- Hepatic metabolism rate is likely slowed, which could lead to an extended therapeutic response.
- Renal excretion is likely slowed, which could lead to an accumulation of the drug in the body and increased risk of adverse effects.

- Determine creatinine clearance prior to drug administration to assess renal function.
- Intentional failure to follow prescribed regimen is a common problem; longer or more extensive patient education may be required.
- Polypharmacy can be an issue with elderly patients; anticipate, assess, and manage drug interactions carefully.

Medication Dosage Calculations

Formulas

Amount to Administer

$$\frac{\text{Dose Ordered}}{\text{Dose on Hand}} = \text{Amount to Administer}$$

Solution Concentration

$$\frac{\text{Dosage in Solution}}{\text{Volume of Solution}} = \text{Solution Concentration}$$

IV Dose Rate Calculation

$$\frac{\text{Dose Ordered}}{\text{Solution Concentration}} = \text{Volume/hour}$$

Oral Medications: Liquids

Use the following formula to calculate dosage for liquids: (Desired/Have) × Quantity = Liquid Dosage

---

Example

Order: amoxicillin 500 mg orally (PO) daily; available: amoxicillin oral suspension 200 mg/5 mL

Use $(D/H) \times Q$:

$(500/200) \times 5 = 2.5 \times 5 = 12.5$ mL

Oral Medications: Tablets & Capsules

There are two types of capsules:
- A capsule with a hard, two-piece gelatin shell that may, in some cases, be opened to release powder or pellets (to be combined with soft food)
- A capsule with a soft gelatin shell

Capsules should never be split, crushed, or altered; scored tablets may be split, but unscored tablets should never be split, crushed, or altered. Use the following formula to find dosage for tablets and capsules:

(Desired/Have) × Quantity = Tablet or Capsule Dosage

Example

Order: ibuprofen 1000 mg PO daily; available: ibuprofen 200 mg tablets

Use $(D/H) \times Q$:

$(1000/200) \times 1 = 5 \times 1 = 5$ tablets

Parenteral Medications (IV, IM & Subcut)

Note: For amounts less than 1 mL, round to the nearest hundredth; for amounts greater than 1 mL, round to the nearest tenth.

Use the following formula to calculate dosage for liquids:

(Desired/Have) × Quantity = Liquid Dosage

Example

Order: oxacillin sodium (Bactocill) 300 mg IM every 8 hours; available: oxacillin sodium (Bactocill) 1 g/3 mL

First, make any necessary conversions: 1 g = 1000 mg

Then use $(D/H) × Q$: (300/1000) × 3 = 0.3 × 3 = 0.9 mL

Because the answer is less than 1 mL, round to the nearest hundredth: 0.90 mL

IV Flow Rate

$$\frac{\text{Volume (mL)} \times \text{Drop Factor (gtt/mL)}}{\text{Time (min)}} = \text{Flow Rate (gtt/min)}$$

Example

Order: nicardipine 10 mg in 25 mL over 1 hour; drop factor = 15

First, convert hours to minutes: 1 hour = 60 minutes

Then calculate rate: $\dfrac{25 \text{ mL} \times 15}{60} = \dfrac{375}{60} = 6.25$

Round to the nearest whole number: 6 gtt/min

Age- & Weight-Adjusted Dosages

Often, doses are adjusted based on weight, especially for pediatric and geriatric patients.

Geriatric Example

An 82-year-old man weighs 174 pounds and is ordered amikacin sulfate. The ordered dose is 7.5 mg/kg IM twice daily (BID); the available dose is amikacin sulfate 250 mg/mL.

Convert weight to kilograms: 2.2 lb = 1 kg, so 174 lb = 79.0909... kg, or 79.1 kg

To find the dose, multiply 7.5 mg/kg by 79.1 kg: 7.5 × 79.1 = 593.3 mg

Then use $(D/H) × Q$:

(593.3/250) × 1 = 2.373 × 1 = 2.4 mL

Pediatric Example

A 14-month-old child weighs 25 pounds and is ordered oxacillin sodium. The ordered dose is 50 mg/kg every 6 hours; available dose is 250 mg/5 mL.

Convert weight to kilograms: 2.2 lb = 1 kg, so 25 lb = 11.3636... kg, or 11.4 kg

To find the dose, multiply 50 mg/kg by 11.4 kg: 50 × 11.4 = 570 mg

Then use $(D/H) × Q$:

(570/250) × 5 = 2.28 × 5 = 11.4 mL every 6 hours

Laboratory Values & Blood Transfusions

Complete Blood Count (CBC) & Differential

CBC Component	Adult	
	Male	Female
RBCs	$4.7–6 \times 10^6$/mcL	$4.2–5.4 \times 10^6$/mcL
Hematocrit (Hct)	42%–52%	37%–47%
Hemoglobin (Hgb)	13.5–18 g/dL	12–16 g/dL
RBC indices		
Mean corpuscular volume (MCV)	78–100 fL	
Mean corpuscular Hgb (MCH)	27–31 pg	
Mean corpuscular Hgb conc. (MCHC)	33–37 g/dL	
WBCs	4K–10.5K/mcL	
Differential WBCs		
Neutrophils	1.5K–6.6K/mcL	
Bands	<1K/mcL	
Eosinophils	<0.7K/mcL	
Basophils	<0.1K/mcL	
Monocytes	<1K/mcL	
Lymphocytes	1.5K–3.5K/mcL	
T lymphocytes	60%–80% of lymphocytes	
B lymphocytes	4%–16% of lymphocytes	
Platelets	150K–300K/mcL	

Lipid Profile

Total cholesterol	<200 mg/dL
High-density lipoprotein	40–60 mg/dL
Low-density lipoprotein	<130 mg/dL
Triglycerides	<150 mg/dL

Comprehensive Metabolic Panel

	Normal Adult Range*	Conditions with Abnormal Findings	
		Increased	Decreased
Blood urea nitrogen (BUN)	6–20 mg/dL	Congestive heart failure (CHF), excessive protein in the GI tract, GI bleeding, heart attack, hypovolemia, kidney disease, kidney failure, shock, urinary tract obstruction	Liver failure, low protein diet, malnutrition, overhydration
Sodium (Na)	135–145 mEq/L	CHF, dehydration, diabetes, diaphoresis, diarrhea, hypertension, ostomies, toxemia, vomiting	Ascites in cardiac failure, bowel obstruction, burns, diarrhea, cirrhosis, emphysema, GI malabsorption
Potassium (K)	3.7–5.2 mEq/L	Acidosis, adrenocortical insufficiency, anemia, anxiety, asthma, burns, dialysis, dysrhythmias, hypoventilation	Alcoholism, alkalosis, bradycardia, CHF, chronic cirrhosis, colon cancer, Crohn disease, diarrhea, diuretics, GI suction, intestinal fistulas, vomiting
Glucose	70–100 mg/dL (fasting)	Prediabetes, diabetes, hyperthyroidism, pancreatic cancer, pancreatitis	Hyperinsulinism, hypopituitarism, hypothyroidism, insulin overdose, malnutrition, transient hypoglycemia
Creatinine	0.6–1.3 mg/dL	ATN, CHF, dehydration, diabetic nephropathy, glomerulonephritis, kidney failure, muscular dystrophy, preeclampsia, pyelonephritis, rhabdomyolysis, shock, urinary tract obstruction	Muscular dystrophy (late stage), myasthenia gravis
Calcium (Ca)	8.5–10.2 mg/dL	ATN, bacteremia, chronic hepatic disease, respiratory acidosis	Alkalosis, burns, cachexia, celiac disease, chronic renal disease, diarrhea, GI malabsorption
Albumin	3.4–5.4 g/dL	Dehydration	Kidney disease, liver disease
Total bilirubin	0.3–1.9 mg/dL	Biliary stricture, cirrhosis, gallstones, Gilbert disease, hepatitis, pancreatic or gallbladder cancer	N/A

Comprehensive Metabolic Panel (*continued*)

	Normal Adult Range*	Conditions with Abnormal Findings	
		Increased	**Decreased**
Aspartate transaminase/ serum glutamic-oxaloacetic transaminase (AST/ SGOT)	10–34 U/L	Acute pancreatitis, cirrhosis, heart attack, hepatitis, kidney failure, liver cancer, mononucleosis	N/A
Alanine aminotransaminase/ serum glutamic-pyruvic transaminase (ALT/ SGPT)	7–56 U/L	Acute pancreatitis, cirrhosis, heart attack, hepatitis, liver cancer, mononucleosis	N/A
Alkaline phosphatase	44–147 U/L	Biliary obstruction, bone cancer, cirrhosis, hepatitis, hyperparathyroidism, Paget disease, leukemia, lymphoma	Malnutrition, protein deficiency, Wilson disease

* Ranges may vary by lab.

Blood Transfusion Reactions

Reaction & Causes	Signs & Symptoms
Transfusion-related lung injury • Antibodies activate granulocytes, causing leakage into lungs	Tachypnea, dyspnea, hypotension, cyanosis, chills, fever, tachycardia
Plasma protein incompatibility • Immunoglobulin A incompatibility	Diarrhea, abdominal pain, dyspnea, fever, chills, flushing, hypotension
Hemolytic • Blood stored improperly • Cross-matching done improperly • Intradonor incompatibility • RH or ABO incompatibility	Dyspnea, flushed face, fever, chest pain, shaking, chills, hypotension, flank pain, oliguria, hemoglobinuria, bloody oozing at surgical incision or infusion site, burning feeling along vein getting blood, shock, renal failure
Febrile • Bacterial lipopolysaccharides • Antileukocyte recipient antibodies directed against donor WBCs	Fever, headache, chills, flushed face, cough, palpitations, increased pulse rate, chest tightness, flank pain
Bacterial contamination • Organisms that can survive cold temperatures (e.g., *Staphylococcus* and *Pseudomonas*)	Fever, chills, abdominal cramping, vomiting, diarrhea, shock, renal failure
Allergic • Donor blood has allergen • Donor blood hypersensitive to certain drugs	Anaphylaxis, nausea, vomiting, fever

Documentation

Documentation is written evidence of:
- The interaction between and among health professionals, patients, families, and health care organizations
- The administration of tests, procedures, treatments, and patient education
- The patient's response to diagnostic tests, procedures, treatments, and interventions

Systematic documentation is critical because it presents the care administered by nurses in a logical manner, as follows:
- Assessment data identify the patient's specific condition or alterations and provide the foundation of the nursing care plan.
- Risk factors and the identified alteration in health patterns direct the formation of the nursing diagnosis and nursing care priorities.
- Identifying the nursing diagnosis promotes the development of the patient's goals (short term and long term) and expected outcomes and triggers the creation of nursing actions or interventions.
- The plan of care identifies the actions necessary to resolve the nursing diagnosis.
- Implementation, or the act of "nursing," is evidenced by actions the nurse performs to assist the patient in achieving the expected outcomes.

Documentation requirements differ depending on the health care facility:
- All nursing documentation must reflect the nursing process, the individualized context of the patient, and the nursing situation.
- Nursing documentation must be logical, focused, and relevant to care and must represent each phase of the nursing process.

> From a legal perspective, if it is not documented, it was not done.

General Documentation Guidelines
- Make sure you have the correct patient record or chart and that the patient's name and identifying information are on every page of the record.
- Document as soon as the patient encounter is concluded to ensure accurate recall of data.
- Date and time each entry accurately.
- Sign each entry with your full legal name and professional credentials.
- Do not leave space between entries.
- If an error is made, use a single line to cross out the error; then date, time, and sign the correction; do not erase or use correction fluid.
- Do not change another person's entry, even if it is incorrect.
- Use quotation marks to indicate direct patient responses.
- Document in chronological order.
- Write legibly.
- Use pens with permanent black ink.
- Document in a complete but concise manner by using phrases and abbreviations (as appropriate).
- Document all telephone calls made or received by you that are related to a patient's care.
- Avoid judgmental language (e.g., "good," "bad," "normal," "abnormal," "appears to be").
- Avoid evaluative statements (e.g., "Patient is uncooperative," "Patient is lazy"); instead, cite specific behaviors or actions that you observed (e.g., "Patient said, 'I hate this place,' and kicked the trash can").
- State time intervals precisely (e.g., "every 3 hours" instead of "occasionally").
- Do not make relative statements (e.g., "a mass the size of an egg"); instead, be specific (e.g., "3 cm × 5 cm mass").

- Draw pictures when appropriate (e.g., location of scars, bruises, skin lesions).
- Refer to findings by using anatomical landmarks, such as LUQ (left upper quadrant).

Methods of Documentation

- **Narrative charting** is done in a story format that describes the patient's status, interventions, and treatment, as well as the patient's response to treatment.
- **SOAP** is a structured method of narrative charting. SOAP stands for:
  - **S**ubjective data (what the patient says)
  - **O**bjective data (assessment findings, such as vital signs and laboratory results)
  - **A**ssessment and analysis (the conclusion reached on the basis of the data collected)
  - **P**lan (actions to be taken to change the status of the patient's problem)
- **PIE** is also a structured method of narrative charting. PIE stands for:
  - **P**roblem
  - **I**ntervention
  - **E**valuation
- **Charting by exception (CBE)** is a method of charting that requires the nurse to document only deviations from preestablished norms.

Contributors

Julie Henry, RN, MPA, is a freelance writer, editor, and project manager who specializes in medical writing. She has written multiple books, articles, and other resources for a number of national health care organizations, including The Joint Commission, the American Academy of Family Physicians, Elsevier, and the Society of Teachers of Family Medicine. Ms. Henry has written extensively in the areas of nursing, patient safety, risk management, accreditation compliance, clinical privileging and credentialing, practice management, medication management, infection prevention and control, transitions of care, cancer, and heart disease. She earned a bachelor of science in nursing from Rockhurst University's Research College of Nursing and a master of public administration degree from the University of Missouri–Kansas City.

Mark D. Jackson, PhD, is a scientist and retired university professor. From 1986 to 2007, he taught chemistry at Florida Atlantic University, where his course offerings ranged from distance learning for nonscience majors to physical and inorganic chemistry for undergraduate chemistry majors and thermodynamics for graduate students. Dr. Jackson specializes in theoretical chemistry, quantum mechanics, and spectroscopy. He is currently an adjunct professor at Lynn University, where he teaches science literacy courses in the Dialogues of Learning core curriculum. In addition, he develops materials for online courses and nontraditional chemistry classes. Dr. Jackson's bachelor's degree in chemistry is from the University of Texas at Arlington; his master's and doctoral degrees (in physics and chemical physics, respectively) are from Harvard University.

Additional Contributors

Cristi Bundukamara, EdD, ARNP
Associate, Senior Professor, School of Nursing, Miami Dade College

Donna C. Maheady, EdD, ARNP
Associate Graduate Faculty, Christine E. Lynn College of Nursing, Florida Atlantic University
Founder of www.ExceptionalNurse.com

Jill E. Winland-Brown, EdD, FNP-BC, DPNAP
Professor, Christine E. Lynn College of Nursing, Florida Atlantic University

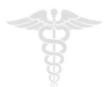

A

Abbreviations, 200–206
  on agencies and organizations, 205
  on blood system, 216
  on cardiovascular system, 213–214
  on diagnostic testing, 202
  "Do Not Use" List of, 200
  on drug therapy, 201–202
  on ears, 221–222
  on endocrine system, 217
  on eyes, 222
  on gastrointestinal system, 215
  on genitourinary system, 210–211, 212
  on health assessment, 203
  on integumentary system, 218
  on laboratory testing, 113, 202
  on locations and directions, 203–204
  on lymphatic and immune systems, 223
  on managed care, 205–206
  on muscular system, 220–221
  on nervous system, 209
  on professional designations, 204–205
  on respiratory system, 219–220
  on skeletal system, 207–208
  on specialized areas and facilities, 205
  on weights and measurements, 110, 111, 112, 113, 200–201
Abdomen
  examination of, 20, 38–39, 259
  as subcutaneous injection site, 150
Abdominal pad, 62
Abducens nerve, 43, 261
Absorbable sutures, 62–63
Absorbed dose of radiation, 94
Absorption of drugs, 120, 122, 158
Absorptive dressings, 61
Accessory muscles of respiration, 28
Accountability, 4, 10
Acetaminophen, 137
Acetone, 101
Acetyl-coenzyme A, 102
Ace wrap, 61
Acids, 85, 95–96
Acoustic stethoscope, 15
Activation energy, 88
Activity in APGAR score, 166, 264

Acute pain, 48, 273
Addison disease, 34
Addition process, 236
  with decimals, 245–246
  with fractions, 242
  with positive and negative numbers, 240
Additive effect in drug interactions, 122
Additives in blood specimen collection, 60
Adenosine triphosphate (ATP), 103
Adhesions, postoperative, 180
Adhesive bandages, 62
Adjusted body weight, 145
Adolescence, growth and development in, 162–163, 264
α-Adrenergic antagonists, 124
β-Adrenergic antagonists, 124
Adventitious breath sounds, 30
Advocacy for patients, 11
Aerobic exercise, 272–273
Afterload, 24
Agency nursing, 226–227
Age-related changes
  in drug therapy, 121–122, 158, 274–275
    dosage calculations in, 146, 147–148, 276
  in growth and development, 162–163, 264–265
  in vital signs, 17
Airborne precautions, 7, 269
Air-entrainment masks, 74
Airway tubes, 31
Alanine aminotransaminase serum levels, 157, 279
Albinism, 34
Albumin
  in blood products, 70
  serum levels of, 156, 278
Albuterol, 128
Alcohols, 85, 99–100
Aldehydes, 85, 101
Aliphatic hydrocarbons, 97
Alkali, 96
Alkali metals, 83, 96
Alkaline earth metals, 83, 96
Alkaline phosphatase serum levels, 157, 279
Alkanes, 85, 98

Alkenes, 85, 98
Alkyl halides, 98
Alkynes, 98
Allergic reactions
  antihistamines in, 135
  in blood transfusions, 71, 279
Alpha-adrenergic antagonists, 124
Alpha particles, 93
Alprazolam, 128
Ambu bag, 74
American Nurses Association Code of Ethics for Nurses, 5
Amides, 85, 104
Amines, 85, 103
Amino acids, 104, 105
Aminoglycoside antibiotics, 138, 168
Amphiprotic materials, 95
Amylose, 104
Analysis in nursing process, 14, 49, 120, 258
Anaphylactic shock, 76
Aneroid manometers, 55–56
Anesthesia, 100, 152, 174–175
Aneurysm of abdominal aorta, 38
Angiogenesis, 233
Angiotensin-converting enzyme inhibitors, 131
Anions, 83
Antagonistic effect in drug interactions, 122
Antianxiety drugs, 128, 168
Antiarrhythmic drugs, 129, 168
Antibiotics, 138–140, 158, 168
Anticholinergics, 122–123, 168, 171
Anticoagulants, 130, 158, 168
Anticonvulsants, 127, 168
Antidepressants, 124–125
Antidiarrheals, 134
Antiemetics, 135, 171
Antihistamines, 135
Antihypertensive drugs, 130–131, 168
Anti-inflammatory drugs, nonsteroidal, 136–137, 168
Antineoplastic agents, 141
Antiparkinsonian drugs, 127
Antipsychotic drugs, 125–126
Antiseptic dressings, 62
Antiulcer drugs, 133–134, 168, 171
Aortic aneurysm, abdominal, 38
Aortic valve sounds, 21, 22

INDEX

APGAR score, 166, 264
Apnea, 28
Apothecary measurement system, 112–113
Application icons, 80
Area measurements, 110
Arm, as subcutaneous injection site, 149
Aromatic hydrocarbons, 97, 98
Arrhenius acid and base, 95
Arrhythmias
  cardioversion in, 74
  defibrillation in, 74–75
  drug therapy in, 129, 168
Arteries
  blood gas analysis, 31, 154
  blood pressure, mean, 26
  blood specimens from, 60–61
  catheterization, 152
  pulse palpation, 27–28
Ascites, abdominal examination in, 38
Aseptic technique, 54
Aspartate transaminase serum levels, 157, 279
Aspirin, 136
Assessment, 14–50, 258–262
  abbreviations in, 203
  analysis and documentation of, 49–50
  of cardiovascular system, 20–28, 260
  conclusion of examination in, 49
  in drug therapy, 120
  of gastrointestinal system, 38–40, 177, 260
  general examination in, 17–20, 259
  of genitourinary system, 40–41, 260–261
  of integumentary system, 32–37, 260
  interview and history-taking in, 16
  of musculoskeletal system, 41–42, 261
  of nervous system, 42–45, 177, 261–262
  of newborn, 17, 166, 264
  of pain, 48, 273
  of peripheral vascular system, 27–28
  postoperative, 176–178

  postpartum, 166
  preoperative, 169–170, 171
  preparation for, 16–17
  psychosocial, 46–48, 262
  of respiratory system, 28–32, 260
    in newborn, 17, 166, 264
    postoperative, 176
  techniques in, 14–15, 258–259
Atelectasis, postoperative, 180–181
Atomic mass, 82–83, 86
Atomic number, 82
Atomic weight, 83
Atoms, 82–83
  bonded, 83–84
Atrial gallop, 22
Atropine, 122
Attributable risk, 115
Auriscope, 19
Auscultation, 15, 259
  in cardiovascular assessment, 21–22
  in gastrointestinal assessment, 38
  in peripheral vascular assessment, 27
  in respiratory assessment, 29–31
Autocratic leaders, 9
Automated external defibrillators, 74
Automatic internal cardiac defibrillators, 74
Autonomy, 4, 266
  in psychosocial development, 163, 265
Avogadro's law, 89
Avogadro's number, 81, 82, 87
Axillary temperature, 55

B

B lymphocytes, 155, 277
Back, assessment of, 19, 259
Background radiation, 93
Bacterial contamination of blood products, 71, 279
Bag-valve-mask, 74
Balance, Romberg test of, 44
Balanced equations, 86
Bandages, 62
Barometers, 88
Barrel chest, 28
Basal thermometer, 55
Bases, 85, 95–96
Basophils, 155, 277
Beneficence principle, 267

Beta-adrenergic antagonists, 124
Beta particles, 93
Bicarbonate serum levels, 31
Bilirubin serum levels, 157, 278
Biochemistry, 104–106
Biomarkers in myocardial infarction, 26
Biot respiration, 29
Birth weight of infants, low, 165, 262
Bladder
  decubitus ulcer risk in incontinence of, 37
  palpation of, 41
Bleeding
  exudates in, 63
  vaginal, in pregnancy, 165, 263
Bleeding time test, 154
Blisters, 34
Blood culture, 154
Blood flow rate, 26
Blood gas analysis, arterial, 31, 154
Blood groups, 215
  incompatibility of, 71, 279
Blood pressure, 55–56, 88, 212
  in hypertension, 20, 130–131, 165, 263
  mean arterial, 26
  in newborn, 17, 166, 264
  normal range for, 17, 20
  systolic and diastolic, 20, 88
Blood specimen collection, 57–61
Blood system, terminology and abbreviations related to, 215–216
Blood transfusions, 69–71, 279
Blood vessels, 212
  formation of, 233
Body mass index, 145–146
Body surface area
  in burns, 117
  in drug therapy, 122, 145, 146
Boiling point, 89
Boltzmann constant, 82
Bonds, 83–84
  hydrogen, 90
  peptide, 105
Bones
  pain in, 42, 261
  terminology and abbreviations related to, 206–208
Bowel obstruction, 38, 181
Bowel sounds, 38

Boyle's law, 89
Brachial artery pulse, 27
Bradypnea, 28
Brand name of drugs, 121
Breast, 211
    examination of, 40
    postpartum, 166, 262
Breast-feeding, drug therapy during,
    121, 274
Breathing. *See* Respiration
Bronchial breath sounds, 29
Bronchodilators, 128–129, 158
Bronchovesicular breath sounds, 29
Brønsted-Lowry acid and base, 95
Bruit
    carotid artery, 21
    femoral artery, 27
Buffers, 95
Bulb drains, 63
Bulla, 34
Burns, 117
Butterfly catheter, 152
Butterfly needles, 60
Butterfly stitches, 63

C

Calcium serum levels, 156, 278
Cancer
    cytotoxic agents in, 141
    screening for, 269
    warning signs of, 35
Capillary refill test, 33
Capsule dosage, 147, 275
Captopril, 131
Carbohydrates, 104
Carbon, 85, 97
Carbon-chain prefixes, 97
Carbon dioxide, 89
    partial arterial pressure, 31
Carboxylic acid, 85, 101–103
Cardiac output, 24
Cardiogenic shock, 76
Cardiovascular system
    assessment of, 20–28, 260
    circulatory care techniques and
        equipment, 74–75
    drugs affecting, 129–131
    function of, 20
    immobility affecting, 42
    nutritional disorders affecting, 39
    peripheral, 27–28, 152
    terminology and abbreviations
        related to, 212–214

Cardioversion, 74
Careers in nursing, 226–228
Caring leaders, 9
Caring relationship with patients, 5,
    16
Carotenemia, 34
Carotid arteries, 21
Case management method of nursing
    care delivery, 8, 266
Case method of nursing care delivery,
    7, 266
Catalysts, 88
Catheters, 152–153
    intravenous, 68–69, 152
    suction, 32
    urinary, 71–72
Cations, 83
Cavities, body, 206
Cefadroxil, 138
Cells, 206
    in nervous system, 208
Cellular respiration, 87
Celsius scale, 54, 80, 81, 82
    conversion to Fahrenheit scale, 54,
        82, 112, 146
Centers for Disease Control and
    Prevention, recommendations on
    infection control and prevention,
    6–7, 268–269
Central nervous system, 42, 177, 208
Central venous catheterization, 152
Cephalosporins, 138–139
Cerebrospinal fluid culture, 154
Certified registered nurse anesthetist,
    174
Chargaff's rule, 105
Charles' law, 89
Charting
    by exception, 50, 281
    narrative, 50, 281
Chemical formulas, 83
Chemical name of drugs, 121
Chemical reactions, 80, 86–87
    acid-base, 96
    of hydrocarbons, 98–99
    rate of, 88
Chemistry, nursing, 79–106
    acids and bases in, 95–96
    alcohols in, 99–100
    aldehydes and ketones in, 101
    amines and amides in, 103–104

atomic structure and periodic table
    in, 82–83
biochemistry in, 104–106
carboxylic acids and derivatives in,
    101–103
compounds in, 83–85
constants in, 82
energy and kinetics in, 87–88
ethers in, 100
measurements in, 80–82
organic, 96–99
radioactivity in, 93–95
reactions in, 86–87
solutions and mixtures in, 90–93
states of matter in, 88–90
thiols in, 100–101
Chest examination, 19–20, 259
    in cardiovascular assessment, 21
    in respiratory assessment, 28,
        29–30
Chest wall deformities, 28
Cheyne-Stokes respiration, 29
Chickenpox, 163, 265
Children, 162–164, 264–266
    age classification of, 162, 266
    coding measurements in, 116
    common diseases of, 163, 265
    drug therapy in, 121–122, 274
        dosage calculations for, 146,
            148, 276
    growth and development of,
        162–163, 264–265
        expected rate of, 162, 266
        milestones in, 162, 266
    immunizations in, 164, 270
    vital signs in, 17
Chloasma, 34
Chlorpromazine, 126
Cholesterol, 157, 277
Chronic pain, 48, 273
Cimetidine, 133, 168
Circulating nurse, 173
Circulation, 212
    assessment of, 27, 176
    nursing care techniques and
        equipment for, 74–75
    postoperative, 176–177
Clark's rule, 146
Clean-catch urine specimens, 57
Clean-contaminated surgery, 168
Cleansers for skin care, 61

INDEX

Clean surgery, 168
Clean technique, 54
Clear-liquid diet, 64, 271
Closed-drainage systems, 63
   urine specimen collection in, 57
Clozapine, 125
Coaching skills of leaders, 10
Coagulation, 215
   and anticoagulant drugs, 130, 158,
      168
   laboratory tests of, 154
Code of Ethics for Nurses of ANA, 5
Coding measurements, 116–117
Coenzyme A, 102
Collaboration, 9
Collagen deposition in wound
     healing, 233
Colloid solutions, 91
Color
   of blood collection tube additives,
     60
   prefixes on, 188
   of skin, 33, 34
   of urine, 41
   of wounds, 64
Colorectal cancer screening, 269
Coma, 45
   Glasgow Coma Scale in, 44–45
Comfort measures, postoperative,
   178
Communication
   in collaborative relationships, 9
   in delegation of tasks, 10
   error prevention in, 267–268
   in mentoring, 11
   patient-nurse, confidentiality of,
     5, 267
   SOLER system for, 170
   in surgical nursing, 175–176
   in team approach to nursing care
     delivery, 8
Community environment assessment,
   46
Competencies of leaders, 10
Complete blood count, 154, 155,
   170, 277
Compounds, 80, 83–85
Compression bandages, 62
Compression stockings, 75
Concentration of solutions, 81, 91
   formula on, 144, 275
Condensation, 89

Conduction system, cardiac, 212
Confidentiality, 5, 267
Confusion, 45
   drugs causing, 158
Congruence valued by leaders, 10
Conjugate acid-base pairs, 95
Conjunctiva, examination of, 18
Consciousness, level of
   decubitus ulcer risk in disorders
     of, 37
   Glasgow Coma Scale on, 44–45
Consent, informed, 170, 267
Constants, 82
   equilibrium, 86
   gas, 82, 89
   rate, 88
Contact precautions, 6, 269
Contamination
   of blood products, 71, 279
   in surgery, 168
Contraceptives, oral, 140–141
Contractility, cardiac, 25
Contraction in wound healing, 233
Controlled substances, 123
Convergence of eyes, 18
Conversion factor, 81
Coordination, testing of, 44
Corticosteroids, 128, 136, 168
Cosmetic surgery, 167
Covalent bonds, 83–84
Crackles, 30, 31
Cranial nerves, 43, 261–262
Creatine phosphokinase/creatine
     kinase myocardial specific
     (CPK/CK-MB2), 26
Creatinine serum levels, 156, 278
Crenation, 92
Critical thinking, 9
Croup, 163, 265
Crusts, skin, 35
Cryoprecipitate, 70
Cultures, 154
Curative surgical procedures, 167
Curie, 94
Cyanosis, 28, 34
Cyclophosphamide, 141
Cysteine, 101
Cytolysis, 92
Cytotoxic agents, 141

D

Dalton's law, 89
Data, scientific, 80

Debriefing, postoperative, 175–176
Decimals, 245–248
   converted to fractions, 248
   converted to percentages, 248
   fractions converted to, 244
   percentages converted to, 249
   rounding of, 245
Decision making
   advocacy for patient in, 11
   in collaborative relationships, 9
   in delegation of tasks, 10
   in ethical issues, 4–5, 267
   in evidence-based practice, 8
   informed consent in, 170, 267
Decomposition, 86
Decubitus ulcers, 35–37
Deep palpation, 14, 39, 258
Defibrillation, 74–75
Dehydration, 86, 91, 99, 100, 104
Delegation, 10
Delirium, 46–48
Dementia, 46–48
Democratic leaders, 9
Denominator, 241
Density measurements, 81
Deoxyribonucleic acid (DNA), 96,
   105
Depression, 46–48
   drug therapy in, 124–125
Despair feelings in psychosocial
     development, 163, 265
Diabetes mellitus
   diet in, 65, 272
   gestational, 165, 263
   insulin therapy in, 131–132, 150
   oral antidiabetic agents in,
     132–133
Diagnosis, nursing, 14, 258
   documentation of, 49
   in drug therapy, 120
Diagnostic procedures, 167, 188
Dialysis, 92
Diaphragm movement in breathing,
   28
Diarrhea, drug therapy in, 134
Diastole, 20
Diastolic blood pressure, 20
Diethyl ether, 100
Diet therapies, 64–65, 271–272
Digital thermometers, 55
Digoxin, 129

Dilution of solutions, 91, 93
Dipeptide, 105
Diphenhydramine, 135
Dipolar molecules, 84, 90
Dipole-dipole interactions, 90
Dipole moment, 84
Directional terms, 187–188
  abbreviations related to, 203–204
Disorientation, 45
Dissociation reactions, 102, 103
Distribution of drugs, 120, 158
Distributive property, 240
Diuretics, 130–131, 168
Division process, 239
  with decimals, 247–248
  with fractions, 243–244
  with positive and negative
    numbers, 240
DNA, 96, 105
Documentation, 280–281
  general guidelines on, 49–50,
    280–281
  methods of, 50, 281
  review of, in preparation for
    assessment, 16
Dorsalis pedis artery pulse, 28
Dosage
  in drug therapy, 144–148, 275–276
  in radiation exposure, 94
Drains, 63
Dressings, 61–62
Droplet precautions, 6–7, 269
Drug therapy, 120–141
  abbreviations used in, 201–202
  administration of, 144–151, 274
  adverse reactions to, 122
  controlled substances in, 123
  dosage calculations in, 144–148,
    275–276
  drug interactions in, 122
  education of patients on, 121
  error prevention in, 267
  life span considerations in,
    121–122, 158, 274–275
    in dosage calculations, 146,
      147–148, 276
  nursing process in, 120
  in pain, 137–138, 273
  potentially dangerous drugs in, 158
  preoperative, 171

rights of patients in, 144, 267
surgical complications related to,
  168–169
Ducts in male reproductive system,
  209
Dullness of percussion sound, 15, 38,
  258, 259
DuoDERM, 62

E

Ears
  examination of, 19
  terminology and abbreviations
    related to, 221–222
Eclampsia, 165, 263
Ectopic pregnancy, 165, 263
Edema, peripheral vascular, 27, 75
Education of patients
  on drug therapy, 121
  for informed consent, 170, 267
  preoperative, 170–171
Ego integrity in psychosocial
  development, 163, 265
Elastoplast, 62
Elderly
  drug therapy in, 122, 274–275
    confusion from, 158
    dosage calculation in, 147, 276
    pharmacokinetics in, 158
  vital signs in, 17
Elective surgery, 167
Electrocardiography, 23–24, 25, 75,
  170
Electrolytes, 91–92, 178
Electronegativity, 84
Electronic manometers, 56
Electronic stethoscope, 15
Electrons, 82
  bonding, 83–84
Elemental enteral formulas, 272
Elementary charge of electrons, 82
Elements, 80, 82–83
  periodic table of, 83, 254
Elimination of drugs, 120, 158
Embolism, pulmonary, 182
Embryonic period, 165, 262
Emergency surgery, 167
Employment in nursing, 226–228
Empowerment skills of leaders, 10
Emulsions, 91

Endocrine system
  drugs affecting, 131–133, 140–141
  terminology and abbreviations
    related to, 216–217
Endogenic processes, 87
Endothermic processes, 87
Endotracheal intubation, 31–32
Energy
  in chemical processes, 87–88
  nutrients providing, 64, 271
English measurement system, 80
Enteral nutrition, 65–68, 272
Enthalpy, 87
Entropy, 87
Enzymes, 88, 105
  as biomarkers in myocardial
    infarction, 26
Eosinophils, 155, 277
Epicardial pacing, 75
Epidural anesthesia, 152, 175
Equations, chemical, 86
Equilibrium, 86
Erb's point, 21
Erikson's stages of psychosocial
  development, 163, 265
Erosion, epidermal, 35
Errors
  in communication, 267–268
  in documentation, 50
  in drug therapy, 267
  in nursing care, 50
  in surgery, 176
    preoperative measures in
      prevention of, 171–172, 268
Erythema, 34
  infectiosum, 163, 265
Erythrocytes, 215
  indices in complete blood count,
    155, 277
  packed, 70
  sedimentation rate, 154
Erythromycin, 139, 168
Esophagus, 214
Esters, 85, 102
Estrogen, 140–141
Ethanol, 100
Ethers, 85, 100
Ethical issues, 4–5, 266–267
Ethylene glycol, 100
Eupnea, 28

INDEX

Evaluation of nursing interventions, 14, 120, 258
Evaporation, 89
Evidence-based practice, 8
Excision of lesions, coding measurements in, 117
Excoriation, 35
Excretion of drugs, 120, 158
Exercise, 272–273
Exogenic processes, 87
Exothermic processes, 87
External cardiac pacing, 75
Extraocular movements, assessment of, 18
Exudates, 63
Eyes
    examination of, 18, 39, 259
    terminology and abbreviations related to, 221, 222

F

Face, examination of, 17
Face masks
    for infection prevention and control, 6, 7, 269
    for oxygen administration, 73–74
Faces pain scale, 48, 273
Facial nerve, 43, 261
Factor-label method, 81
Fahrenheit scale, 54, 80, 81, 82
    conversion to Celsius scale, 54, 82, 112, 146
Fallopian tubes, 211
Falls, prevention of, 268
Faraday's constant, 82
Fats, 106
Fatty acids, 101, 106
Fecal occult blood, 154
Feeding tubes, 65–68, 272
Female reproductive system
    assessment of, 40
    terminology and abbreviations related to, 211–212
Femoral artery pulse, 27
Fetal period, 165, 262
Fetal stethoscope (fetoscope), 15
Fever, 88
    postoperative, 179
    in transfusion reactions, 71, 279
Fiber, dietary, 65
    in enteral formulas, 65
    in high-fiber diet, 65, 272

in low-residue diet, 65, 271
Fidelity principle, 266
Fifth disease, 163, 265
First-order reactions, 88
Fissures, cutaneous, 35
Flail chest, 28
Flatness of percussion sound, 15, 258, 259
Flowmeters, respiratory, 32
Flow rate
    of blood, 26
    of intravenous solution, 153–154, 276
Fluids
    in burns, Parkland formula on, 117
    in enteral formulas, 272
    measurement of, 111–112
    postoperative status, 178
Fluoxetine, 125
Fluticasone, 128
Foam dressings, 62
Forearm, as intradermal injection site, 149
Formulas
    chemical, 83
    in drug dosage calculations, 144, 275
    in enteral nutrition, 65, 272
    on organic compounds, 97
Formula weight, 87
Fractions, 241–244
    converted to decimals, 244
    converted to percentages, 244
    decimals converted to, 248
    percentages converted to, 249
Fremitus, 29
Friction rubs, pleural, 30, 31
Fried's rule, 146
Friendships, 6
Full-term infants, 165, 262
Functional model of nursing care delivery, 7, 266
Funduscopic examination, 18

G

Gallop, atrial and ventricular, 22
Gamma rays, 93
Gases, 88, 89
    in arterial blood, 31, 154
    constants for, 82, 89
    elemental, 84
    laws on, 89

in periodic table, 83
Gastrointestinal system
    assessment of, 38–40, 177, 260
    decubitus ulcer risk in disorders of, 37
    drugs affecting, 133–135
    functions of, 38
    immobility affecting, 42
    nutritional disorders affecting, 39
    obstruction of, 38, 181
    postoperative, 177–178, 181
    terminology and abbreviations related to, 214–215
Gastrostomy tube, 66, 272
Gauze, 62
General anesthesia, 100, 174
Generativity stage in psychosocial development, 163, 265
Generic name of drugs, 121
Genitalia, examination of, 40, 260
Genitourinary system
    assessment of, 40–41, 260–261
    decubitus ulcer risk in disorders of, 37
    immobility affecting, 42
    terminology and abbreviations related to, 209–212
Gentamicin, 138
Geriatrics. See Elderly
Gestational diabetes, 165, 263
Gestational hypertension, 165, 263
Glands
    in endocrine system, 216, 217
    in integumentary system, 217
    in male reproductive system, 209
Glasgow Coma Scale, 44–45
Glossary on medical terminology, 190–199
Glossopharyngeal nerve, 43, 262
Glove use
    in clean and aseptic techniques, 54
    for infection prevention and control, 6, 7, 268–269
Glucose, 104, 156, 278
Glue for skin closure, 63
Glutamic-oxaloacetic transaminase, serum, 157, 279
Glutamic-pyruvic transaminase, serum, 157, 279
Glyburide, 132
Glycerol, 99, 100

Glycine, 104
Glycopyrrolate, 168
Gown use for infection prevention and control, 6, 269
Granulation in wound healing, 233
Grimace in APGAR score, 166, 264
Groshong catheter, 152
Growth and development, 162–163, 264–265
  expected rate of, 162, 266
  milestones in, 162, 266
  psychosocial, 163, 265
  terminology related to, 206
Guilt feelings in psychosocial development, 163, 265

H

Hair, 217
  examination of, 33, 260
Half-life of radioactive emissions, 94
Halides, 83, 85
  alkyl, 98
Halogenation reactions, 99
Hand, foot, and mouth disease, 163, 265
Hand hygiene, 6–7, 268–269
  in clean and aseptic techniques, 54
Happiness, 167
Head, examination of, 17, 259
  and HEENT assessment, 17–19
Healing process, 232–233
Health care operating indicators, 114
Hearing assessment, 19
Heart, 212
  assessment of, 21–26
Heart failure, 26
Heart sounds, 21–22
Heave of chest, 21
HEENT (head, eyes, ears, nose, and throat) assessment, 17–19
Hematocrit, 155, 277
Hematoma, postoperative, 182
Hemoconcentration, 57, 58
Hemodynamic parameters, 24–25
Hemoglobin, 155, 277
  glycosylated, 154
  mean corpuscular, 155, 277
  mean corpuscular concentration, 155, 277
Hemolysis, 57, 58
  in transfusion reactions, 71, 279
Hemorrhage
  exudates in, 63

vaginal, in pregnancy, 165, 263
Hemostasis, 232
Hemovac drains, 63
Henry's law, 91
Heparin, 130
Hess's law, 87
High-density lipoproteins, 91, 157, 277
High-fiber diet, 65, 272
Histamine 2 receptor antagonists, 133–134, 168, 171
History-taking, 16
Home environment assessment, 46
Hormones, 216
  estrogen and progestin, 140–141
  thyroid, 133, 169
Hospital administration, finding employment in, 227
Household measurement system, 112, 113, 146
Hydration reactions, 99
Hydrocarbons, 96, 97–99
Hydrochloric acid, 96
Hydrochlorothiazide, 130
Hydrocolloid dressings, 62
Hydrogenation, 86, 99, 101
Hydrogen bonds, 90, 100
Hydrohalogenation, 99
Hydrolysis, 102
Hydrophilic materials, 84
Hydrophobic materials, 84
Hyperbaric oxygen therapy, 91
Hyperpnea, 28
Hyperresonance of percussion sound, 15, 38, 258, 259
Hypertension, 20
  drug therapy in, 130–131, 168
  gestational, 165, 263
Hypertonic solutions, 92, 152
Hyperventilation, 28
Hypodermic syringe, 148
Hypoglossal nerve, 43, 262
Hypothesis, 80
Hypothyroidism, 133
Hypotonic solutions, 92, 152
Hypoventilation, 28
Hypovolemic shock, 76, 182–183

I

Ibuprofen, 137
Ideal body weight, 144
Identification of patient, preoperative, 171–172, 268

Identity development, 163, 265
Ileus, paralytic, 181
Imipramine, 124
Immobility
  decubitus ulcer risk in, 37
  physiologic effects of, 42
Immune system, terminology and abbreviations related to, 222–223
Immunizations, recommended schedule of, 164, 270–271
Immunoglobulin A incompatibility in transfusions, 71, 279
Immunosuppression, corticosteroids in, 136
Impetigo, 163, 265
Implantable cardioverter-defibrillators, 74
Implementation of nursing interventions, 14, 258
  documentation of, 49
  in drug therapy, 120
  postoperative, 176–178
Incontinence, decubitus ulcer risk in, 37
Industry stage in psychosocial development, 163, 265
Infants, 162, 266
  coding measurements in, 116
  drug therapy in, 121
  full-term, 165, 262
  growth and development of, 162, 264
  with low birth weight, 165, 262
  premature, 162, 165, 262, 266
Infarction, myocardial, biomarkers and serum enzyme levels in, 26
Infections
  antibiotics in, 138–140, 158, 168
  in children, 163, 265
  pathogens in, 188
  prevention and control of, 6–7, 268–269
  immunizations in, 164, 270–271
  respiratory, postoperative, 180
  of wounds, postoperative, 178
Inferiority feelings in psychosocial development, 163, 265
Inflammation, 232
  corticosteroid therapy in, 136
  nonsteroidal anti-inflammatory drugs in, 136–137

INDEX

Informed consent, 170, 267
Inhalation of drugs, 144, 274
  corticosteroid, 128
Inorganic substances, 84
  in nutrients, 64, 271
Inotropic drugs, 129–130
Inspection, 14, 258
  in cardiovascular assessment, 20, 21
  in gastrointestinal assessment, 38, 39
  in genitourinary assessment, 40
  in integumentary assessment, 32–33, 34
  in musculoskeletal assessment, 41
  in respiratory assessment, 28–29
Insulin therapy, 131–132, 168
  syringe for, 148
  types of insulin in, 131, 150
Integumentary system
  assessment of, 32–37, 260
  components of, 32
  functions of, 32
  immobility affecting, 42
  nutritional disorders affecting, 39
  terminology and abbreviations related to, 217–218
Intensity, radiation, 94
Intercostal retractions in breathing, 28
Intermolecular forces, 90
Interview, nursing, 16
Intimate relationships in psychosocial development, 163, 265
Intradermal injections, 144, 274
  needle length and gauge in, 148
  sites of, 149
Intramuscular injections, 144, 274
  needle length and gauge in, 148
  sites of, 151
Intraoperative period, 172–176
Intrathecal injections, 144, 274
Intravenous access, 144, 274
  dose rate in, 275
  flow rate in, 153–154, 276
  line insertion in, 68–69
  taping of site, 69
  types of solutions in, 152
Intuition of leaders, 10
Ion, 83
Ionic salts, 85, 91
Ionizing radiation, 94

Iris, examination of, 18
Isolation feelings in psychosocial development, 163, 265
Isolation precautions, 7, 269
Isomers, 97
Isopropanol, 99
Isotonic solutions, 92, 152, 272
Isotopes, 83
IUPAC nomenclature, 97, 98, 104

J

Jackson-Pratt drains, 63
Jaundice, 33, 34
Jejunostomy tube, 66, 272
Jobs in nursing, 226–228
Joints, 206–207
  assessment of, 41, 42, 261
  pain in, 42, 261
Jugular veins, inspection of, 20
Justice principle, 266

K

Kelvin scale, 80, 81, 88
Ketones, 85, 101
Kinetics, 87–88
Kussmaul respiration, 29
Kyphosis, 28

L

Labor, 166, 262
  preterm, 165, 263
Laboratory procedures, 154–157, 277–279
  abbreviations in, 113, 202
  preoperative, 170
Laceration repair, coding measurements in, 117
Laissez-faire leaders, 9
Lanosterol, 106
Laparotomy pad, 62
Large intestine, 214
  screening for cancer of, 269
Laryngoscope, 32
Laws, scientific, 80
Laxatives, 134–135
Leadership, 9–10
Least common denominator, 241
Le Chatelier's principle, 95
Legal issues
  accountability in, 4
  documentation in, 49, 280
Length measurements, 110
  household units in, 146
  metric units in, 80, 110, 113, 146

Lethal dose of radiation, 94
Lethargy, 45
Leukocytes, 215
  count of, 155, 277
Levodopa, 127
Levothyroxine, 133
Lewis acid and base, 95
Lewis structure, 84
Lichenification, 35
Life span considerations
  in drug therapy, 121–122, 158, 274–275
    dosage calculations in, 146, 147–148, 276
  in growth and development, 162–163, 264–265
  in vital signs, 17
Light palpation, 14, 39, 258
Limiting reagent in chemical reactions, 87
Line formula, 97
Lipids, 106
  blood tests for, 91, 157, 277
Lipoproteins, blood tests for, 91, 157, 277
Liquids
  in diet, 64, 271
  medications as, 146–147, 275
  solutions and mixtures, 90–93
  as state of matter, 88–89
Liver, 214
  function tests of, 154
Local anesthesia, 174
Lochia, postpartum, 166, 262
London force, 90
Loop diuretics, 130
Loperamide, 134
Lotions in skin care, 61
Low birth weight infants, 165, 262
Low-density lipoproteins, 91, 157, 277
Lower extremity
  assessment of, 20, 259
  as intramuscular injection site, 151
  as subcutaneous injection site, 150
Low-residue diet, 65, 271
Lungs
  sounds of, 29–31
  transfusion-related injury of, 71, 279
  volume and capacity values, 31

Lupus erythematosus, 34
Lymphatic system, terminology and abbreviations related to, 222–223
Lymphedema pumps, 75
Lymphocytes, 155, 277

M

Macrolide antibiotics, 139–140
Macules, 34
Male reproductive system
    assessment of, 40
    terminology and abbreviations related to, 209–210
Mammograms, 269
Managed care, abbreviations on, 205–206
Management job opportunities, 228
Manometers for blood pressure measurement, 55–56
Manual defibrillators
    external, 74
    internal, 75
Markovnikov's rule, 99
Masks
    for infection prevention and control, 6, 7, 269
    for oxygen administration, 73–74
Mass
    of electron, 82
    metric units for, 80
    molar, 87, 92
    of neutron, 82
    of proton, 82
Mass number, 82
Mathematics, 110–117, 236–250
    addition process in, 236. See also Addition process
    in coding, 116–117
    decimals in, 245–248, 249
    division process in, 239. See also Division process
    fractions in, 241–244, 248, 249
    health care operating indicators in, 114–115
    measurements in, 110–114, 116–117
    multiplication process in, 237–238. See also Multiplication process
    percentages in, 244, 248, 249
    positive and negative numbers in, 240
    proportions in, 249–250

rates in, 250
ratios in, 249
reimbursement calculations in, 114
risk calculation in, 115
subtraction process in, 236–237. See also Subtraction process
symbols in, 236
Matter, 80
    states of, 88–90
Maturation phase of wound healing, 233
Mean arterial blood pressure, 26
Mean corpuscular hemoglobin, 155, 277
Mean corpuscular hemoglobin concentration, 155, 277
Mean corpuscular volume, 155, 277
Measurements, 110–114
    abbreviations in, 110, 111, 112, 113, 200–201
    apothecary system, 112–113
    in coding, 116–117
    English system, 80
    household system, 112, 113, 146
    in laboratory, 113
    of length, 80, 110, 113, 146
    metric system. See Metric system
    of temperature. See Temperature measurement
    of volume, 80, 81, 88, 113, 146
    of weight. See Weight measurements
Medical terminology, 186–199
    on body systems, 206–223
    glossary on, 190–199
Medicare physician fee schedule, 114
Medications. See Drug therapy
Melting point, 89
Membranes, 92
    lipids in formation of, 106
Menstrual cycle, 211
Mental status examination, 46
    in depression, delirium, and dementia, 48
Mentoring, 11
Mercury manometers, 56
Mercury thermometers, 55
Metabolic panel
    basic, 154
    comprehensive, 154, 156–157, 278–279

Metabolism, 87
    of drugs, 120, 122, 158
Metalloids, 83
Metals, 83
Methanol, 99, 100
Metric system, 80, 113
    abbreviations in, 110
    conversion to other systems, 110, 111, 113
    household equivalents of, 146
    prefixes in, 81, 110
Mid-deltoid injection, 151
Minimally invasive surgery, 167
Mitral valve sounds, 21, 22
Mixtures, 80, 90–93
Moisture barrier creams, 61
Moisture scale in wound care, 64
Molar mass, 87, 92
Mole, 81, 86–87, 92
Molecules, 83
    dipolar, 84
    and intermolecular forces, 90
    properties of, 84
    small, 85
Monocytes, 155, 277
Monomers, 84
Monosaccharide, 104
Montgomery strap, 62
Mood
    in depression, delirium, and dementia, 47
    in mental status examination, 46
Moral distress, 5
Morphine, 137
Motor assessment, 44
Mouth, 214
    examination of, 19, 39
    temperature measurement in, 55
Multiplication process, 237–238
    with decimals, 247
    distributive property in, 240
    with fractions, 243
    with positive and negative numbers, 240
Multisample venipuncture needles, 59
Murmurs, 21, 22
Muscles
    pain in, 42, 261
    of respiration, 28
    strength testing, 41, 44

strength training, 273
terminology and abbreviations related to, 220–221
Musculoskeletal system
assessment of, 41–42, 44, 261
components and function of, 41
immobility affecting, 42
nutritional disorders affecting, 39
pain in, 42, 261
terminology and abbreviations related to, 206–208, 220–221
Myocardial infarction, biomarkers and serum enzyme levels in, 26
Myoglobin, 26

N

Nails, 217
examination of, 33, 260
Narrative charting, 50, 281
Nasal cannula for oxygen delivery, 73
Nasogastric tube, 66, 67, 272
Nasointestinal tube, 272
Nasopharyngeal tube, 32
Nebulizers, 74
Neck, examination of, 17, 259
blood vessel assessment in, 20–21
Needles, 58, 59–60, 148
Negative numbers, 240
Neonates, 162, 266
assessment of, 17, 166, 264
Nerve block, 174
Neurogenic shock, 76
Neurologic system
assessment of, 42–45, 177, 261–262
central, 42, 177, 208
drugs affecting, 122–124, 127–128
immobility affecting, 42
nutritional disorders affecting, 39
peripheral, 43–44, 122–124, 208
postoperative, 177
terminology and abbreviations related to, 208–209
Neutralization reactions, 102, 103
Neutrons, 82, 93
Neutrophils, 155, 277
Newborn, 162, 266
assessment of, 17, 166, 264
Nitrogen, 85
organic molecules based on, 103–104

Nondirective leaders, 9
Nonmaleficence principle, 267
Nonrebreather mask for oxygen delivery, 74
Nonstick pads, 62
Nose, examination of, 19
Nothing by mouth (NPO), 64, 271
Nuclear medicine, 94–95
Nuclear reactions, 80, 93–94
Nucleic acids, 105
Nucleotides, 105
Nucleus of atoms, 82
Nuclide symbol, 93
Numbers. *See also* Mathematics
positive and negative, 240
prefixes for, 188
and roman numerals, 114
Numerator, 241
Numerical pain scales, 48, 273
Nursing assessment. *See* Assessment
Nursing care delivery models, 7–8, 266
Nursing home administration, finding employment in, 227
Nursing organizations, professional, 11
ethical codes of, 5
Nursing practice
evidence-based, 8
standard of care in, 8
Nursing procedures, 53–76
blood specimen collection, 57–61
blood transfusions, 69–71
in circulatory care, 74–76
clean and aseptic techniques in, 54
indwelling catheter insertion, 71–72
for nutrition, 64–69
ostomy bag replacement, 72–73
oxygen administration, 73–74
urine specimen collection, 56–57
vital signs measurement, 54–56
wound care, 61–64
Nursing process
analysis or diagnosis in, 14, 49, 120, 258
assessment in. *See* Assessment
components of, 14, 258
documentation of, 49–50, 280–281
in drug therapy, 120
evaluation of interventions in, 14, 120, 258

implementation of interventions in, 14, 49, 120, 176–178, 258
planning in, 14, 49, 120, 258
Nutrition, 64–69, 271–272
carbohydrates in, 104
decubitus ulcer risk in disorders of, 37
diet therapies in, 64–65, 271–272
energy nutrients in, 64, 271
enteral, 65–68, 272
evaluation of, 39
inorganic nutrients in, 64, 271
organic nutrients in, 64, 271
parenteral, 65, 272
physiologic basics of, 64, 271

O

Obesity, abdominal examination in, 38
Obstetrics, 164–166, 262–264. *See also* Pregnancy
Obtundation, 45
Occlusive dressings, 62
Octet rule, 84
Oculomotor nerve, 43, 261
Ointments, 61
Olfactory nerve, 43, 261
Ondansetron, 135
Open drainage systems, 63
Ophthalmoscopic examination, 18
Opiates, 169
Opioids, 137–138, 169, 171
Optic nerve, 43, 261
Oral administration of drugs, 144, 274
antidiabetic, 132–133
contraceptive, 140–141
dosage calculations in, 146–147, 275
syringe for, 148
Oral cavity, 214
examination of, 19, 39
temperature measurement in, 55
Organic compounds, 84, 85, 96–104
in nutrients, 64, 271
Organism, 206
Organizations
abbreviations on, 205
nursing, 5, 11
Organs, 206
Oropharyngeal airway, 32
Oscillometric method of blood pressure measurement, 56

Osmosis, 92
Osmotic pressure, 92
Ostomy
  bag changing procedure in, 72–73
  gastrostomy, 66, 272
  jejunostomy, 66, 272
Otoscopic examination, 19
Ovaries, 211
Over-the-needle catheter, 152
Oxidation, 86, 100, 101
Oxygen, 83, 85
  administration of, 73–74, 91
    pressure measurement in, 89
    pressure regulator in, 32
  arterial saturation, 31
  in inhaled air, 89
  partial arterial pressure, 31

P

Pacemakers, cardiac, 75
Pacing, cardiac, 75
Pads and dressings, 62
Pain
  acute and chronic, comparison of, 48, 273
  assessment of, 48, 273
  drug therapy in, 137–138, 169, 171, 273
  musculoskeletal, 42, 261
  postpartum, 166, 262
Palliative surgical procedures, 167
Palpation, 14, 258
  in cardiovascular assessment, 21
  deep, 14, 39, 258
  in gastrointestinal assessment, 39–40
  in genitourinary assessment, 40, 41
  in integumentary assessment, 33
  light, 14, 39, 258
  in musculoskeletal assessment, 42
  in peripheral vascular assessment, 27–28
  in respiratory assessment, 29
Pancreas, 214
Pap tests, 269
Papules, 34
Paralytic ileus, 181
Parenteral administration
  of drugs, 147, 276
  of nutrition, 65, 272
Parkinsonism, drug therapy in, 127
Parkland formula, 117
Participative leaders, 9

Pastes in skin care, 61
Paternalistic leaders, 9
Pathogens, prefixes on, 188
Patient care technicians, 226
Patient-nurse interactions
  advocacy for patient in, 11
  in caring relationship, 5, 16
  confidentiality of communication in, 5, 267
  professional boundaries in, 5
  respect in, 11, 17
Pectus carinatum, 28
Pectus excavatum, 28
Pediatrics, 162–164, 264–266. See also Children
Penicillins, 138
Penis, 209
Penrose drain, 63
Peptide bonds, 105
Percentages, 249
  converted to decimals, 249
  converted to factions, 249
  decimals converted to, 248
  fractions converted to, 244
Percussion, 14–15, 258–259
  in cardiovascular assessment, 21
  in gastrointestinal assessment, 38
  in respiratory assessment, 29
  types of sounds in, 15, 258–259
Percutaneous endoscopic gastrostomy, 66, 272
Pericardium, assessment of, 21–26
Perinatal period, 165, 262
Perineum, postpartum, 166, 262
Periodicity, 83
Periodic table of elements, 83, 254
Peripherally inserted central catheter, 152
Peripheral nervous system, 43–44, 208
  drugs affecting, 122–124
Peripheral vascular system
  assessment of, 27–28
  catheterization of, 152
Peripheral venous catheter, 152
Permanent cardiac pacing, 75
PERRLA (pupils equal, round, reactive to light and accommodation), 18, 259
Personal protective equipment for infection prevention and control, 6–7

Personnel, friendships with, 6
Pertussis, 163, 265
Petechiae, 34, 58
Petrolatum gauze, 62
pH, 96
  of arterial blood, 31
  buffers of, 95
Pharmacodynamics, 120
Pharmacokinetics, 120, 158
Pharmacology, 120–141. See also Drug therapy
Pharmacotherapeutics, 120
Pharynx, 214
Phenol, 99
Phenytoin, 127
Phosphoesters, 102, 103
Phospholipids, 106
Phosphoric acid, 103
Physical examination, 14–15. See also Assessment
PIE format, 50, 281
Pinard stethoscope, 15
Placenta previa, 165, 263
Planck's constant, 82
Planes, 206
Planning in nursing process, 14, 258
  documentation of, 49
  in drug therapy, 120
Plasma, 215
  fresh frozen, 70
Plasma protein incompatibility in transfusions, 71, 279
Platelets, 215
  count of, 155, 277
  transfusion of, 70
Pleural friction rubs, 30, 31
Pneumonia, postoperative, 180
Point of maximum impulse (PMI), 21
Polar covalent bonds, 84, 90
Polybasic chemicals, 95
Polycythemia vera, 34
Polymers, 84
Polyprotic chemicals, 95
Polysaccharides, 104
Polyunsaturated fat, 106
Popliteal artery pulse, 28
Port or Port-A-Cath, 153
Positions, 206
Positive numbers, 240
Postoperative period, 176–183
  team debriefing in, 175–176

Postpartum period, 165, 166, 262
Potassium serum levels, 156, 278
  in diuretic therapy, 130
Potentiation in drug interactions, 122
PQRST mnemonic on symptom
    analysis, 16
Prazosin, 124
Preeclampsia, 165, 263
Prefixes, 186
  carbon-chain, 97
  metric, 81, 110
  substituent, 97
Pregnancy, 164–166, 262–264
  common complications in, 165,
      263
  drug therapy in, 121, 274
  ectopic, 165, 263
Prehypertension, 20
Premature infants, 162, 165, 262, 266
Prenatal period, 165, 262
Preoperative period, 169–172
  identification of person and
      surgical site in, 171–172, 268
  team briefing in, 175
  time-out in, 172, 268
Preschool children, growth and
    development of, 162, 264
Prescribed as needed (PRN)
    medications, 273
Pressure dressings, 62
Pressure measurements, 81, 88
Pressure sores, 35–37
Preterm labor, 165, 263
Preventive care, 269–271
  immunizations in, 164, 270–271
Primary intention, 232
Primary nurse model, 8, 266
Privacy
  and confidentiality of patient-nurse
      communication, 5, 267
  in nursing assessment, 14, 17
PRN (prescribed as needed)
    medications, 273
Procainamide, 169
Product of chemical reactions, 86
Professional boundaries between
    nurse and patient, 5
Professional designations,
    abbreviations on, 204–205
Professional nursing organizations, 11
  Code of Ethics for Nurses of ANA, 5

Progestin, 140–141
Proliferative phase of wound healing,
    232–233
2-Propanol, 100
Proportions, 249–250
Propranolol, 124, 169
Prostate cancer screening, 269
Protective skin barriers, 61
Protein, 104, 105
  in enteral formulas, 65
  total serum, 155
Protons, 82
Psychosocial status
  assessment of, 46–48, 262
  Erikson's stages of development,
      163, 265
  immobility affecting, 42
Psyllium, 134
Puerperium period, 165, 262
Pulmonary valve sounds, 21, 22
Pulmonary vascular resistance, 24
Pulse, 56, 212
  in newborn, 17, 166, 264
  normal range for, 17, 27, 56
  in peripheral vascular assessment,
      27–28
Pulse pressure, 20
Pupils, examination of, 18, 259
Pure substances, 80
Pursed-lip breathing, 28
Purulent exudates, 63
Pustules, 34

Q

Quality improvement specialist,
    finding work as, 228
Quantum mechanics, 83
Quaternary ammonium salts (QASs),
    103
Quinidine, 129

R

Radial artery pulse, 27, 56
Radiation, 93–95
Radioactive emissions, 94
Radioactivity, 83, 93–95
Radiocarbon dating, 94
Radioisotopes, 83
Rain, acid, 96
Rales, 30
Range of motion in musculoskeletal
    assessment, 41, 261

Rate, 250
Rate constant, 88
Ratio, 249
Reactants, 86
Rebreather mask for oxygen delivery,
    73
Reconstructive phase of wound
    healing, 232–233
Rectum
  examination of, 39–40
  as route of drug administration,
      144, 274
  temperature measurement in, 55
Red blood cells, 215
  indices in complete blood count,
      155, 277
  packed, 70
  sedimentation rate, 154
Redox reactions, 100
Reduction reactions, 86, 100
Reflex testing, 44
Regional anesthesia, 174–175
Registered nurse first assistant,
    173–174
Reimbursement
  Medicare physician fee schedule
      in, 114
  resource-based relative value scale
      in, 114
Relative biologic effect of radiation,
    94
Relative risk, 115
Reliability of data, 49, 82
Resonance of percussion sound, 15,
    258, 259
Resource-based relative value scale,
    114
Respect for patients, 11, 17
Respiration, 87
  assessment of, 17, 28–32, 56, 176
  lung sounds in, 29–31
  rate of, 17, 56
  in newborn, 17, 166, 264
Respiratory distress, signs of, 28
Respiratory syncytial virus
    infections, 163, 265
Respiratory system
  assessment of, 28–32, 260
  in newborn, 17, 166, 264
  postoperative, 176

drugs affecting, 128–129
function of, 28
immobility affecting, 42
postoperative, 176, 180–181, 182
terminology and abbreviations related to, 218–220
Responsibility, 4, 10
Restorative surgical procedures, 167
Reverse osmosis, 92
Rh incompatibility, 71, 279
Rhonchi, 30, 31
Ribonucleic acid (RNA), 96, 105
Ribose, 105
Rights of patients, 4
advocacy for, 11
in drug therapy, 144, 267
Risk assessment for decubitus ulcers, 37
Risk calculations, 115
Risk management, 267–268
finding job in, 228
RNA, 96, 105
Roentgen, 94
Roentgen equivalent in man (rem), 94
Role confusion in psychosocial development, 163, 265
Roman numerals, 114
Romberg test, 44
Rosenbaum chart, 18
Rounding decimals, 245
Rule of nines, 116

S

Safety issues
in delegation of tasks, 10
in nuclear medicine, 94
in surgery, 171–172, 182
in syringe needles, 59
Saline, physiological, 91
Saponification, 103
Saturated fat, 106
Saturated hydrocarbons, 98
Saturated solutions, 91
Scales, epidermal, 35
Scarlet fever, 163, 265
Scars, 35
School-age children, growth and development of, 162, 264
Science, definition of, 80
Scientific method, 80

Sclera, examination of, 18
Scoliosis, 28
Scopolamine bromide, 169
Screening procedures for preventive care, 269
Scrotum, 209
Scrub nurse, 173
Secondary intention, 232
Second-order reactions, 88
Sedative drugs, 128, 169, 171
Seizures, anticonvulsant drugs in, 127
Selective serotonin reuptake inhibitors, 125
Self-understanding of leaders, 10
Sensitivity of test, 49
Sensory system
assessment of, 44
terminology and abbreviations related to, 189, 221–222
Septic shock, 76
Sequential compression devices, 75
Serology, 155
Serotonin reuptake inhibitors, selective, 125
Serous exudates, 63
Shock, 76
hypovolemic, 76, 182–183
Sibilant rhonchi, 30
Situational leaders, 9
SI units, 80
Skeletal system
pain in, 42, 261
terminology and abbreviations related to, 206–208
Skin, 217
assessment of, 32–37, 260
functions of, 32
immobility affecting, 42
nutritional disorders affecting, 39
preparation for surgery, 172
wounds of, 61–64. See also Wounds
Small intestine, 214
Snellen chart, 18
Soap, 61, 103
SOAP format, 50, 281
Sodium
dietary restriction of, 65, 272
serum levels of, 156, 278
Soft diet, 64–65, 272

SOLER system for good communication, 170
Solids, as state of matter, 88
Solubility, 91
Solutes, 90, 91–92
Solutions, 90–93
concentration of, 81, 91, 144, 275
dilution of, 91, 93
intravenous, 152
pH of, 96
Solvents, 90, 91
Sonorous rhonchi, 30
Sounds
auscultation of, 15, 259. See also Auscultation
in percussion, 15, 258–259. See also Percussion
Specialty nursing, 160–183
finding job in, 226
obstetrical, 164–166
pediatric, 162–164
surgical, 167–183
Specific gravity, 81
Specificity of test, 49
Specimen collection
blood, 57–61
urine, 56–57
Speech
in depression, delirium, and dementia, 47
in mental status examination, 46
Sphygmomanometers, 55
Spinal accessory nerve, 43, 262
Spinal anesthesia, 174–175
Spine, assessment of, 41, 42
Spiritual assessment, 46
Sponge dressings, 62
Spring evacuator drains, 63
Staging of decubitus ulcers, 36
Stagnation in psychosocial development, 163, 265
Standard precautions, 6, 268–269
Standards of practice, 8
Staples, surgical, 63
Stearic acid, 102
Steri-Strips, 63
Steroids, 106
Stethophone, 15
Stethoscopes, 15
in heart sound auscultation, 21–22
in lung sound auscultation, 29

INDEX

Stomach, 214

Strength testing, 41, 44

Strength training, 273

Stridor, 30, 31

Stroke, symptoms of, 26

Structural formula, 97

Stupor, 45

Subcutaneous injections, 144, 274
  needle length and gauge in, 148
  sites of, 149–150

Sublingual route of drug
  administration, 144, 274

Subscapular region, as intradermal
  injection site, 149

Substituent prefixes, 97

Substituted hydrocarbons, 98

Subtraction process, 236–237
  with decimals, 246
  with fractions, 242–243
  with positive and negative
    numbers, 240

Suction catheters, 32

Suffixes, 186

Sugars, 104

Supersaturated solutions, 91

Surgical procedures, 167–183
  drug complications in, 168–169
  intraoperative period in, 172–176
  medical terminology related to,
    188
  postoperative period in, 175,
    176–183
  preoperative period in, 169–172,
    175, 268
  prevention of errors in, 171–172,
    268
  types of, 167–168

Suspensions, 91

Sutures, 62–63

Swan-Ganz catheter, 153

Sweating, 87

Symbols in mathematics, 236

Synonyms, 189

Syringes, 148

Systemic vascular resistance, 24

Systems, 206

Systole, 20

Systolic blood pressure, 20

T

T lymphocytes, 155, 277

T tube drainage, 63

Tablet dosage, 147, 275

Tachypnea, 28

Tape, 62
  for venous access site, 69

Team approach to nursing care
  delivery, 8, 266
  in operating room, 175–176

Tegaderm, 62

Telemetry, 75

Temperature measurement, 54–55,
  80, 81, 82, 88, 112
  Celsius scale in, 54, 80, 82, 112,
    146
  conversion formulas in, 54, 82,
    112, 146
  Fahrenheit scale in, 54, 80, 81, 82,
    112, 146
  Kelvin scale in, 80, 81, 88
  in newborn, 17, 166, 264
  normal range for, 17, 55
  postoperative, 177, 179

Temporary cardiac pacing, 75

Tertiary intention, 232

Tetracyclines, 139

Theoretical yield in chemical
  reactions, 87

Thermodynamics, 87

Thermometers, 55, 88

Thiazide diuretics, 130

Thigh, as subcutaneous injection site,
  150

Thioesters, 102

Thiols, 100–101

Thorax
  anterior, examination of, 19–20,
    259
    in cardiovascular assessment, 21
    in respiratory assessment, 28,
      29–30
  posterior, examination of, 19, 259

Thrill, in murmurs, 21

Throat, examination of, 19, 39

Thrombocytes, 215

Thromboembolism, 75, 182

Thrombophlebitis, postoperative, 183

Thyroid hormones, 133, 169

Tibial artery, posterior, pulse
  assessment, 28

Time, metric units for, 80

Time-out, preoperative, for error
  prevention, 172, 268

Tissues, 206

Titration, 96

Total parenteral nutrition, 65, 272

Tracheal intubation, 31–32

Tranquilizers, 169, 171

Transcutaneous cardiac pacing, 75

Transfusions, 69–71, 279

Transition metals, 83

Transvenous cardiac pacing, 75

Travel nursing, 227

Tricuspid valve sounds, 21, 22

Tricyclic antidepressants, 124–125

Trigeminal nerve, 43, 261

Triglycerides, 106, 157, 277

Trochlear nerve, 43

Troponins, cardiac, 26

Trust, in psychosocial development,
  163, 265

Tube feedings, 65–68, 272

Tuberculin syringe, 148

Tuning fork in hearing assessment,
  19

24-hour urine collection, 57

Tympanic membrane
  examination of, 19
  temperature measurement, 55

Tympany of percussion sound, 15,
  38, 258, 259

U

Ulcers, 35
  decubitus, 35–37
  of stomach and duodenum, drug
    therapy in, 133–134, 168,
    171

Umbilical catheters, arterial and
  venous, 153

Units of measurement, 80
  prefixes for, 80, 81

Unsaturated fat, 106

Unsaturated hydrocarbons, 98

Upper extremity
  assessment of, 19, 259
  as intradermal injection site, 149
  as intramuscular injection site, 151
  as subcutaneous injection site, 149

Urea nitrogen in blood, 156, 278

Urgent surgery, 167

Urinalysis, 170
  urine specimen collection for,
    56–57

Urinary system
  assessment of, 40–41, 260–261
    postoperative, 177
    preoperative, 170
  catheter insertion, 71–72
  decubitus ulcer risk in disorders
    of, 37
  immobility affecting, 42
  postoperative, 177, 179
  postpartum, 166, 262
  terminology and abbreviations
    related to, 210–211
Urine
  color of, 41
  retention of, postoperative, 179
  specimen collection, 56–57
Uterine tubes, 211
Uterus, 211
  postpartum, 166, 262

V

Vagina, 211
  bleeding from, in pregnancy, 165,
    263
  as route of drug administration,
    144, 274
Vagus nerve, 43, 262
Valence electrons, 82
Validity of test, 49

van der Waals force, 90
Vascular resistance, systemic and
  pulmonary, 24
Vastus lateralis injection, 151
Veins
  blood specimens from, 57–60
  catheterization of, 68–69, 152
Venipuncture, 57–60
Ventricular gallop, 22
Ventricular stroke work index, left
  and right, 25
Ventrogluteal injection, 151
Venturi mask, 74
Veracity principle, 267
Vesicles, 34
Vesicular breath sounds, 29
Vestibulocochlear nerve, 43, 262
Visual acuity, 18
Visual analog pain scale, 48, 273
Vital signs, 17, 54–56
  in newborn, 17, 166, 264
Vitiligo, 34
Volume measurements, 80, 81, 88
  conversion factors in, 146
  household units in, 146
  metric units in, 113, 146
Volunteer positions, 226
Vomiting, antiemetics in, 135, 171

W

Water, 90
  in acid-base chemistry, 95
  body content, 90
Weight measurements, 111
  adjusted body weight, 145
  conversion formulas for, 111, 146
  in drug therapy, 144–146,
    147–148
  household units in, 146
  ideal body weight, 144
  metric units in, 111, 113, 146
Wet dressings, 62
Wheals, 34
Wheezing, 30, 31
White blood cells, 215
  count of, 155, 277
Whiteboard use in operating room,
  176
Whooping cough, 163, 265
Winged infusion kits, 60
Wounds, 61–64
  coding measurements on, 117
  healing of, 232–233
  postoperative, 177, 178–179

Z

Z-track technique in intramuscular
  injections, 151
Zaitsev's rule, 100
Zwitterions, 104

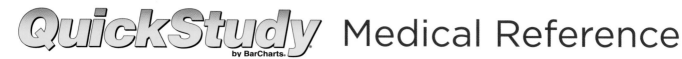

QuickStudy
by BarCharts®

Medical Reference

Laminated Reference Guides

Since 1997, our **laminated nursing guides** have become a staple among nurses, students, and instructors because of their **accurate**, **clear**, and **concise** information.

» 8 1/2" × 11" format with 1, 2, or 3 panels
» Fluff-free
» Textbook's worth of information
» Detailed illustrations help reinforce learning
» Over 450 titles available
» Over 50 million in print
» **Only $4.95–$6.95**

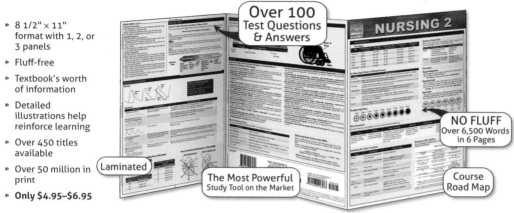

Over 100 Test Questions & Answers

NO FLUFF
Over 6,500 Words in 6 Pages

Laminated

The Most Powerful Study Tool on the Market

Course Road Map

Posters

Highly detailed anatomical posters that enhance the learning process.

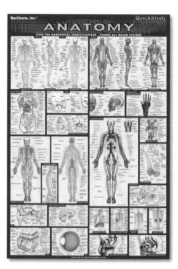

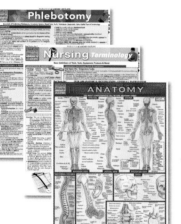

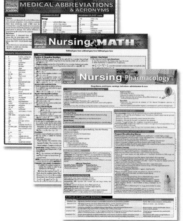

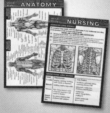

Also in **pocket form!**

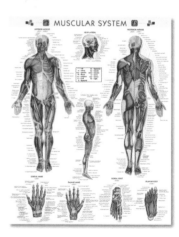

MUSCULAR SYSTEM

Books & Flash Cards

More ways to reference and study.

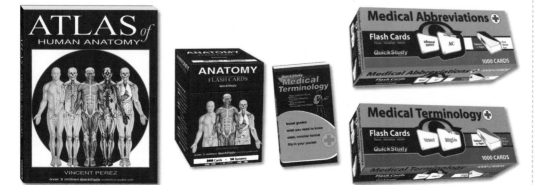

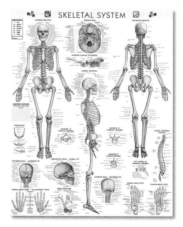

SKELETAL SYSTEM